CW00944381

THE
★REAL
MEAL
REVOLUTION

LOW-CARB
COOKING

ROBINSON

realmealrevolution.com

therealmealrevolution1

@realmealrevolution

therealmealrevolution

THE REAL MEAL REVOLUTION

LOW-CARB COOKING

REAL HEALTH IN 50 WORDS

EAT VEGETABLES, MEAT, NUTS, SEEDS, LITTLE FRUIT AND MINIMAL STARCH. **EAT REAL FATS.** AVOID SUGAR, GRAINS, SEED OILS **AND PROCESSED FOOD. TASTE NEW DISHES.** PROTECT YOUR GUT. EAT WHEN HUNGRY. **DRINK WHEN THIRSTY. FAST OCCASIONALLY.** EXERCISE. **SOCIALISE.** RELAX. **SLEEP WELL.** LISTEN TO YOUR BODY. ESCAPE ROUTINE. **SEEK ADVENTURE. KEEP IMPROVING.**

ABOUT THE AUTHOR

Jonno Proudfoot is a food expert, entrepreneur and adventurer, and the driving force behind the Real Meal Revolution brand. He conceptualised and co-authored the bestselling *Real Meal Revolution*, *Superfood For Superchildren* and *Real Meal Revolution 2.0* books, which have sold in excess of 400,000 copies between them.

With his friend Thane Williams, he holds the world record for the longest unassisted open-ocean stage swim, having swum 459 kilometres from Mozambique to Madagascar between 28 February and 23 March 2014.

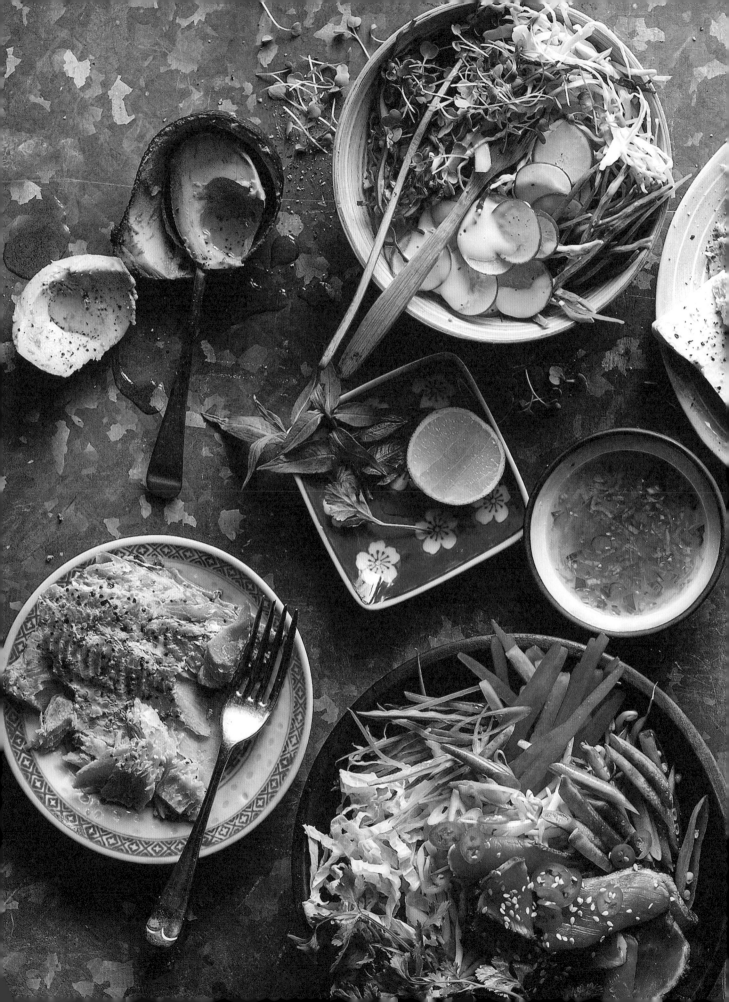

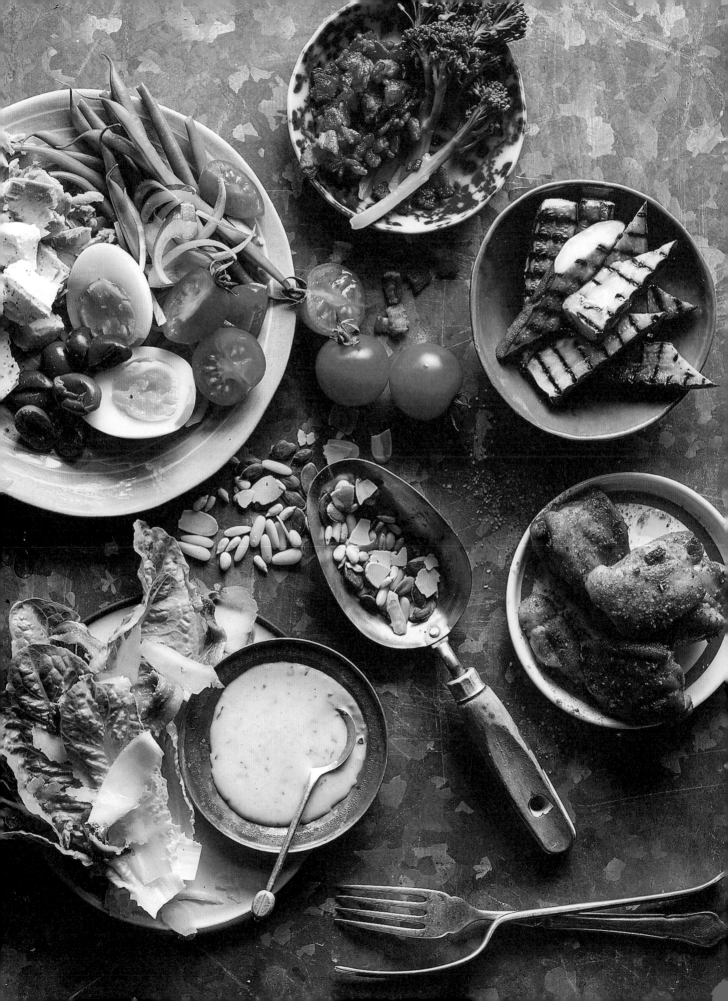

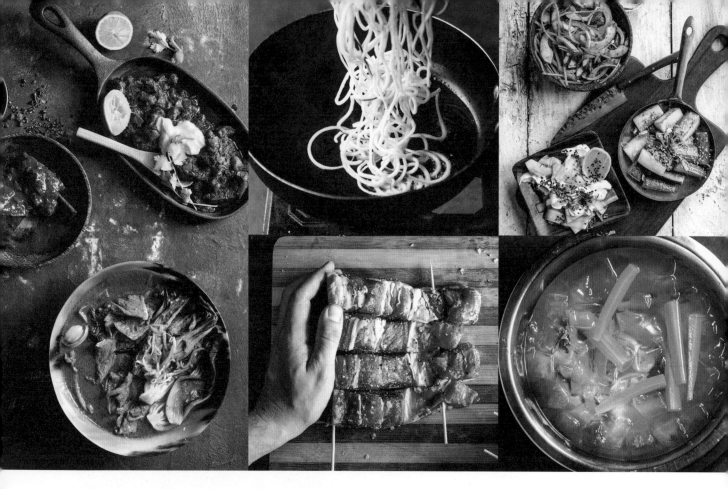

CONTENTS

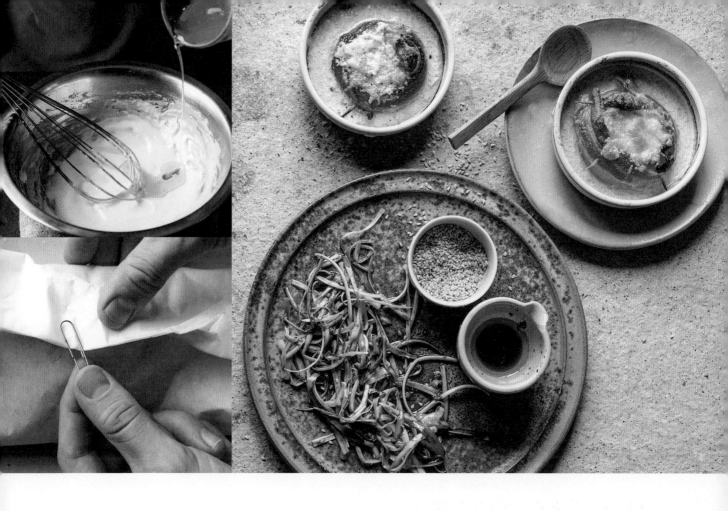

LESSONS

INTRODUCTION

The first time I developed a firm, professional opinion on anything food-related was back in 2004. I was a junior chef in a rather fancy restaurant in Cape Town. Ferran Adrià had just been voted best chef in the world, and a new wave of molecular gastronomy was sweeping the globe, led by crazy-talented individuals inspired by Adrià's restaurant in Catalonia, El Bulli.

For those who may not know, the dishes at El Bulli (which closed in 2011) were created with a combination of ingredients you've probably never heard of and certainly wouldn't have thought of eating, and were prepared using methods you'd need a million-dollar kitchen to produce. Think *sous vide duck tongue with eucalyptus sphere* or *coral made from chocolate and raspberry powder*, and you'll get a sense of what I'm talking about.

All of a sudden chefs everywhere were conjuring up caviar from roasted peppers and egg yolks from pumpkin purée. Things like soy lecithin, guar gum, xanthan gum, alginate and – one that stuck with me – a chemical called sodium citrate were appearing in kitchens, before ending up in the mouths of diners.

While the skill, beauty and novelty of turning a purée into delicate caviar was not lost on me, it occurred to me at the time that we had gone full circle. Humans had learned how to cook however many thousands of years ago. We had that nailed until about the middle of the 20th century. Then we developed manufacturing techniques to produce pretty much anything from anything: including faux caviar and miscellaneous foams in fine restaurants, and mass-produced artificially thickened sauces, ready-made meals and salad dressings that would never split in everyday supermarkets.

Those who cared about the food they ate continued to eat at fancy restaurants, which were fancy because they served up the best ingredients money could buy, cooked by the best in the business. Those who didn't care about the food they ate bought the convenience option off the shelf.

In 2004, I found myself staring at a bunch of chefs who were trying to master the art of using a whole bunch of ingredients that factories and food manufacturers had been using for years, to serve to people who were paying top dollar to eat the best of the best. We were going the wrong way, and I was of the opinion that these spheres, foams, gels, airs and emulsions were just paint for pretty plates – and far from anything we could call food.

I realised that molecular gastronomy, in whatever form, wasn't for me. And with that, my quest for real food began.

Some time later I came to understand the dietary benefits of low-carb eating, and after conceptualising the *The Real Meal Revolution* in 2013, I was fortunate enough to help launch a genuine eating and health revolution in South Africa, which would go on to make a significant contribution to the global low-carb movement. I take much pride in the three books I have authored or co-authored to date – it has been a helluva journey, to say the least!

Today, while I am grateful to be able to assist so many of our Real Meal Revolution members in their journeys to better health, I gain the greatest satisfaction in hearing that people who never used to cook are now cooking all the time and, as a result, are spending more time with their families at the table chatting and enjoying meals. The key to this, I believe, is in being able to prepare and cook delicious, good food from the best ingredients and basic principles.

With that realisation, this is the book I've been itching to publish since 2004.

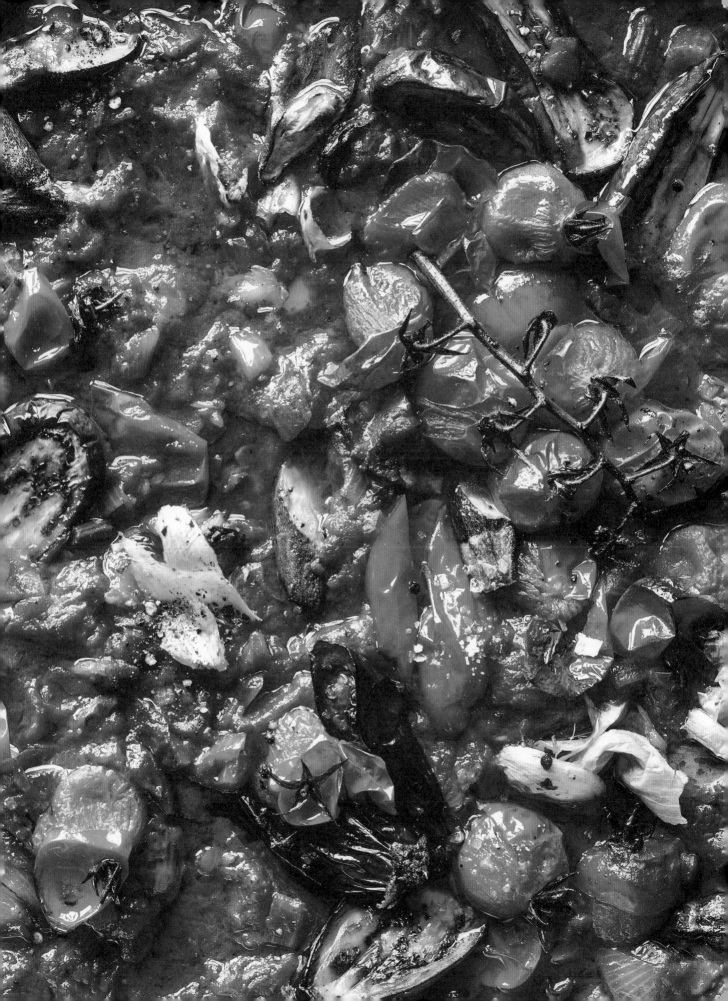

WHO AM I?

I call myself a lifestyle entrepreneur but I'm not always sure I know what that really means. I certainly enjoy my lifestyle, and yes, I own a business.

What I do know is that I'm obsessed with self-improvement, and I love setting ambitious goals like getting another degree while working full time, or entering impossible-sounding endurance events.

All goals worth achieving are tough, but I believe the hardest thing on earth is balancing life, work and having a family. To me, living itself is a professional sport. It is an art and science that fascinates me. When I say I'm a lifestyle entrepreneur, I think I'm actually saying that I will go into any business that helps people to do better at life.

For me, winning at life is having all six of my Tony Robbins needs satisfied, as often as possible and in as many areas of my life as possible. Those needs are certainty, variety, significance, connection, contribution and growth. Any activity in life will satisfy one of those needs.

- ★ Watching the same movie again will provide certainty.
- ★ Wine tasting will provide variety.
- ★ Getting Facebook likes will provide significance.
- ★ Calling a friend will provide connection.
- ★ Giving your money away will make you feel like you've contributed.
- ★ Reading a self-help book will help you grow.

I believe there are many activities in life that tick the right boxes, but I'm constantly looking to maximise the utility of every minute. For me, that means doing fewer things, but ensuring those things satisfy most, if not all of those needs at once. Because, as Dr Seuss would say, 'These things are fun and fun is good.'

It turns out that cooking is one of the easiest things to do that satisfies all of those needs. And it is something we can do every single day.

Simply eating low-carb will most likely make you thinner. It will make you feel significant, and you may grow through exercising self-discipline. If you're buying pre-made meals, or packaged food products, I can almost guarantee you certainty too.

Not just eating low-carb, but cooking low-carb really is the next level in bettering yourself as a whole. Cooking a simple, healthy supper for yourself, friends or family offers you an opportunity to contribute, and experience variety, connection and growth (especially if you mess it up) – and significance when you see people licking their plates.

So, sure, I can teach you to cook low-carb. And if you eat the food from these recipes, like others, your doctor might take you off your diabetes meds, and you might perform better on the sports field or at work. But if after a few months of eating this food, all you can say is that you're off your meds and you're thinner than ever, I will only be partially satisfied.

What will really rev my motor is if you tell me you've fallen in love with food again, and that eating and cooking are now things that you get excited about, that inspire you. That it has helped you grow, improve your relationships and, better yet, fills an immovable slot in your daily routine.

If you ask me, that's winning at life. And it's what I'm here to help you do.

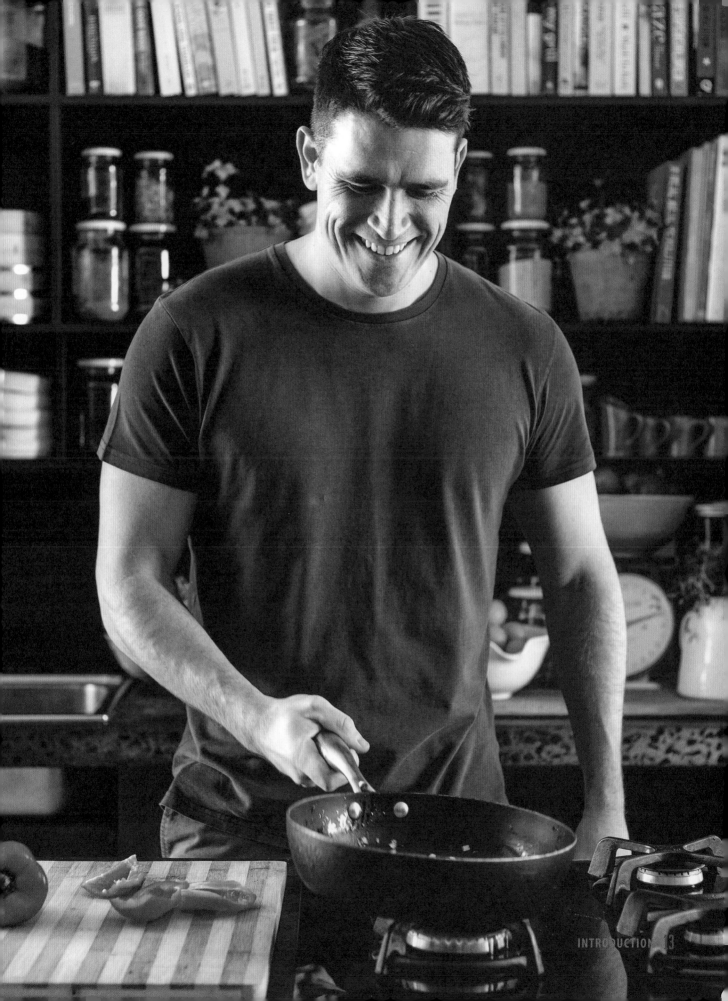

MASTER THY KITCHEN. MASTER THYSELF.

Aikido, the Japanese martial art, describes its three phases of mastery as Shu Ha Ri.

★ During the Shu stage, you learn to follow the rules until they sink in.
★ During the Ha stage, you reflect on the rules and look for exceptions.
★ And when you reach the Ri stage, the rules are forgotten as you have developed mastery and grasped the essence of the underlying forces.

More simply put: *Follow the rule. Break the rule. Be the rule.*

In that regard, Aikido is not dissimilar from health, business or cooking.

With health, in particular, the Shu stage could be simply following a diet or exercise regime. This will help you, but only as long as you're 'on the plan'.

Learning the rules and reflecting on why they work or don't work for you would be the Ha stage. This stage brings you a certain level of control over your health.

But learning many sets of rules, and trying them all, over and over again, will push you into a state of what I call Self Mastery, or Ri. At this stage, you don't even think about DOs and DON'Ts because they've become second nature. You're constantly manipulating your mood, your physique and your health by taking conscious actions that are driven by the knowledge and habits that you have drilled into your subconscious through wide-ranging research and repetitive effort.

Your health journey is one you have to travel on your own, because it is different for everyone.

Cooking, however, is the same for everyone. And low-carb cooking is even easier. To master low-carb cooking, or to achieve Ri, you must learn the most common cooking methods, in conjunction with the most common flavour combinations, and you must learn to cook all of these things without the addition of high-carb ingredients. It's really not that complicated.

To work out how this book will help you do this, it will help to understand how it was made and what the underlying principles are.

Chocolate and almond cake sweetened with xylitol may be lower in carbs than the real thing, but that right there is the problem. It's not the real thing (and I just can't handle the taste of artificial sweeteners). I'd rather eat the real thing and hate myself for a day than eat a fake carb and hate eating it.

Nut flours, artificial sweeteners, low-carb breads, low-carb baked goods and other carb substitutes don't feature in this book. They are *lower* carb, not low-carb. There is a misconception that because a treat has been labelled low-carb, it's okay to have after a meal or instead of a meal. They are certainly less unhealthy, but I still see them as treats rather than mealtime staples.

On my company's website, realmealrevolution.com, we have lists of ingredients that are appropriate to eat at different stages of your journey. You can download them for free – go check it out.

The most important of these lists is the Green List, which is made up of foods you can eat without restriction and still lose weight and feel great. That list has guided me in what to write for this book.

I took the 100-odd ingredients on the green list and researched more than 40 cuisines to find the flavour combinations and methods that bring out the best in each of them. I then matched the ingredients with appropriate methods and flavours, avoiding repetition of either, being sure to provide options that were more affordable, less affordable, more difficult, less difficult, with varied flavours, textures, colours and cooking times for each Green List ingredient.

Damn, was it a mission.

I also wrote a bunch of lessons to help explain the way I cook. Some you may know, but perhaps not all – they all offer great ways to enhance flavour, specifically when cooking low-carb. (They also allowed me to avoid repeating myself in recipe methods.)

The methods and the lessons really do impact the entire flavour of each dish, and I do recommend following them the way I have written them – at least before you reach the Ri stage of low-carb cooking.

The book was created in a way that if you practise every lesson and cook every recipe in this book just once, you will have cooked food from more than 40 countries and tried every major culinary technique.

In case you're wondering, there are also no specialised pre-workout, post-workout keto bars or shakes. There are no fancy supplements.

I've made no mention of how to store things or whether to cover them in cling wrap, foil or hessian. There is no mention of non-stick pans. No mention of organic, green-reared, sustainably farmed and all that. In general, I've tried to stay agnostic in all areas other than those where your enjoyment of food is concerned. I've also avoided pushing an environmental agenda. I care about the environment, but there are many views on many things, and I trust you to do what you can.

I am not knocking on your door, praying for you to join my low-carb cult. Low-carb is not a religion. It is a tool, and a jolly useful one at that.

The same way low-carb is a tool for weight loss, high-carb is a tool for weight gain, or fuelling. Hell, pizza and doughnuts are tools for pleasure, and alcohol is a tool for sterilising wounds, or lubricating social occasions. There is no morality here. Just a means to an end.

The goal for which this book was designed was the achievement of mastery, or Shu Ha Ri, in my favourite tool, low-carb cooking. It was designed to bring you closer to food and to help you win at life.

Please dig in.

MY LIST OF LOW-CARB FOODS

Ah, low-carb food lists. A contentious issue on the internet as it is around the dinner tables of biohackers, paleolites, keto warriors and nutritionists everywhere.

My Green List, in particular, has been compiled and repeatedly revised over the course of five years. The first iteration was based largely on the Dukan Diet list of 100 foods you can eat. Through trial and error, heaps of member feedback from the Real Meal Revolution website, and as much common sense as possible, my team and I arrived at the ultimate 'eat your fill' Green List on the page opposite. Along with the Orange, Red and Grey lists, it has been downloaded from realmealrevolution.com over a million times.

While we have counted carbs, we've found that going strictly on carb count just isn't efficient. If the idea of going low-carb is to keep your *total* carbs low, there are ingredients that are technically high in carbs that really shouldn't be ruining your day. For instance, some herbs and spices, and garlic in particular, are high in carbs – more than 50 percent carb in some cases. But, you'd struggle to consume enough of any of them to actually make an impact on your blood sugar or your weight. Meanwhile, onions – a favourite topic of mine – have a similar carb content to apples. But you don't walk past the fruit bowl and smash an onion on a whim. When you're cooking dinner for four, you might only use one – a quarter each – which, in my book, means onions make the Green List cut.

There is an explanation, and often a lengthy debate, behind each ingredient on the Real Meal lists, and my hope is that, over time, as you do your own research, you will develop your own list, whether consciously or not. This Green List has worked well for me and many of the realmealrevolution.com members, but you will become aware, if you're not already, of what foods do and don't agree with you.

Please note a critical observation: the majority of foods on the Green List are vegetables. This is not a coincidence, and it is reflected in the recipes in this book. If it is not evident through the book, please hear me now: eat your vegetables! Personally, I stick to a ratio of two veg dishes to one meat.

If some of the ingredients in this book are not available in your area, feel free to replace them with your favorite local veggies, meats and fish. Many of our chicken dishes would work equally well with turkey, for example, and some of the beef recipes that involve long, slow cooking would be good ways of preparing goat. If you have any questions, please email me or my team through the website, realmealrevolution.com.

Download the full, printable Green, Orange, Red and Grey lists for free from realmealrevolution.com.

THE GREEN LIST

FRUIT & VEGETABLES

- All green leafy vegetables
- Artichoke hearts (p)
- Asparagus (p)
- Aubergine (n)
- Avocado (p)
- Bean sprouts
- Beans (whole in pods, such as green, runner, broad) (p)
- Broccoli (p)
- Brussels sprouts (p)
- Cabbage (p)
- Cauliflower (p)
- Celery (p)
- Chard (p)
- Courgettes
- Cucumber
- Endive (p)
- Fennel (p)
- Garlic (p)
- Gem squash
- Kale (p)
- Leeks (p)
- Lemons and limes
- Lettuce
- Mange tout (p)
- Mushrooms
- Olives
- Onions (p)
- Okra
- Palm hearts (p)
- Peppers (all kinds) (n)
- Radicchio (p)
- Radishes (p)
- Rhubarb
- Rocket (p)
- Shallots (p)
- Spinach (p)
- Spring onions
- Sugar-snaps (p)
- Tomatoes (n)
- Turnips
- Watercress (p)

DRINKS

- Caffeine-free herbal teas (with real slices of fruit and herbs)
- Flavoured waters from RMR recipes or other recipes that follow the lists
- Water – sparkling or still

PROTEINS

Free-range, organic and as natural as possible

- All meats, poultry and game
- All naturally cured meats like pancetta, parma ham, coppa, bacon, salami, biltong, jerky
- All offal (highly recommended)
- All seafood
- Eggs

CONDIMENTS

- All vinegars, flavourings and condiments are okay provided they are free from sugar, gluten, preservatives or vegetable oils
- Tamari/fermented soy sauce

FERTILISERS

- All homemade bone broths
- Coconut yoghurt
- Coconut kefir
- Kefir butter/cheese
- Kimchi
- Milk kefir
- Naturally fermented pickles
- Sauerkraut

FATS

- Any rendered animal fat (lard, tallow, duck and bacon fat)
- Avocado oil (cold-pressed is best) (e)
- Butter or ghee
- Coconut oil (e)
- Firm cheeses like Cheddar, Emmental and Gouda
- Hard cheeses like Parmigiano Reggiano and Pecorino
- Macadamia oil (e)
- Mayonnaise, free from preservatives and seed oil
- Nut oils like groundnut oil (as long as they're not heated during extraction or cooking)
- Olive oil (extra-virgin) (e)
- Seeds (p)

For those sensitive to nightshades, we've marked them with (n). If you're keen on getting more prebiotics (fibre) into your diet, we've marked prebiotics with (p). And, if you're searching for more digestive enzymes, look out for foods marked with (e).

THE FOUR PILLARS OF FLAVOUR

When you taste something really delicious, that deliciousness is usually the result of four vitally important forces coming together. Conversely, when you taste something uninspired or average, it's often because one or more of these critical factors have been neglected or misused. I call these forces the Four Pillars of Flavour, and they are Produce, Seasoning, Heat and Time.

PRODUCE

When I was still a student, my head chef conferred on me words of great wisdom. He told me that the best chefs in the world aren't any more skilled at actually cooking than most chefs with five years' experience. What sets them apart is their phenomenal appreciation and understanding of ingredients.

Take a winemaker's approach to harvesting as an extreme example. Harvesting grapes two weeks early might create a lower-alcohol, almost sour, low-colour wine, while harvesting them two weeks late might result in a 'flabby', overly fruity wine, lacking acidity, with a high alcohol content.

Much as a master winemaker knows the exact date to harvest his grapes, a great cook must know the nuances of every ingredient, and what each one looks, feels and smells like on the exact date on which it is ready to eat. In my opinion, great cooks are ingredient connoisseurs, and their job should be to use as few techniques as possible to showcase the brilliance of what they've scored at the market.

Great produce is half the battle won, and you can learn to win more often by simply smelling, feeling and tasting your ingredients while you're cooking them. Make an effort to remember what tasted good, and consider whether it was good just because the ingredients were good, and not because of any fancy thing you did to them.

You'll soon be that person at the store smelling the melon, fingering the avocado or, eventually, asking the fishmonger for a sliver of raw fish.

SEASONING

Sometimes all an average dish needs to elevate it to OMG greatness is a squeeze of lime or a tablespoon of soy. But be warned: as simple as seasoning may sound, it is the killer of many a potentially great meal.

Every cuisine from around the world has its own nuances, and those nuances come from the produce available and the ingredients used to season them. But there are common traits that make all food delicious.

Humans have an obvious affinity for sweetness. But our palates are most excited when all parts of our tongues are stimulated in the right proportions. We like our food to be a little bit sweet, a little bit salty, a little bit sour (acid) and, sometimes, a little bit bitter. Then, some humans like it hot.

Each cuisine has its own ways of adding sweetness, saltiness and acidity. And although adding the right pinch of salt, twist of lemon, splash of olive oil and sprinkling of sugar will add this balance to just about anything, knowing the right things to use for different types of cuisines will make your food taste authentic and, in general, better.

Some examples of acids would be lemon juice (anywhere west of India), vinegar (most of Europe), lime and yuzu (southeast Asia). But because they carry a lot of acid, these sour flavours can alter the consistency of some foods; they might split a cream-based sauce, for instance. There are also dry sour flavours like amchoor powder, which is powdered dried green mango, and sumac, both of which are used from Israel to Myanmar.

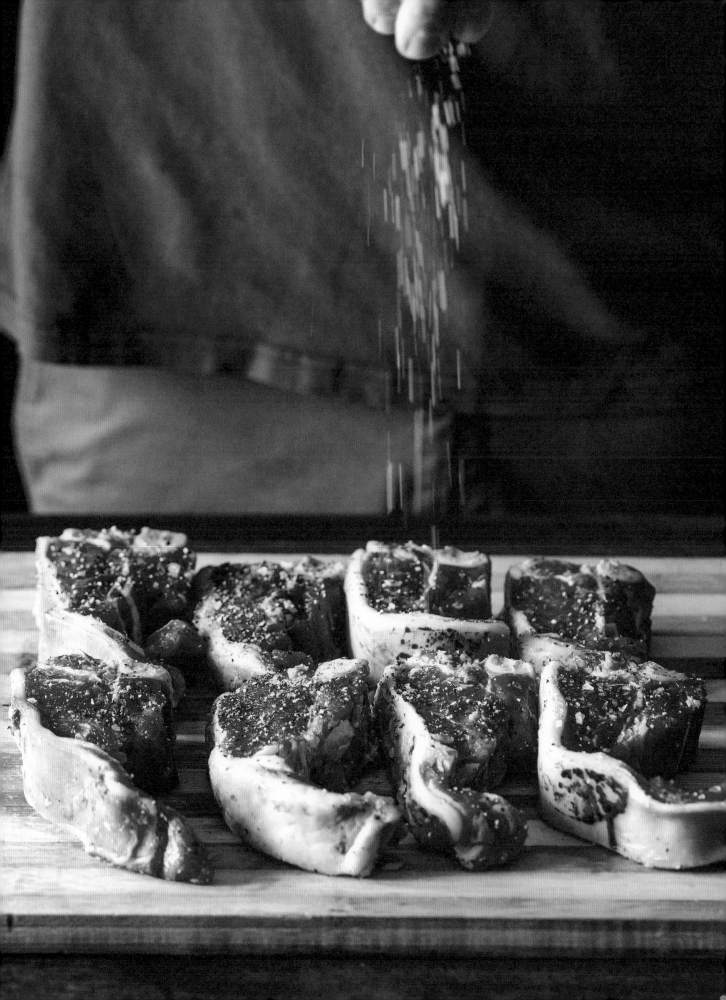

Saltiness can be found in good old sea salt, soy sauce (most of eastern Asia) and fish sauce (southeast Asia and some places in India).

Bitterness is actually more popular than you might think. Olive oil adds bitterness to most meals eaten west of India on a daily basis. In the Far East there are literally thousands of fermented pastes and delicacies that add the bitter edge, but the one we are most familiar with is fermented shrimp paste.

My final note on seasoning is this: remember that you don't add seasoning to add the flavour of salt / pepper / lime juice / fish sauce / whatever. You add these things to enhance the flavour of the hero ingredients in whatever it is you are cooking.

You'll know when you're seasoning like a master when your food tastes perfectly balanced, and the flavours explode in your mouth, but you can't actually taste any of the individual seasonings.

HEAT

Proteins, carbs and fats all work together in mysterious ways in the pan. Carbs cooked in lots of fat at the right temperature can get very crispy. Protein cooked in anything at the right temperature coagulates (solidifies) eventually, while fats soften and harden when warmed or cooled. Cooking in fat is also considered a dry cooking method, which is easy to understand if you consider the fact that you can burn something in fat, but you can never burn something in water.

At the bottom of all of these reactions is heat. It is heat that causes these things to crisp up, melt down or coagulate, and the misapplication of heat to even the best ingredient can ruin it. The sinewy cuts require low temperatures which, over time, break down the sinews. The likes of green vegetables and leaner, more tender cuts of meat require high heat, in shorter bursts, to bring out the best in them.

Heat and time also have a huge impact on texture, which is not a flavour, but plays a large role in how flavour is carried.

There are some basics that you will pick up as you cook your way through this book. It won't take you long before you appreciate the huge difference that a hotter or cooler pan can make to the ingredients that you're cooking.

TIME

Time and heat are intimately related; in fact, they can't really be considered independently of each other. When something is cooked at a ferocious heat, it is generally cooked for a shorter period. Likewise, when something is cooked at a very low heat, it will most likely be cooked for a long time. Time is often an element of cooking in the absence of heat, as in fermentation, pickling or curing. Time is the secret ingredient that can be applied to any curry, stew, dressing or marinade that will allow the flavours to intensify and the colours to darken. You will know you have achieved true mastery when you forget cooking times, you intuitively know that your lamb shanks need two hours at 180 °C, or your courgettes two minutes at a high heat, and when to add minutes on or take them away.

In life, time is your most valuable resource, and mastering this pillar will not only enhance your skills as a cook, but deliver more wealth in an age of time-poverty.

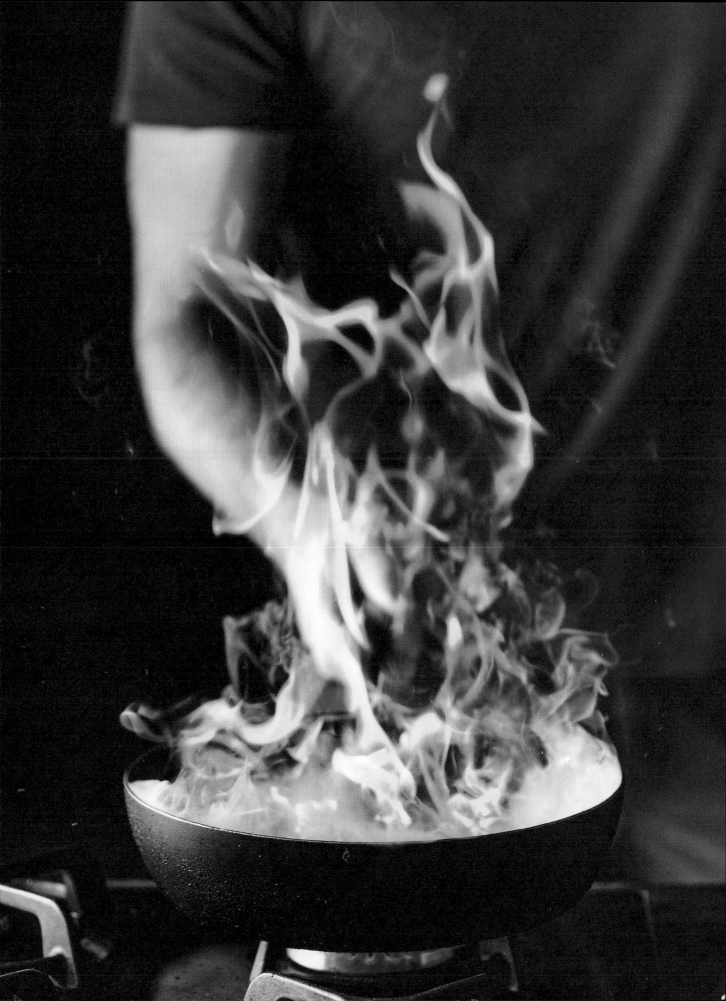

ALL THE GEAR AND NO IDEA

My lecturer at college, a chef of the old era, drilled into us that 'We don't need machines. We are machines.'

For the most part, I've taken this good advice to heart. Apart from the stick blender, the food processor and a good quality spiralizer, he is most certainly correct.

In my experience, industrial knives, boards, bowls, pots and the like are often cheaper than the fancy branded versions you get in homeware shops, and they work better and are more durable.

My thoughts on the basics are as follows.

Glass and ceramic cutting boards should all be milled into sand, or used as decorations. There is nothing worse to cut on, except for rock. Wood and plastic are the way to go.

Spend as much as you can on the best heavy-based pans, pots and casseroles you can afford. But more importantly, don't waste a cent on cheap thin-based anything. They will warp. But before they do, they will suck to cook with.

To elaborate on heavy versus thin-based pans, you will discover as you work through the recipes in these pages that most methods start with medium, medium-high or high heat. If you're cooking with a thin-based pan, the temperature of the pan will drop immediately when you add whatever it is you're cooking. With a heavy-based pan, the base of the pan retains its heat no matter what you add.

If you're a novice, you may be thinking, 'Yes, but it will heat up again, my stove is awesome.' That cold period will make or break your meal, because when food is heated from a cold pan, its juices often leach out into the pan, and the thing you were trying to fry, or sear, ends up boiling in its own juices. Which is bad.

So basically you need wood or plastic to cut on, some heavy-based cookware and some (sharp) industrial knives. These will improve your odds of making things more delicious.

That all said, we do need to chat about knives in a little more detail. So please turn the page.

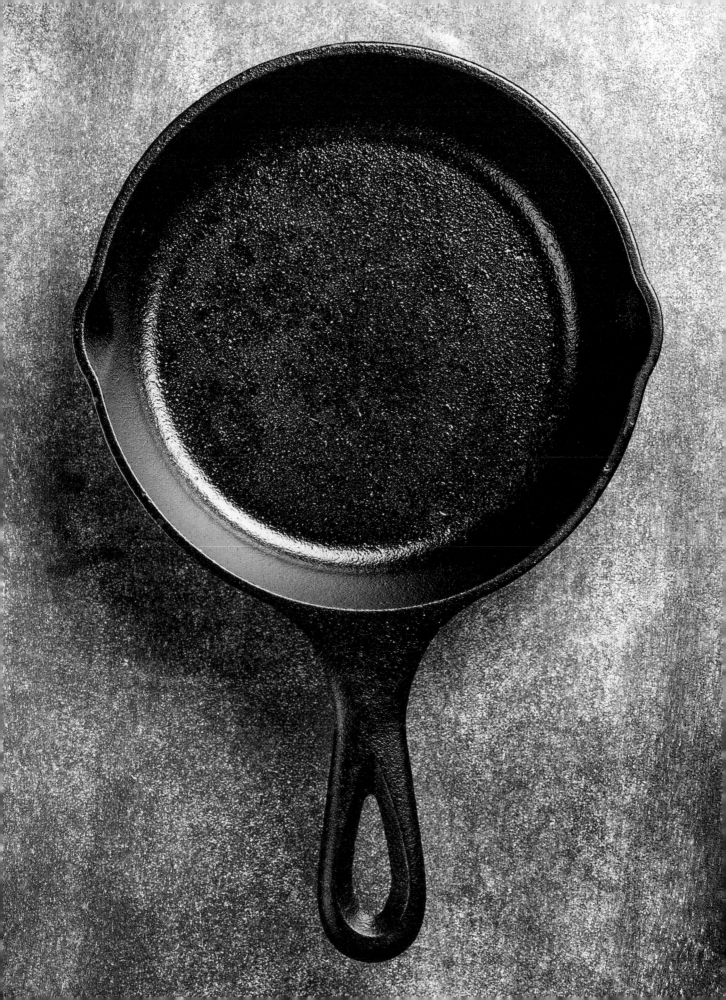

Those are my knives on the opposite page. What should be immediately obvious is I don't simply go for the most expensive of everything. The two points I consider when choosing a knife are comfort and ease of sharpening. If a knife can't be sharpened easily, it will only be sharp for the first few weeks you have it.

Sharpening a knife erodes the blade over time. For a carving knife or a boning knife, which you would use on a meat joint, that's fine. For a chef's knife or santoku, which requires the knife to be flush with the board to do its job, the erosion will end up creating an arch between the blade and the board, rendering the knife useless… unless your blade doesn't have a butt.

If you look at the point where a carving knife is joined to the handle, you will see the whole piece of metal thickens before it is attached to the handle. If you compare that to the base of the chef's knife and the santoku, the blade is the blade all the way to the end. What this means is that when you are sharpening it, you can run the sharpener all the way to the end of the blade, so the whole blade erodes at the same pace.

These are the knives (and sharpeners, tweezers, grater and peeler) you need:

1 Pin-boning tweezers You could use long nose pliers too. These ones have a super-flat edge and are very strong, which helps when pulling out tough fish bones.

2 Microplane The only thing you should ever grate Parmigiano Reggiano with. Also great for minced garlic and ginger.

3 Smooth paring knife Great for finicky veg work like cutting florets from cauliflower and broccoli.

4 Serrated paring knife Same as above but the serrated edge is better for cutting through tomatoes and aubergines.

5 Tomato knife My favourite of the little knives. I use this for everything, including as a steak knife, which annoys my wife no end.

6 Sharpening steel It takes some practice, but as long as your knife still has an edge, you should be able to get it back to the sharpness it had on the day you bought it by using this guy.

7 Chef's knife For any amount of laborious chopping, even breaking through small bones, and cutting big things in half, this is my go-to blade.

8 Santoku Much the same as above, though the one pictured is my wife's, so I only get to use it when she's not cooking.

9 Carving knife Obviously used for carving meat but superb for cutting sashimi and other very neat stuff.

10 Filleting knife This one has a bendy blade that makes it perfect for getting between a fish fillet and its bones.

11 Boning knife Honestly, you should get this knife just to see how easy it is to debone a chicken. It's also great for portioning any meats with bones in them.

12 Peeler Obviously you need a peeler, but this peeler is the best and probably the only peeler you should ever have. When it was invented everyone else who makes peelers should have packed up and gone home. Light, perfectly balanced, cheaper than a block of butter. Look no further.

13 Sharpener/edge-maker When you can't get your blade any sharper using a steel, it usually means your edge has gone. This tool actually scrapes an entirely new edge on your blade. After using this, all you'll need is a minute on the steel and you should have your blade back in showroom condition.

That's literally everything you need. Probably more than you need. In my first two years as a professional chef all I had was a tomato knife and a chef's knife, and I still managed to get promoted.

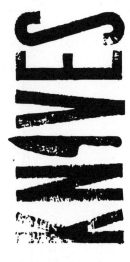

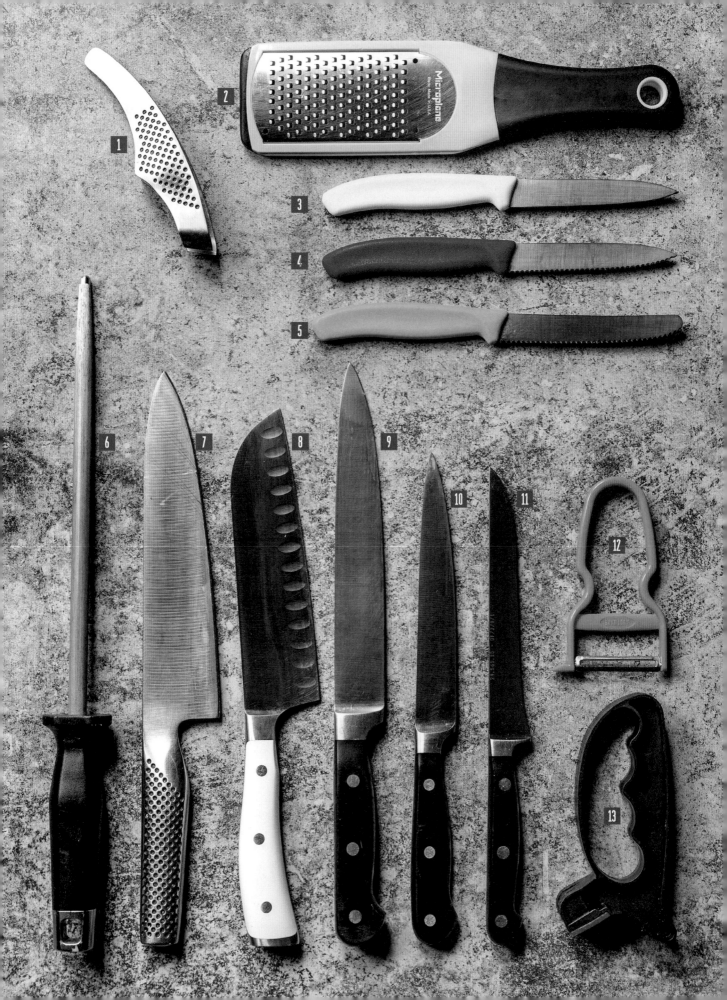

SPEAKING JONNO

While you may already know how to cut stuff, this page is here to show you what I mean when I describe things in my methods. Not all chefs speak the same dialect of chef, so here are some translations from Jonno into English.

1 Garlic, roughly chopped I like chunks of garlic so they can turn bitter on the outside but stay soft and sweet on the inside.

2 Finely grated ginger and

3 Finely grated garlic Usually how I prep these two for dressings and marinades, where I need them to infuse flavour. Use a microplane.

4 Snipped chives Longer than chopped chives. They look prettier. And they're easier to do.

5 Roughly chopped parsley, coriander and oregano This is how I like to chop any herbs that get thrown into a dish as a finishing touch. There's no need to finely chop them; my way they still release their flavours – and they stay pretty.

6 Cucumber grated on the large grater That's the large grater look – how I do cucumber for tzatziki, as well as courgettes for courgette cakes, and my preferred way for carrots.

7 Julienne I hardly ever call for this one, but that's what it looks like.

8 Smashed or cracked black pepper and

9 Smashed or cracked spices I'll call for either of these when I want a little more texture in a dish, along with the flavour, or when it will be cooked for so long that the spices will disintegrate.

10 Shredded cabbage What you buy a mandolin for – but easily done with a chef's knife.

11 Sliced ginger I call for this in long cooking methods where it will either be broken down or strained off at the end. You could leave the peel on if you want.

12 Sliced onion Used everywhere. Something you really should practise.

13 Roughly chopped onion I use this in recipes that get cooked for hours because the neatness of your chopping will be lost when the onions disintegrate in the sauce.

14 Finely chopped or minced onion What you need when you'll see the onion in the finished product and it needs to look neat. Gravies, dressings and other quick sauces get this treatment.

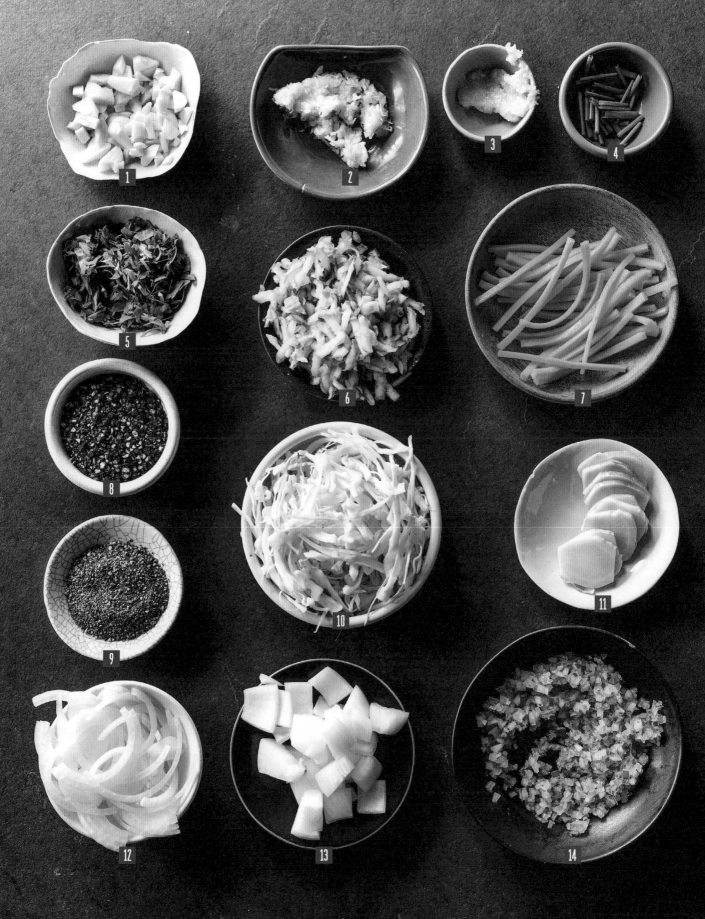

A FEW MORE JONNOISMS:

A thumb of ginger, or anything else: look at your thumb, and cut a piece as big as that. The same rule applies to one finger and two fingers.

And then handfuls of herbs. I usually use 'handful' when I'm talking about fresh parsley, coriander or oregano. See below for what I mean by a large, medium and small handful.

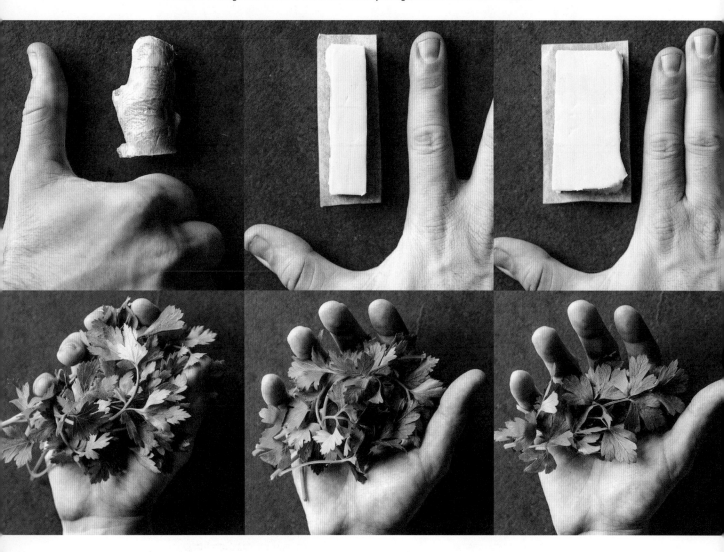

Note: some of the recipes in this book include exact measurements – see the conversion table on page 320 if you prefer using 'cups'. There is no need to be too scientific – please adjust according to your taste!

WHEN YOU ACQUIRE COOKING SKILLS AND TACKLE FOOD HEAD-ON, RATHER THAN FEARING IT, EATING BECOMES MORE PLEASURABLE AND REWARDING.

WEIGHT LOSS AND AWESOME HEALTH ARE SIDE EFFECTS.

CARAMELISATION
THE GOLDEN KEY OF COOKERY

If you've ever wondered why we're wired to prefer the taste of grilled foods over boiled foods, prepare to have your mind blown.

You may already know that we humans are prone to developing an addiction to sugar. And though we love pure white sugar, what we love even more is the flavour of burnt sugar, or caramel as we call it in the kitchen. The best example of a caramel that everyone loves is Coca-Cola, which is basically water, sugar and caramel, with bubbles. The billions of servings of Coke products that are consumed every week around the world might represent a lot of poor beverage-choice decision-making, but they do teach us something valuable. We love sugar and, more than that, we love the bittersweet flavour of caramel.

As it turns out, almost all of the foods that we eat have some natural sugar in them. Even your steak. And the reason your steak goes brown when it's cooked on a high heat is because the natural sugar in it is caramelising. In fact, the reason any of your food goes brown when cooked is because of the caramelisation of its natural sugars.

But don't freak out. Caramelising food doesn't make it higher in sugar than it was before; it only makes it more delicious.

This caramelisation process is called the Maillard reaction and it occurs when sugar reaches about 160°C in the absence of water. In other words, you will need a dry pan and a high heat if you ever want some of this action.

Which leads me to my next subject: onions.

I had always wondered why we add onions in the beginning of so many recipes, and it turns out onions have the same sugar content as apples. Add caramelisation to that, and you're basically adding a caramel bittersweetness to everything you're cooking. That's right, onions add a natural sweetness, and the longer you sauté them, the sweeter they get and the more roasted or grilled caramel flavour they add.

Opposite you can see four phases of onion caramelisation that I regularly refer to in the book: from lightest to darkest they are softened, lightly caramelised, well caramelised and very dark.

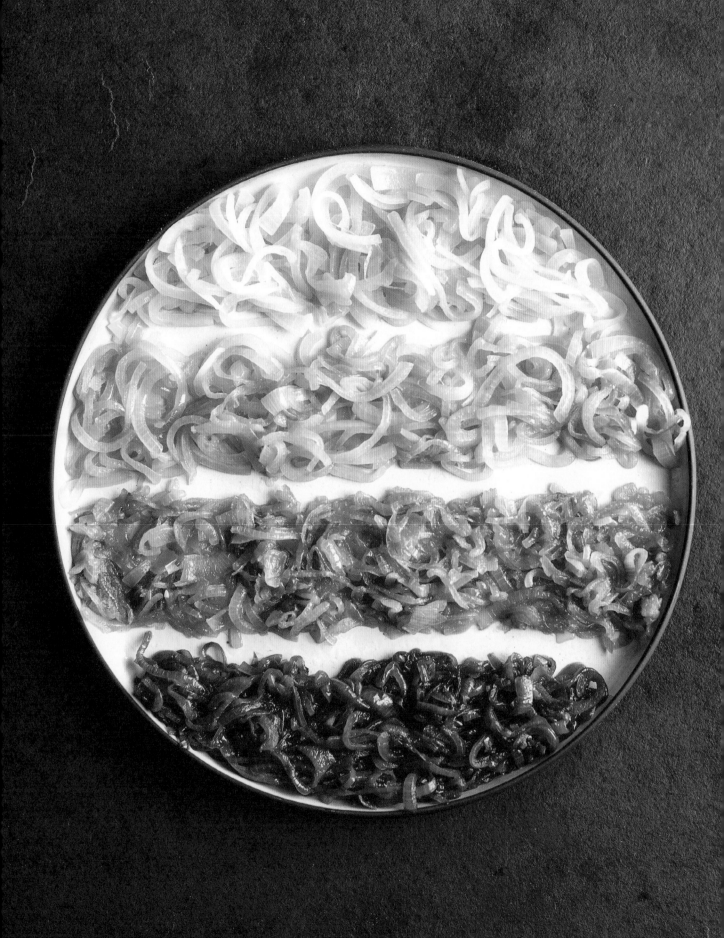

HOW DO YOU LIKE YOUR STEAK?

Following our lesson on caramelisation, it should be no surprise that grilling meat is next. This is believed by most to be the oldest cooking technique known to humankind – which is why it is so sad to see people with grills behaving badly.

The basics of grilling are easy. The more complex stuff like rare, medium rare and medium will come with practice. People do the thumb test but it depends on the size of the piece of meat, the cut and of course the type of meat you're cooking.

There are only two things you are trying to accomplish when you grill, and these are:

★ Delicious grilled flavour
★ Perfect juicy texture

The same rules apply for grilling most cuts:

Make sure your pan is hot The oil should be smoking a bit and the meat you put in the pan needs to sizzle aggressively when it hits the pan. If it doesn't, the meat will release its juices into the pan (see image 1 opposite) – and that will really ruin your day.

Make sure your meat is well seasoned Use salt and pepper, or an invincible spice rub that can withstand high heat without burning and going bitter. If you do opt for a rub, use only enough to bring out the flavour in the meat. If you taste more rub and less meat, you went in too hard.

Use the 2-minute rule A little trick we learned in restaurants, to make sure everyone's meat came out perfectly and at the same time, was to seal the meat off in a pan in advance, then finish it in the oven just before serving. Every piece of meat got two minutes in a very hot pan to get colour all over it. Then each steak was placed in the oven, in separate trays until they were exactly 2 minutes away from being perfectly cooked. This required constant checking and touching and lots of practice. Once each piece was 2 minutes from the perfect rarity we would remove it from the oven and place it on a tray to wait for the hostess to call the kitchen to begin preparing mains. As we got the hostess's call, we'd just pop the whole tray in

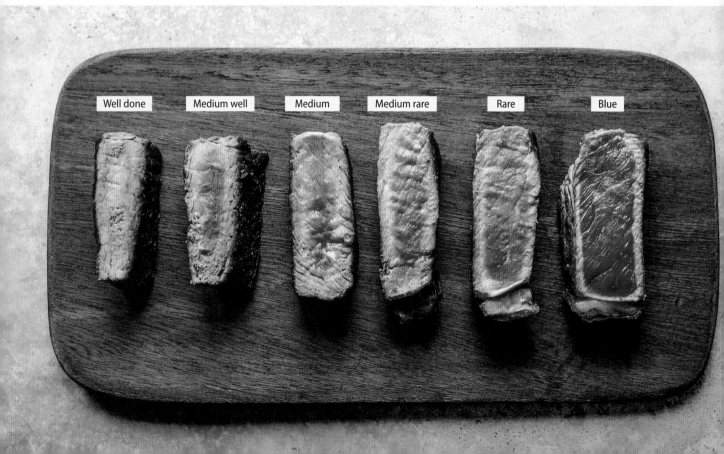

Well done · Medium well · Medium · Medium rare · Rare · Blue

the oven for 2 minutes and – voila! – all the steaks came out perfectly cooked, together. Use this trick and you won't be stressing about rarities while you should be warming veg or pouring drinks. Another benefit is that finishing in the oven creates a lot less smoke than cooking everything in a hot smoking pan. Happy guests all round.

Baby steps If you really have no clue how to cook steak, do this. Preheat your oven to as hot as it can get on the thermofan or convection setting. Cook the steak in a stinking-hot pan for two minutes on each side and place it on a roasting pan. Poke it with your finger, and slice a piece off to see what it looks like inside. Then put it in the oven for two minutes and take it out quickly again. Let it rest for a minute, poke it with your finger again, and slice another piece off to see what it looks like. Repeat this until you either run out of steak or hit well done (dry, grey and awful). Take note of how many minutes it took you, in your oven, to get what you need. Repeat this technique with each different cut you cook and you will soon be an expert.

Courage is being afraid of something but doing it anyway – be brave.

The numbered shots below show you the difference a hot pan can make. In the first shot **1** you can see what happens when you drop an unseasoned steak into a cold pan (or a hot thin-based pan for that matter). The juices aren't sealed inside and they leak out into the pan. The meat comes out grey and dry and you have a bad meal and feel sad.

In the centre shot **2** you can see I'm grilling the fat first so that it's crispy when we get to eating it. Remember, when cooking the actual steak the fat is often not cooked long enough for it to get crispy and tasty, so giving it some love in the beginning can really up your steak game. Also note the seasoning.

Once the fat has rendered, place the steak on its side (bottom image **3**) and let it sizzle. Smoke is essential at this point. No smoke is a bad sign.

Finally, once you've given colour to the one side, flip it and do the other side (main pic **4**). Note that the heat stays the same the whole time. There is never any moisture in the pan. And it looks grilled even though it was cooked in a pan.

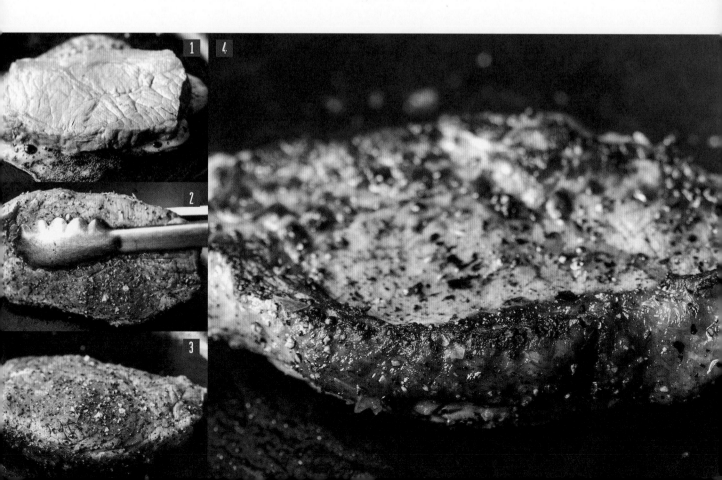

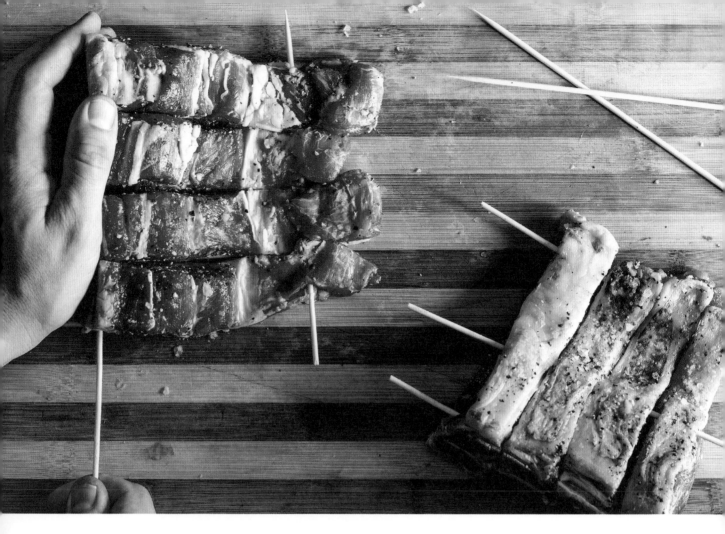

COOKING LAMB CHOPS

If you remember the benefits of grilling the fat from the steak lesson, you'll understand why lamb chops need extra-special attention. The fat-to-meat ratio is almost equal and if you were to cook the meat to medium, or medium rare, the fat would be medium to medium rare too – not ideal, because we all know lamb fat is best when it's crispy, or well done.

Here's how you can cook the fat to well done without overcooking the tender meat.

★ Lay the chops down on a board, fat side down. If possible, try to reassemble them into the order they would have been in when they were still the whole loin.

★ Then push two or three skewers through all of
★ them to rebuild the loin.

★ To crisp up this fat, just place the whole 'loin' fat side down on any grill, griddle or frying pan on a medium heat for about 10 minutes. The fat will drip off, leaving each chop with a delicious
★ crispy layer.

★ Then, separate them and continue grilling, braaiing or barbecuing as usual.

THE ONLY THING YOU NEED TO KNOW ABOUT FIRE

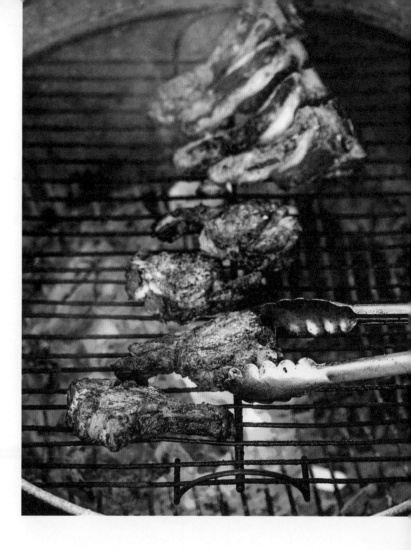

There are thousands of tricks of the trade when it comes to the grill. I believe all of them come with time and practice. For many people, managing the heat on a grill is stressful and can often end in burnt meat, or uncoloured, uncharred, dry meat.

The end goal we are all aiming for is enough char to add flavour without burning the food, and meat (or vegetable) that is cooked to your liking.

Here's one trick that has made my life around the fire a thousand times easier. Only ever build a fire on one side of the grill. Literally, make a half-fire. And you can make it as hot as you like.

What you get from this is a sliding scale of heat. If you look at the picture above, you will see outrageously hot coals on the left and zero ash or coals on the right. There are some flames in the middle, but those are from the fat dripping off the lamb.

What I do then is barbecue down the middle, moving things closer to the heat when I want them to char, and further away when I want them to keep cooking, but without burning.

The fire picture is in a Weber – I turn the coal grid upside down because it helps the coals stay to one side – but you could do this with any grill. It really is a genius manoeuvre.

I also find that knowing there is a safe zone with no direct heat gives me the confidence to position my meat over the hottest part of the fire. This way, there's no need to waste your drink to dampen (or mistakenly extinguish) flaming coals; you can simply slide the goods to the safe zone, breathe a sigh of relief and get excited about the deliciousness to come.

AND THEN THERE'S THE
GRIDDLE PAN

That griddle pan over there is my personal pan. It's made of thick cast iron and I've had it since my early 20s. I use it to put black lines on everything from fish and steaks to courgettes and aubergines.

The same principles from the grilling lesson apply, with two additional rules:

★ There is no 'too hot' for a griddle pan. Only 'too cold'. I leave this thing on the gas hob at full blast for about 10 minutes before I go near it with food. If I don't, I won't get my perfect black lines, but worse, whatever I am cooking on it will stick. The fat that comes off the food creates a ton of smoke, and I either use this when there's a wind pumping through my house, or I just fire this up on a gas burner outside. If you have an extractor, great.

★ Oil the ingredient, not the pan. Whatever you are cooking, make sure you toss it in a bowl with a light coating of oil before placing it on the griddle. Remember, the point of the griddle pan is to get the griddle lines and chargrilled flavour. You will get this by doing the above. If you add oil to the griddle pan, especially if you have obeyed rule one, not only are you going to run a serious fire risk, but you will also be dealing with spitting hot oil as an additional hazard.

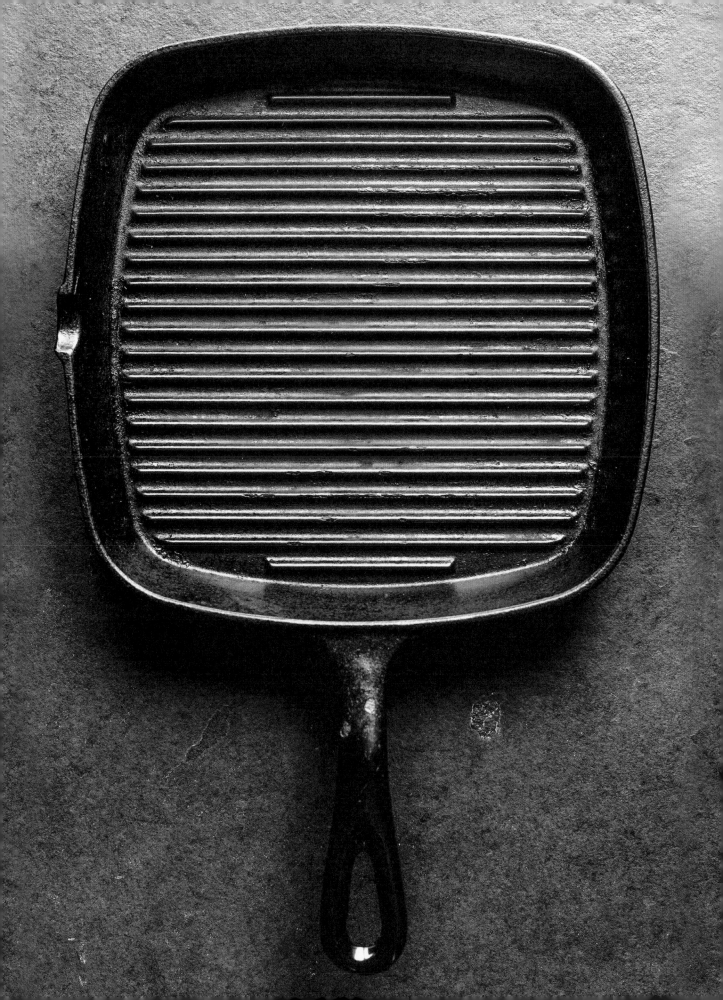

STEAMING & BLANCHING

Throughout the book I make references to blanching and steaming.

I usually say something like 'blanch the ingredient then refresh it in iced water'. Here is the longer explanation.

Blanching could also be described as parboiling. There is no fixed time for blanching all ingredients, but the basic idea is that they are boiled until they are 'just cooked'. Not mushy, not raw.

Carrots could be blanched for five minutes. Asparagus could be blanched for two minutes. The real value in this technique is in the next step, which is to 'refresh'.

Refreshing is what happens when you take these blanched vegetables and drop them into an ice bath – basically a bowl with water and lots of ice. The freezing cold water rushes the food straight back down to an icy temperature, stopping the cooking process dead in its tracks. For some greener veg, refreshing also enhances the colour.

The steps for steaming and blanching are also quite similar.

STEAMING

★ Bring about 4cm of water to a rolling boil in a medium-sized pot.
★ Place the vegetables in a colander that will fit snugly into the pot.
★ Pop the pot lid, or a smaller lid, into the colander to create a steamer.
★ After the specified time has passed, drop the vegetables straight into an ice bath.
★ Once they are cool, remove them from the water, pat them dry with a cloth and keep them out (short term) or in the fridge until you need them.

BLANCHING

★ Bring a pot of water to a rolling boil and throw in a tablespoon of salt.
★ Drop the vegetables into the water and wait until the prescribed time has passed.
★ Use a slotted spoon to transfer the vegetables into an ice bath.
★ Once they are cool, remove them from the water, pat them dry with a cloth and keep them out or in the fridge until you need them later.

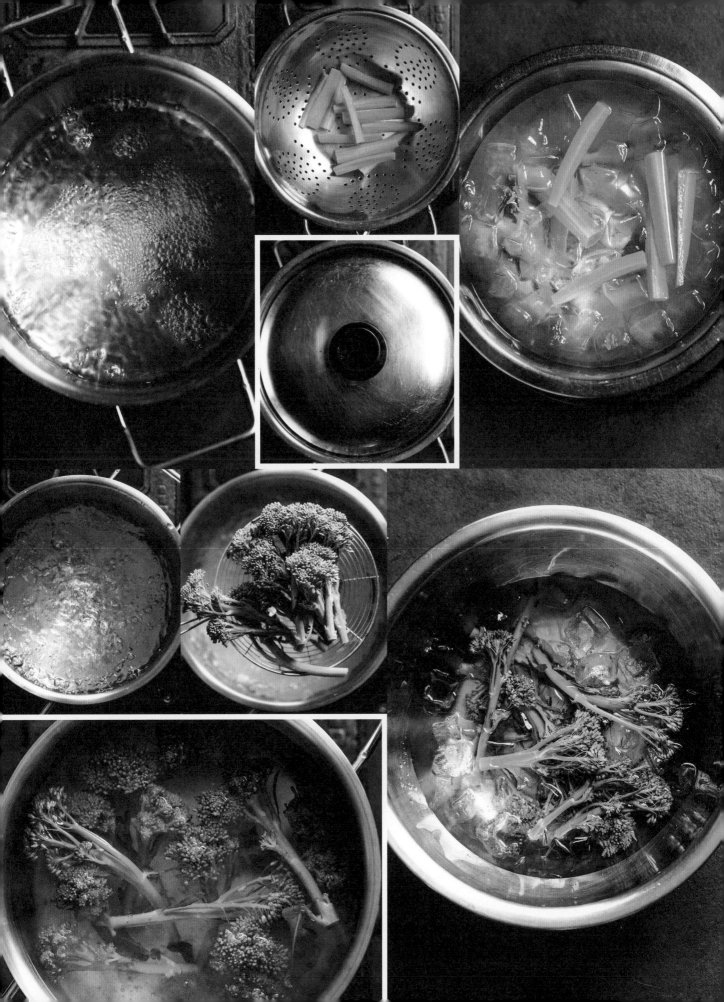

VEGETABLES

The vegetable section, including the numbers of servings, was built around the idea of a dinner or lunch that is made up of the classic 'meat and two veg'. So if you're only having one side, rather than two, you will need to double the recipe for the same yield.

You'll notice that there are about three or four recipes for most vegetables. I've tried to marry different flavour profiles with each vegetable to suit different palates, levels of proficiency in the kitchen and budgets – and, of course, the different protein recipes that you'll see later in the book.

One of the happy challenges of eating good low-carb food is coming up with exciting vegetable dishes. I hope you'll step out of your comfort zone and try something new.

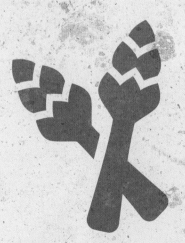

CLEANING AN ARTICHOKE

Whole artichokes can look terrifying if you've never cleaned them before. There's nothing to be afraid of.

Make sure you have a bowl of water handy with some lemon juice in it. Once you expose the meat of artichokes, they oxidise (go brown) at lightning speed. If you cut them in half lengthways, you will see some fibreglass-like hairs in the middle. You can scoop those out with a teaspoon and discard them, as they're not great to eat.

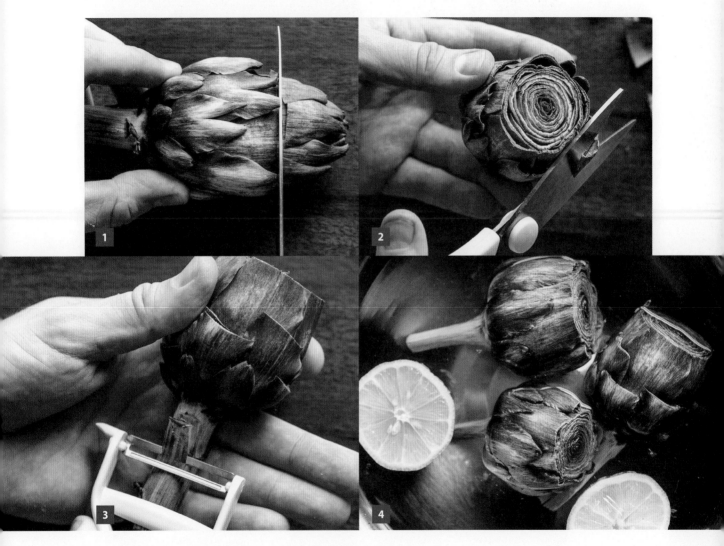

1 First, cut off the top of the artichoke, using a very sharp knife.
2 Then use kitchen scissors to cut away the spiny leaves around the outside.
3 Use a peeler to shave the furry skin from the stem.
4 And drop them straight into the lemon water.

After these steps, you should be able to follow any artichoke recipe like a pro.

ROASTED ARTICHOKES WITH LEMON AND DILL VINAIGRETTE

Serves 4

4 large artichokes

1 solid glug of olive oil

8 garlic cloves, peeled

100ml basic vinaigrette (see page 272)

Juice of 1 fat lemon

½ red onion, finely sliced

2 tbsp capers, roughly chopped

2 tbsp roughly chopped fresh dill

Salt and pepper

Parmigiano Reggiano, to serve

GOES WELL WITH: Chicken Parmigiana, Caprese Salad.

1   Heat your oven up to 200°C.

2   Clean the artichokes as per the cleaning lesson on page 41, then cut them in half lengthways and remove the fibres with a teaspoon.

3   Place the artichoke halves on a large, lightly oiled piece of foil. Season liberally with salt, pepper and a glug of olive oil.

4   Place a clove of garlic in the middle of each artichoke, then fold the foil over to make a large parcel.

5   Place the parcel on a tray and roast the artichokes in the oven for about 40 minutes.

6   While they're roasting, mix the vinaigrette and the lemon juice with the red onion, capers, dill. Season to taste.

7   Once the artichokes are done, leave them to cool for about five minutes before smothering them in the dressing.

8   Tip the artichoke halves onto a platter and serve with a liberal shaving of Parmigiano Reggiano, using a microplane or a peeler.

CARCIOFI ALLA ROMANA – ITALIAN BRAISED ARTICHOKES

Serves 4 to 6

6 artichokes, cleaned as per lesson on
  page 41

250ml dry white wine

250ml olive oil

250ml water

1 small handful fresh parsley,
  finely chopped

1 small handful fresh oregano,
  finely chopped

1 big handful fresh mint,
  finely chopped

Juice of 1 large lemon

2 cloves garlic, minced

Salt and pepper

1   Remove all the hard leaves from the artichokes, then cut them in half lengthways.

2   Place the artichokes face down in a medium-sized pot and cover with the wine, oil and water.

3   Bring the mix to a gentle simmer and leave it to tick away for 20 minutes. The artichokes should be very tender.

4   At this point, add the remaining ingredients and leave the mix to simmer for an additional 5 minutes.

5   Before serving, give the mix a liberal sprinkling of salt and pepper, then transfer the artichokes to a serving plate and drizzle with some of the cooking liquid.

6   These keep well in the fridge for about two weeks – useful if you want to make them in advance.

GOES WELL WITH: Courgetti with Basil, Mint and Pine Nuts, Romesco Chicken Tray Bake.

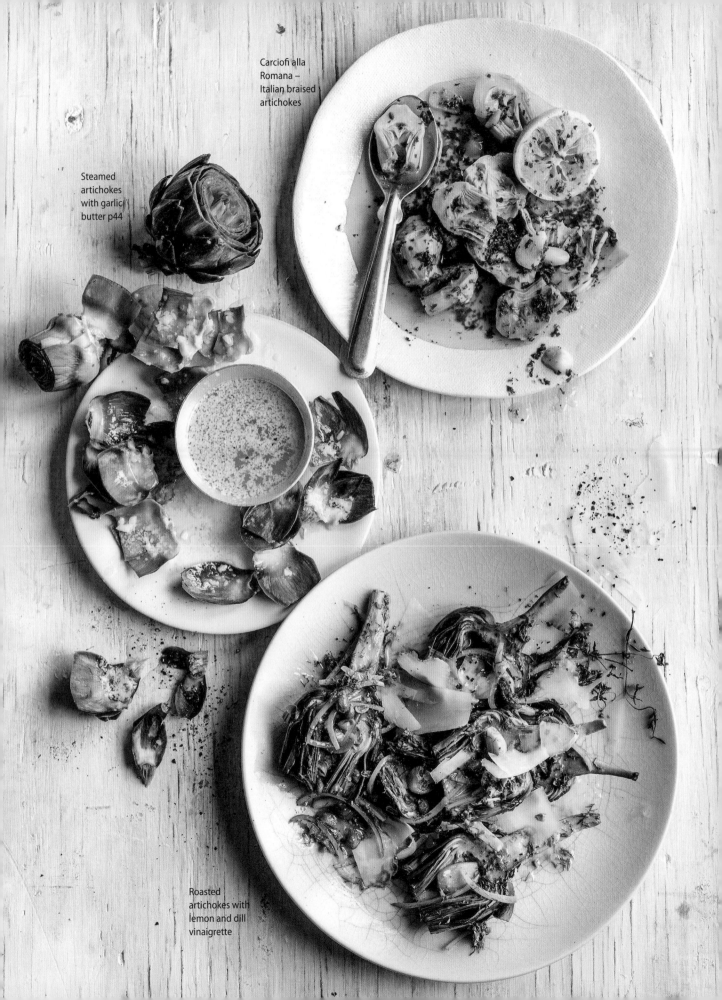

Carciofi alla Romana – Italian braised artichokes

Steamed artichokes with garlic butter p44

Roasted artichokes with lemon and dill vinaigrette

STEAMED ARTICHOKES WITH GARLIC BUTTER

See page 43

Serves 4

My wife makes these for us when artichokes come into season. If you're looking for an ice-breaker on a first date, you'll nail it with this. Nothing screams 'marry me' more than garlicky artichoke all over your face and buttery fingerprints all over your glass of Puligny-Montrachet.

4 artichokes, cleaned as per lesson on page 41
500ml water
350g butter, melted
2 garlic cloves, roughly chopped
3 tbsp fresh lemon juice
Salt and pepper

GOES WELL WITH: Beans with Caper Dressing, Roasted Cherry Tomato Caprese.

1 Place the artichokes in a heavy-based pot that has a fitted lid.
2 Pour about 3cm of water into the pot, pop the lid on and fire it up to as hot as it can go.
3 Leave the artichokes to steam for about 25 minutes.
4 While they're steaming away, melt the butter with the garlic and lemon juice in a small pot.
5 Get it bubbling and spitting hot, then remove it from the heat, season with heaps of salt and pepper and separate it into four dipping bowls.
6 Serve each person an artichoke with a bowl of the garlic butter and let them get their hands dirty.

Best eaten like this: Peel off each leaf and dunk it into the butter. Use your teeth to scrape the meaty bits and the butter off the base of each leaf. The deeper you get into the artichoke, the meatier the bites get. When you finish eating the leaves, use a teaspoon to scrape out and discard the hairy, fluffy stuff. Pour the rest of your butter over the heart of the artichoke and finish the job.

SAUTÉED ASPARAGUS WITH GRIBICHE DRESSING

See page 47

Serves 4

1 hard-boiled egg, yolk and white
   separated, white finely grated
1 tsp Dijon mustard
1 tsp white wine vinegar
4 tbsp olive oil
4 tbsp avocado oil
2 cornichons (baby gherkins),
   finely chopped
½ tbsp capers, finely chopped
1 tsp chopped fresh tarragon
1 tsp chopped chervil
1 tsp chopped flat-leaf parsley
400g asparagus spears, trimmed
Salt and black pepper

1. Place the egg yolk, mustard and white wine vinegar in a small bowl and whisk together until smooth.
2. Slowly whisk in a tablespoon of olive oil (as in the vinaigrette lesson on page 272), adding it in gradually so that it is completely incorporated (emulsified).
3. Once the oil has been whisked in, you should have a creamy-looking mayonnaise.
4. Fold in the remaining ingredients and the grated egg white and leave it to infuse for a couple of hours.
5. For the asparagus, heat a large, heavy-based, non-stick frying pan up to a medium-high heat and add 3 tablespoons of olive oil.
6. When the oil is hot, chuck in the asparagus spears and sauté them for 6 minutes, stirring them around gently from time to time.
7. They should caramelise nicely on the outside while becoming soft, or at least tender, on the inside.
8. Once they're done, tip them onto a platter and spoon over the gribiche dressing along with a liberal sprinkling of salt and a crack of black pepper.

GOES WELL WITH: Tarragon Roasted Chicken, and any meat or fish dish with European flavours.

BUTTERED ASPARAGUS

See page 47

Serves 4

400g asparagus, trimmed
750ml ice
2 tbsp butter
Salt and black pepper

1. Blanch the asparagus spears for 2 minutes, then refresh them in an ice bath as per the lesson on blanching on page 38.
2. Melt the butter over a medium heat in a medium-sized frying pan. Once it starts bubbling, add the asparagus and season with salt and pepper. Toss the spears gently to warm them through and give them an even coating of butter before serving.

GOES WELL WITH: Poached Eggs, Hollandaise/Béarnaise.

CHARRED ASPARAGUS WITH LEMON AND WHOLEGRAIN MUSTARD

Serves 4

Juice and zest of 1 large lemon
1 tbsp wholegrain mustard
4 tbsp olive oil (and extra for drizzling)
400g thick asparagus, trimmed
Salt and black pepper

1 Light up a barbecue to a medium heat or get a griddle pan super-hot.

2 Whisk together the lemon juice, zest, mustard and olive oil, and season with salt and pepper.

3 In a small tray or mixing bowl, drizzle the asparagus with some extra olive oil, season with salt and pepper, and get your hands in there to make sure the spears are all evenly coated.

4 Grill them on the hottest part of the fire or the griddle pan, making sure you get some charred bits on each one.

5 Use your tongs to transfer them back into the mixing bowl, toss them in the lemon-mustard dressing and serve immediately.

GOES WELL WITH: Any grilled meat, fish or poultry, Ratatouille.

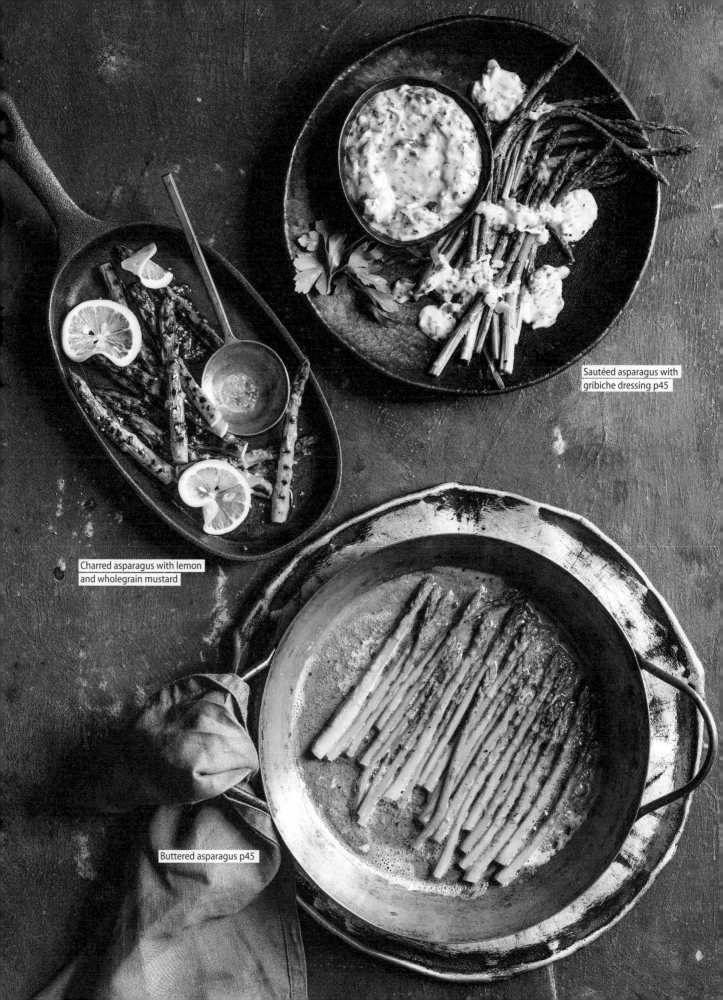

Sautéed asparagus with gribiche dressing p45

Charred asparagus with lemon and wholegrain mustard

Buttered asparagus p45

SPICY AUBERGINE

Serves 4

125ml chicken broth (see page 232)

1 tbsp soy sauce

2 tsp rice vinegar

4 tbsp coconut oil

500g aubergines, cut into 2cm-thick finger lengths (soldiers)

1 garlic clove, finely chopped

1 thumb ginger, grated

2 tsp chilli bean paste

1 tsp chilli flakes

Sesame oil

2 small spring onions, finely sliced

1. Make the sauce by mixing the chicken broth, soy sauce and vinegar in a bowl.
2. Heat the coconut oil up to a high heat in a heavy-based pan and then add the aubergine soldiers.
3. In batches that cover one layer of the surface of the pan at a time, fry the soldiers for about 5 minutes until they are caramelised on the outside and soft on the inside, then tip them into a bowl.
4. In the same pan, with extra oil if needed, add the garlic and ginger to caramelise.
5. Then, add the chilli bean paste, chilli flakes, aubergines and the chicken-broth sauce, and crank up the heat for about 3 minutes for the juices to boil into the soldiers.
6. Give them a splash of sesame oil and a good toss, then tip them onto a platter and scatter with spring onions before serving.

GOES WELL WITH: Lime, Chilli and Sesame Stir-Fried Mange Tout, Fried Garlic Green Beans, Szechuan Boiled Beef.

HOT AUBERGINE SALAD

Serves 4

80ml olive oil

2 tbsp sherry vinegar

1 tbsp smoked paprika

½ tsp ground cumin

4 garlic cloves, peeled and chopped

2 large aubergines, cut into 3cm cubes

2 tbsp fresh lemon juice

½ red onion, finely chopped

1 handful flat-leaf parsley, roughly chopped

1 handful fresh mint, roughly chopped

Salt and black pepper

20g flaked almonds, toasted (smoked is even better)

100g feta or creamy goat's cheese

1. Preheat your oven to 200°C and line and grease a medium-sized baking tray.
2. To make the marinade, whisk together the olive oil, vinegar, smoked paprika, cumin and garlic, and toss the aubergine cubes in it.
3. Spread the cubes out on the baking tray and roast in the oven until golden-brown and tender, about 30 minutes.
4. When they are done, tip them into a bowl and add the lemon juice, red onion, parsley, mint and season with salt and pepper. Mix gently to combine everything.
5. Spoon onto a flat platter or plate and scatter over the almond flakes and crumbles of feta or goat's cheese.

GOES WELL WITH: Greek Pork Chops, Charred Okra with Coriander and Lemon Dressing, Turnip Skordalia.

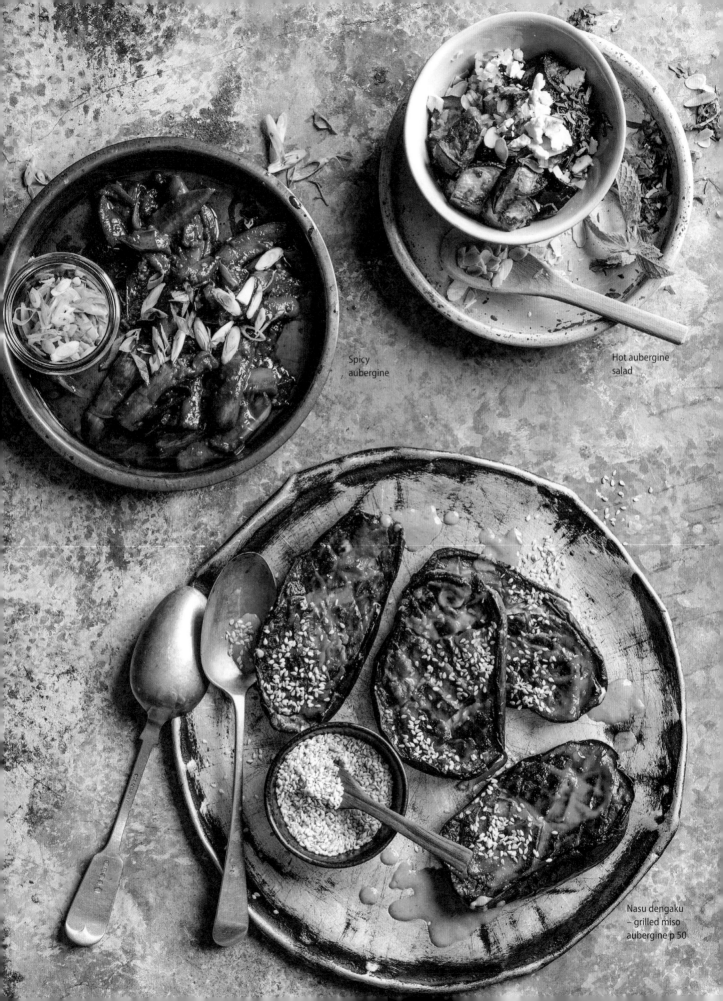

Spicy
aubergine

Hot aubergine
salad

Nasu dengaku
– grilled miso
aubergine p 50

NASU DENGAKU – GRILLED MISO AUBERGINE

See page 49

Serves 4

2 large aubergines, cut in half
  lengthways
2 tbsp coconut oil
4 tbsp yellow miso paste
1 tbsp sake
2 tbsp mirin
2 tbsp toasted sesame seeds

1 Get a barbecue fired up and aim for a medium to high heat – in a Weber, if possible. You can do this in a large, heavy-based pan too.

2 Score the meat of the aubergines in a diamond pattern as deeply as possible without cutting through the skin.

3 Pop the aubergines, skin-side down, on a relatively high heat for about 5 minutes to cook and crisp. If you do this in the pan, throw in a splash of coconut oil to help spread the heat.

4 Flip the aubergines over and cook the fleshy part for another 5 minutes. Put the lid on for this, whether you're using a pan or a Weber.

5 While you're doing this, turn on the oven to the grill setting if you're doing the pan method. Whisk the miso, sake and mirin together for the glaze.

6 When the aubergines are cooked through, pop them on a baking tray with the flesh facing up and give them each a generous glaze of the miso mixture.

7 Grill in the oven or cook indirectly on the Weber (see page 35) for 5 minutes or until they are slightly caramelised and bubbling.

8 Sprinkle with sesame seeds and serve.

GOES WELL WITH: Takeaway Chicken, Kale and Cabbage Salad.

'TO COOK FOR THE PLEASURE OF IT, TO DEVOTE A PORTION OF OUR LEISURE TO IT, IS TO DECLARE OUR INDEPENDENCE FROM THE CORPORATIONS SEEKING TO ORGANISE OUR LIVES INTO YET ANOTHER OCCASION FOR CONSUMPTION.'

– MICHAEL POLLAN

JUST EAT AN AVOCADO

Makes 2 halves

It may seem bizarre that there is a recipe for this, because it is such a simple thing, but it's getting an inclusion because a good avo, served as is, beats anything.

1 avocado
Squeeze of lemon juice
Tabasco sauce (optional)
Salt and pepper

1   Cut the avocado in half (toss the stone), then give it a splash of lemon juice, a drop or two of Tabasco, a liberal salting and peppering, and eat it with a spoon.

GOES WELL WITH: Rough Seed Crackers, Fried Egg, anything with cream cheese.

CHILLED SUGAR SNAP AND AVOCADO SOUP

Serves 2

2 avocados, cut into cubes
1 tbsp fresh lemon juice
1 pinch dried chilli flakes
125ml crème fraîche
125ml Bulgarian yoghurt
250g raw sugar snap peas in their pods
1 handful mint leaves
Salt and black pepper

1   Combine all the ingredients in a food processor and whizz them until everything is super-smooth.
2   Strain the soup through a sieve, chill and serve.

GOES WELL WITH: This is a superb starter before any fish or light poultry dish. Serve with seed crackers.

BILTONG-FILLED AVOCADO

Makes 4 halves

2 avocados
1 tbsp fresh lemon juice
60g biltong powder
4 tbsp cream cheese
1 pinch paprika
1 pinch cayenne pepper
1 tsp finely chopped spring onions
Salt and black pepper

1   Slice the avocados in half and remove the stones, leaving the skins on.
2   Mix the remaining ingredients together in a mixing bowl, season to taste.
3   Divide the mixture between the four avocado halves and serve immediately.

GOES WELL WITH: Charred Asparagus with Lemon and Wholegrain Mustard.

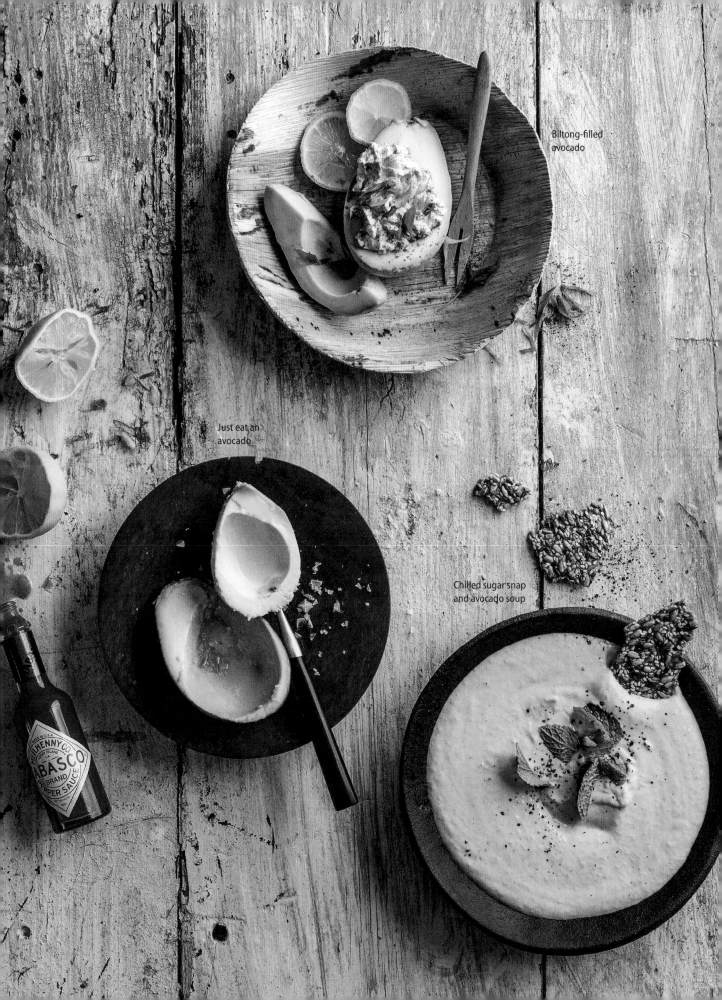

Biltong-filled
avocado

Just eat an
avocado

Chilled sugar'snap
and avocado soup

ROASTED BROCCOLI

Serves 4

1 head broccoli, cut into florets
3 tbsp olive oil
1 tsp salt
1 tsp black pepper
90g Parmigiano Reggiano shavings
½ tsp dried chilli flakes

1 Preheat your oven to 220°C.
2 Mix the broccoli florets, olive oil, salt and pepper in a mixing bowl before laying them, evenly spaced, on a baking tray.
3 Pop them into the oven and roast for about 10 minutes, giving them a good toss at the 5-minute mark.
4 Remove from the oven and serve immediately, sprinkled with Parmigiano Reggiano shavings and dried chilli flakes.

GOES WELL WITH: Courgetti with Mint, Basil and Pine Nuts, Garlic, Thyme & Truffle Mushroom Sosaties.

BROCCOLINI IN OYSTER SAUCE

Serves 4

400g broccolini
1 tbsp coconut oil
1 garlic clove, thinly sliced
4 tbsp oyster sauce
2 tbsp vegetable or chicken broth
   or stock
1 tsp sesame oil
2 tbsp toasted sesame seeds

1 Blanch the broccolini for 3 to 4 minutes and refresh it in ice-cold water as per blanching lesson on page 38.
2 Heat the coconut oil in a large, heavy-based pan over a medium-high heat and fry the garlic and the broccolini for about a minute.
3 Add the oyster sauce and cook for another minute.
4 Add the stock and the sesame oil, and cook until everything is heated and mixed well.
5 Serve immediately with a sprinkling of sesame seeds.

GOES WELL WITH: Confit Duck, Stir-fried Spring Onions and Pak Choi, Gyu Tan Don Chinese Ox Tongue.

BUTTERED BROCCOLI

Serves 4

1 head broccoli, cut into florets
2 tbsp butter
Salt and black pepper

1 Blanch the broccoli for 3 to 4 minutes and refresh it in ice-cold water as per blanching lesson on page 38.
2 Heat the butter in a pan over a medium heat and add the broccoli.
3 Warm the broccoli through, season with salt and pepper, and serve immediately.

GOES WELL WITH: Any grilled meat, fish or poultry, Wet Jerk Spiced Chicken, Romesco Chicken Tray Bake.

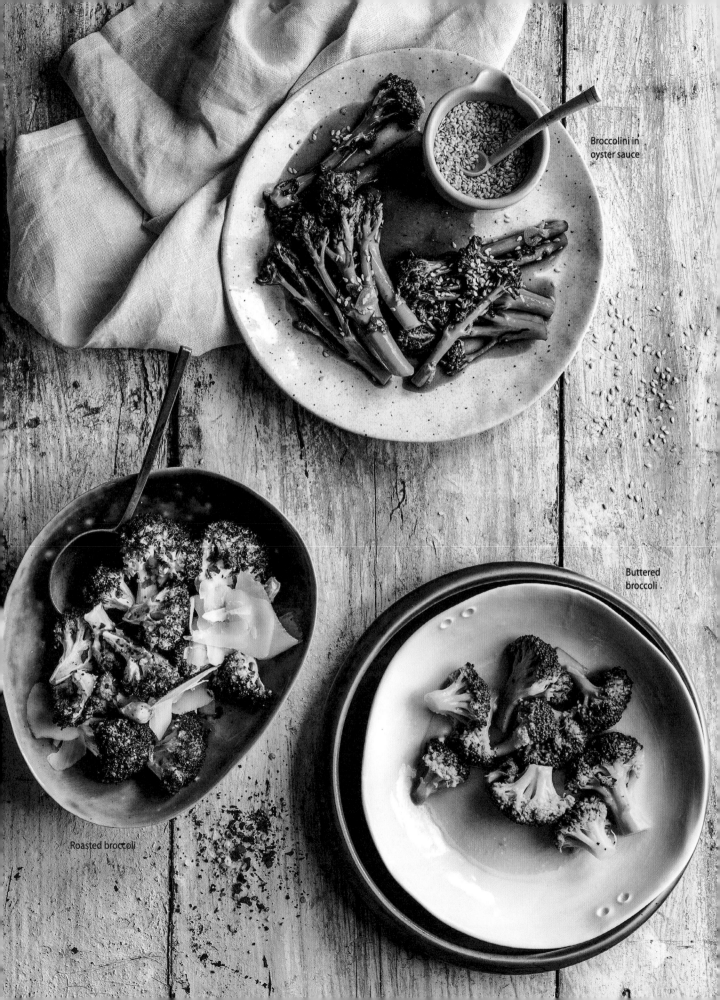

Broccolini in oyster sauce

Buttered broccoli

Roasted broccoli

ROASTED BRUSSELS SPROUTS

Serves 4

400g Brussels sprouts, cut in
  half lengthways
1 white onion, cut into 12 wedges
2 garlic cloves, roughly chopped
1 solid glug of olive oil
Salt and black pepper
Lemon

1 Preheat your oven to 180°C.
2 In a medium bowl, mix all of the ingredients together.
3 Tip the mix into a roasting tray and pop it in the oven for about 30 minutes until everything is nice and brown.
4 Serve immediately with a squeeze of lemon.

GOES WELL WITH: Sole Meunière, Marinated Endive with Pecorino and Walnuts and Blue Cheese Dip, Rémoulade Sauce.

CREAMY BRUSSELS SPROUTS

Serves 4

400g Brussels sprouts
1 red onion, finely chopped
2 tbsp butter
3 sprigs thyme, destemmed
  and finely chopped
250ml cream
180g grated Gruyère or Cheddar
1 pinch ground nutmeg
Salt and black pepper

1 Preheat your oven to 180°C.
2 Cut the sprouts in half and blanch them for 4 minutes before refreshing them in iced water, as per the blanching lesson on page 38.
3 Soften the onion in butter over a medium heat in a large, heavy-based pan, then mix in the thyme and cream and bring to the boil.
4 When the mixture starts to boil, remove it from the heat and stir in half of the cheese, nutmeg and salt and pepper to taste.
5 Mix the sprouts in the sauce and tip them into a gratin dish. Cover loosely with foil and place in the oven for about 35 minutes.
6 Remove the foil, top the bake with the remaining cheese and pop it under the grill until the cheese forms a golden-brown crust. Serve immediately.

GOES WELL WITH: Tarragon Roasted Chicken, Kale, Bacon and Sweet Onions with Roasted Garlic, Charred Leeks with Almond Noisette Dressing and Crème Fraîche.

BUTTERED BRUSSELS SPROUTS

Serves 4

300g Brussels sprouts, cut in half
2 tbsp butter
Salt and black pepper

GOES WELL WITH: Casablanca Chicken Casserole, Kttbular.

1 Blanch the sprouts for 5 minutes as per the blanching lesson on page 38.
2 While they're simmering, melt the butter in a medium-sized pan.
3 Once the sprouts are blanched, use a slotted spoon to tip them straight from the water into the pan.
4 Pump up the heat and sauté the sprouts until they are slightly caramelised, then season them with salt and pepper and serve immediately.

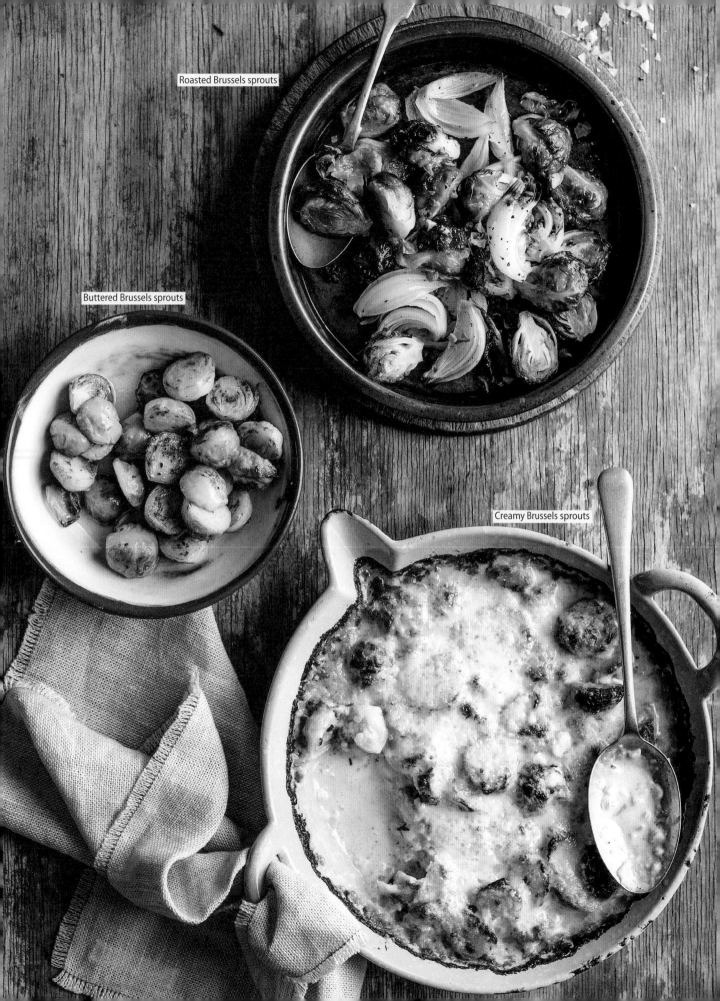

Roasted Brussels sprouts

Buttered Brussels sprouts

Creamy Brussels sprouts

FRIED CURRY CABBAGE

Serves 4

4 tbsp butter

2 garlic cloves, finely sliced

1 large onion, sliced as fine as cabbage

½ head cabbage, shredded

½ tsp ground turmeric

6 curry leaves

½ tsp dried chilli flakes

Salt and black pepper

1 lime, cut into 4 cheeks

1 Melt the butter in a large pan over a high heat.

2 The moment it starts to bubble and sizzle, drop in the garlic, giving the mix a quick stir before adding the onion, cabbage, turmeric and curry leaves.

3 Sauté this mix until the cabbage is well cooked and beginning to caramelise – this could take up to 10 minutes.

4 Once it is cooked, stir through the chilli flakes, add salt and pepper to taste, and serve with lime cheeks.

GOES WELL WITH: Wet Jerk Spiced Chicken.

SPICY ROASTED CABBAGE WEDGES

Serves 4

4 tbsp olive oil

1 garlic clove, minced

4 sundried tomatoes, finely chopped

¼ tsp dried chilli flakes

1 tbsp Dijon mustard

½ head cabbage, cut into 4 wedges

small handful basil, finely chopped

small handful flat-leaf parsley, finely chopped

Salt and black pepper

1 Heat your oven to 200°C.

2 Mix the olive oil, garlic, sundried tomatoes, chilli flakes and mustard in a large bowl.

3 Stir the cabbage wedges through the dressing in the bowl and pop them onto a baking tray, reserving whatever dressing is left in the bowl.

4 Cover the tray with foil and roast for 40 minutes, then remove the foil and pop the tray back for another 15 minutes so the wedges get crispy and brown.

5 Remove from the oven, turn the wedges out into the mixing bowl with the leftover dressing. Add the basil, parsley, season and give it a good toss before serving.

GOES WELL WITH: Chocolate Mole Chicken, Blackened Swordfish with Guacamole.

CLASSIC SLAW

Serves 4

125ml sour cream

250ml mayonnaise (see page 274)

1 tsp apple cider vinegar

1 tsp Dijon mustard

¼ white cabbage, shredded

¼ red cabbage, shredded

1 carrot, peeled and grated

¼ red onion, thinly sliced

Salt and black pepper

1 To make the dressing, whisk together the sour cream, mayonnaise, vinegar and mustard in a small bowl.

2 In another bowl, mix the cabbages, carrot and red onion.

3 Pour the dressing over the vegetables, add a liberal seasoning of salt and pepper, and get your hands in there to give it a proper mix.

4 Leave the slaw in the fridge for about an hour so the flavours can infuse before serving.

GOES WELL WITH: Dry-Rubbed Brisket, Bourbon and Miso Chicken Wings, Crunchy Pigs Ears.

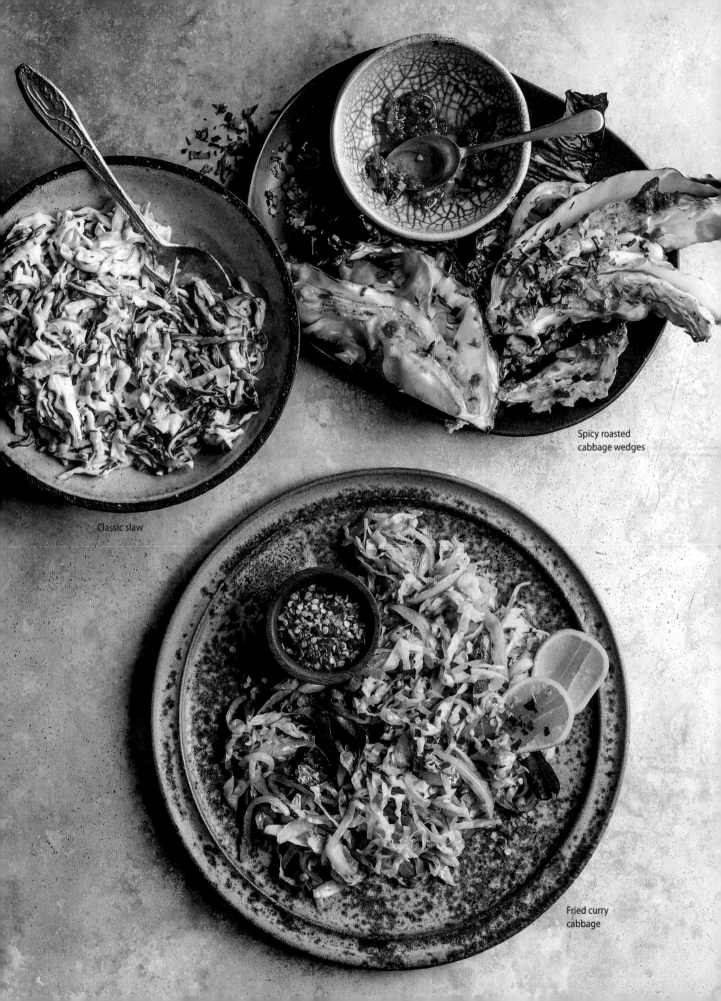

Classic slaw

Spicy roasted
cabbage wedges

Fried curry
cabbage

'DIET FOOD IS
FOR LAZY PEOPLE.'
– ICE T

BERBERE CAULIFLOWER WITH TARATOR

See page 63

Serves 4

4 tbsp tahini

1 tbsp lemon juice

½ clove garlic, minced

1 large pinch salt

Water

1 large head cauliflower, cut
  into florets

120ml melted butter

1½ tbsp ground cinnamon

2 tbsp ground cumin

1 tsp ground allspice

1 pinch ground cardamom

1 pinch ground nutmeg

1 tbsp sumac

1 small handful fresh coriander,
  roughly chopped

1 small handful flat-leaf parsley,
  roughly chopped

2 tbsp toasted pine nuts

Salt and black pepper

1   Heat your oven to 180°C.

2   Whisk the tahini, lemon juice, garlic and salt together.

3   While continuing to whisk, slowly add water, 2 tablespoons at a time, until the tarator has reached the desired consistency. (It should be the consistency of drinking yoghurt, if you remember what that was like.)

4   Place the cauliflower florets into a large mixing bowl.

5   Add the butter, cinnamon, cumin, allspice, cardamom, nutmeg, sumac and season with salt and pepper. Tip the whole lot into a large roasting tray. The florets should be well spaced.

6   Pop them in the oven for 20 minutes, until they are dark and caramelised.

7   Return them back to the mixing bowl, with as much of the butter from the tray as possible, then add the coriander and parsley and mix well.

8   Place them on a platter and scatter with the pine nuts, lashings of tarator and extra herbs.

GOES WELL WITH: Baba Ganoush, Persian-style Stuffed Fish Bake.

For the full recipe for Tarator, see page 298.

CAULIFLOWER COLCANNON

Serves 4

1 head cauliflower

¼ head green cabbage,
  finely shredded

4 tbsp butter

3 tbsp double cream

12g spring onions, chopped

1 small handful dill, finely chopped

Salt and black pepper

1 Steam the cauliflower as per the steaming lesson on page 38.
2 While the cauliflower is steaming, sauté the cabbage in half the butter in a large pan until it is soft and translucent.
3 Once the cauliflower is soft, pour off the water, and add the cream and the remaining butter with some salt and pepper, then purée with a stick blender to make mash.
4 Mix the cauli mash with the cabbage along with the spring onions, dill and a last round of seasoning.
5 Serve immediately.

GOES WELL WITH: Oxtail Stew, Sole Meunière, Hobochokes.

WHOLE ROASTED JERK CAULIFLOWER

Serves 4

2 tbsp salt

2 tsp onion powder

2 tsp ground allspice

2 tsp garlic powder

1 tsp dried red chilli flakes

1 tsp freshly ground black pepper

1 tsp ground nutmeg

1 tsp dried chives

1 tsp paprika

1 tsp ground ginger

½ tsp dried thyme

½ tsp ground cloves

½ tsp ground cinnamon

1 head cauliflower, trimmed
  of leaves and destemmed

2 tbsp coconut oil, melted

Lemon wedges

1 Preheat your oven to 180°C.
2 To make the jerk spice rub, mix all the dry ingredients together.
3 Rub the cauliflower head with the coconut oil, then the jerk rub until it is evenly coated.
4 Pop the head onto a baking tray and cover the tray with foil.
5 Roast in the oven for 1 hour, then remove the foil and roast, uncovered, for another 20 minutes. The cauliflower should be almost black.
6 Serve straight out of the oven with lemon wedges.

GOES WELL WITH: Kale and Cabbage Salad, Wet Jerk Spiced Chicken.
For the full recipe for Dry Jerk Rub, see page 303.

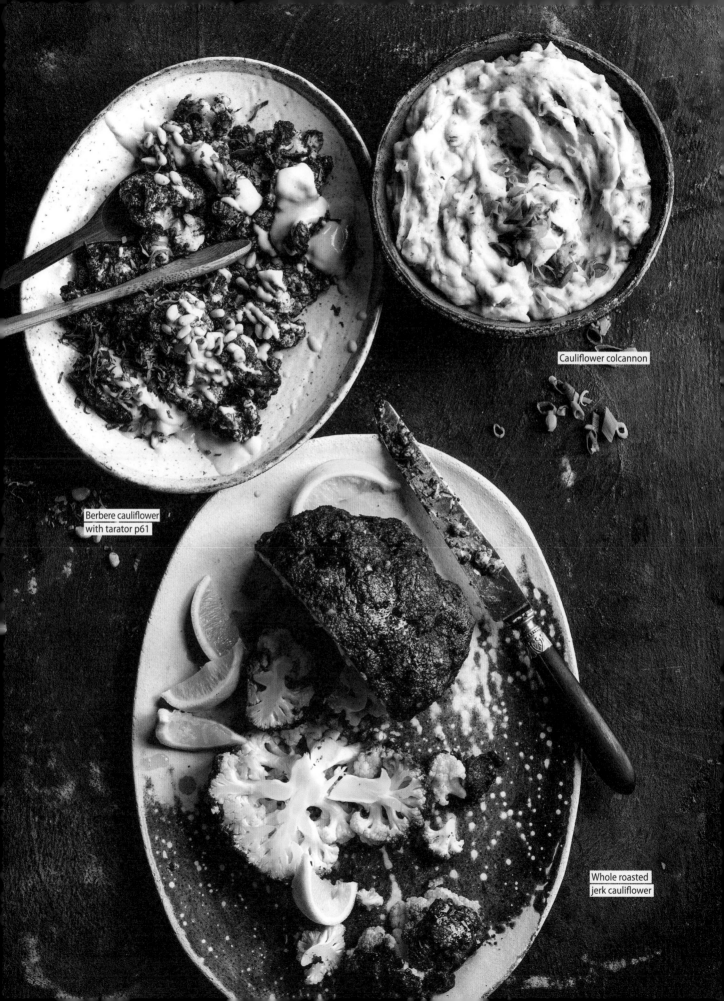

Cauliflower colcannon

Berbere cauliflower
with tarator p61

Whole roasted
jerk cauliflower

PERI-PERI CHARD

Serves 4

2 tbsp olive oil
1 medium onion, roughly chopped
1 red pepper, cored, seeded and
   roughly chopped
1 mild red chilli, finely chopped
1 clove garlic, minced
400g Swiss chard, washed, destemmed
   and roughly chopped
Juice of 1 small lemon
Salt and black pepper

1. Heat the olive oil to a medium heat in a large pan, then toss in the onion and pepper, stirring until they begin to caramelise.
2. Add the chilli and garlic and stir until they become fragrant.
3. Then add the chard and stir it constantly until it has wilted. Pop the lid on and leave it to steam for 3 or 4 minutes to cook through.
4. Take the lid off, give it a squeeze of lemon and some seasoning and serve it hot.

GOES WELL WITH: Takeaway Chicken, Harissa Chicken Wings.

SAUTÉED CHARD AND ALMONDS

Serves 4

3 tbsp olive oil
2 garlic cloves, thinly sliced
40g toasted flaked almonds
400g Swiss chard, washed, destemmed
   and roughly chopped
1 tbsp fresh lemon juice
Salt and black pepper

1. Heat the olive oil in a large saucepan over a medium heat, add the garlic and almonds and sauté for about 2 minutes.
2. Add the chard and stir until it has completely wilted, then continue to stir, while on the heat, until all of the excess moisture in the pan evaporates – this could take up to 5 minutes.
3. Remove from the heat, season with lemon juice, salt and pepper.

GOES WELL WITH: Moreish Pork Fillet Skewers, Romesco Chicken Tray Bake, Persian Baked Fish.

BUTTERED CHARD

Serves 4

2 tbsp butter
400g Swiss chard, washed, destemmed
   and roughly chopped
Salt and pepper

1. Heat the butter in a pan over a medium heat, add the chard, pop the lid on and let it cook for about 3 minutes.
2. Remove the lid and stir the chard until the moisture has evaporated, then season to taste and serve.

GOES WELL WITH: Cocoa and Fennel Pork Loin with Green Sauce, Köttbular, Sardines with Warm Chorizo and Tomato Dressing.

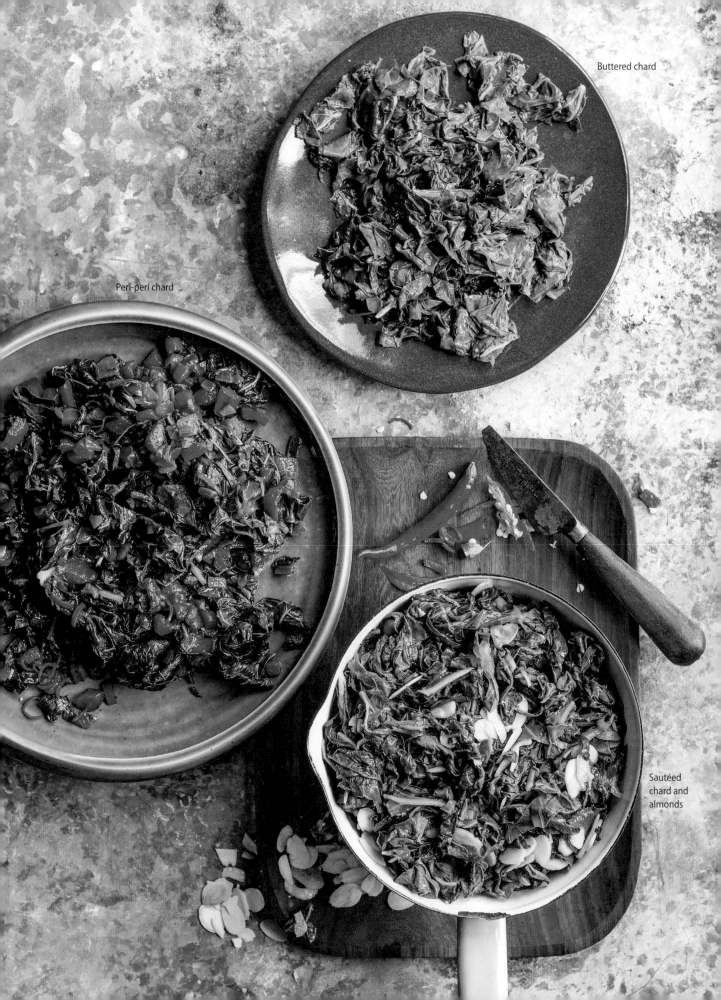

Buttered chard

Peri-peri chard

Sautéed chard and almonds

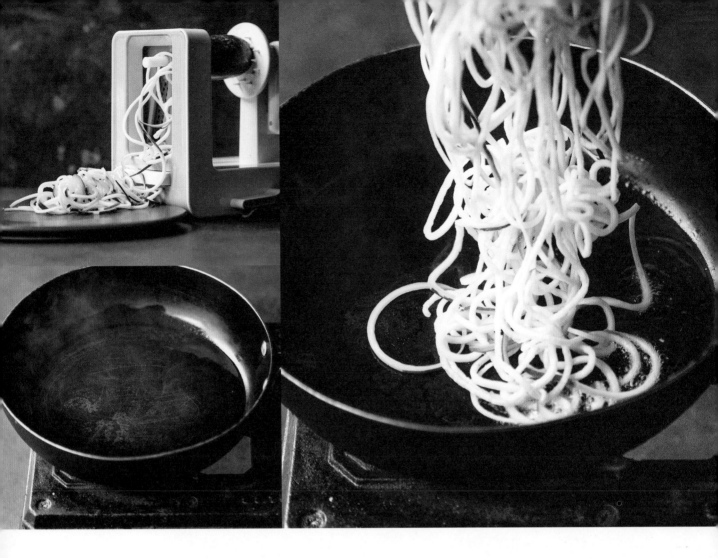

SPIRALISING COURGETTES/MARROWS/ZUCCHINI

Courgetti – Baby Marrow Noodles – Zucchinilini – Spiralised Marrows… Call them what you will, since my first book came out in South Africa, these noodles have been available, pre-packed, on the shelves of all major supermarket chains. It's great that they're widely available, but the store-bought variety can't compare to the ones you make yourself.

It comes back to time, and heat.

The courgetti in the stores have often spent days in the warehouse and on the shelf, and by the time they get to your pan will have released liquid and gone a little mushy. This has a massive impact on the end result. Courgettes have the same reaction to a cold pan and moisture that steaks do – read the lesson on grilling on page 32. For that reason alone, I encourage you to make your own and cook them within hours of cutting them.

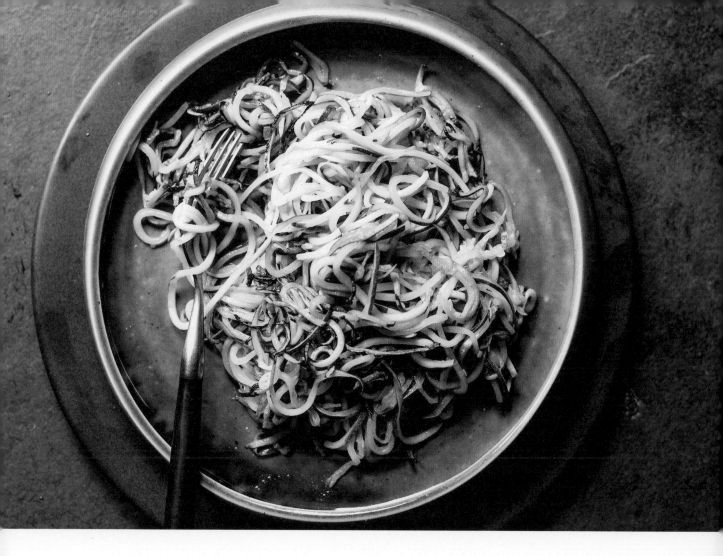

★ Get a decent spiralizer. The handheld ones are cheaper, but they suck. The shape and size of the one in the picture is the only one I'd bother using. There are many brands; that choice is up to you.

★ Spiralise your courgettes into courgetti.

★ Now, the key is to cook your courgetti in batches, so they never crowd the pan and start leaching their juices. You want a really hot pan throughout the cooking process.

★ Get a heavy-based pan really, really hot and drop in some oil (usually coconut or olive – it depends what you're serving them with).

★ Drop the courgetti into the pan – if they don't sizzle, remove them. This means the pan isn't ready.

★ Don't move the pan, just use tongs or a wooden spoon to mix them around gently.

★ Once they have a little colour and have wilted, remove them from the heat and serve.

If any moisture leaches from your courgetti during cooking, one or more of these things is happening. They are too old, your pan isn't hot enough or you've put too many into the pan at once – or all of the above.

WALNUT AND SAGE COURGETTES WITH STILTON

Serves 4

400g large courgettes, sliced

2 tbsp olive oil

3 tbsp butter

1 handful sage leaves, shredded

60g toasted walnuts

50g Stilton

Salt and black pepper

1. Get a griddle pan smoking-hot.
2. Mix the sliced courgettes with olive oil until each slice is coated evenly.
3. Grill the slices on each side until the edges are charred, then leave them to cool, preferably tightly packed so they keep softening in the residual heat.
4. In another pan, heat the butter until it goes brown and nutty. The moment it turns brown, toss in the sage and walnuts. Remove from the heat and stir vigorously until it stops sizzling.
5. To serve, tip the charred courgette disks onto a platter and drizzle them with the nutty butter. Crumble the Stilton over the top and dig in.

GOES WELL WITH: Steak – and a ferocious red wine.

COURGETTI WITH BASIL, MINT AND PINE NUTS

Serves 4

2 garlic cloves, finely chopped

½ handful fresh basil, roughly chopped

½ handful fresh mint, roughly chopped

2 tbsp capers, roughly chopped

2 tsp apple cider vinegar

3 tbsp olive oil

400g courgetti (see lesson on spiralising on page 67)

3 tbsp toasted pine nuts

Salt and black pepper

1. In a bowl, mix the garlic, basil, mint, capers and vinegar.
2. Get a pan ridiculously hot and add the olive oil.
3. Cook the courgetti as per the instructions on page 67. I would recommend doing this in two batches to avoid them leaching their juices.
4. Once both batches of courgetti are cooked, keeping the pan on the heat, add the first batch back to the pan, add the dressing and toss it together until everything has warmed through and the herbs are mixed.
5. Now, tip the courgetti onto a platter and sprinkle them with pine nuts, salt, pepper and a glug of olive oil.

GOES WELL WITH: Carciofi alla Romana, Roasted Broccoli, Takeaway Chicken.

BUTTERED COURGETTES

Serves 4

400g small baby marrows, cut in half lengthways

3 tbsp butter

2 sprigs thyme

Salt and black pepper

1. Steam the courgettes as per the lesson on steaming on page 38.
2. Heat a pan to a medium heat and sauté the courgettes until they begin to caramelise.
3. Season with salt and pepper, sprinkle with thyme and serve immediately.

GOES WELL WITH: Chicken and Mushroom Casserole, Gribiche, Provençal Mushrooms.

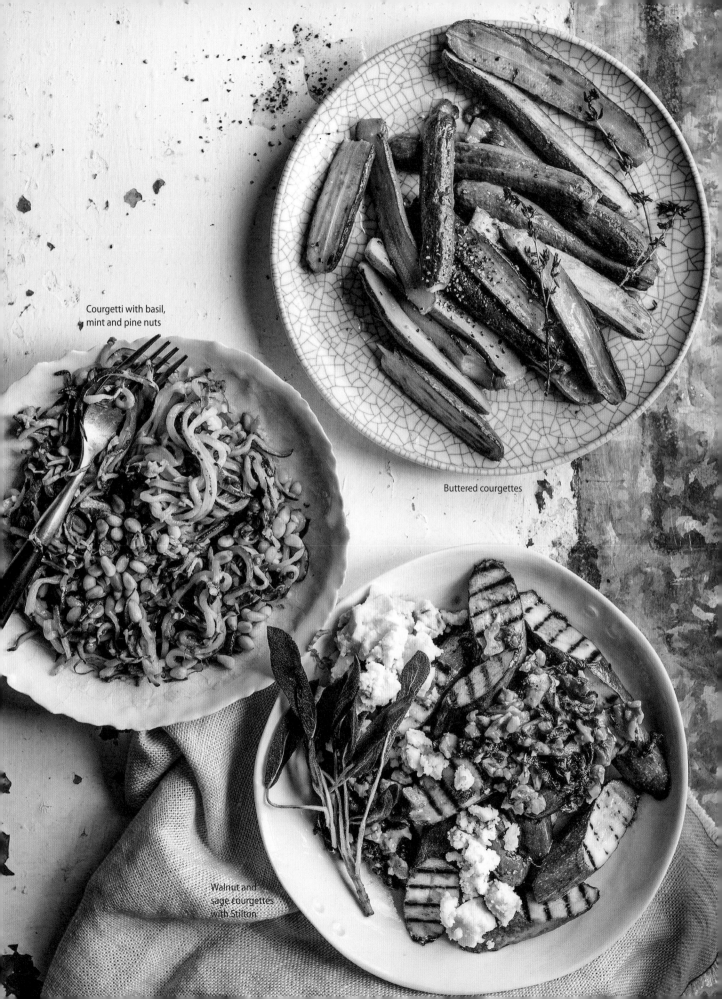

Courgetti with basil, mint and pine nuts

Buttered courgettes

Walnut and sage courgettes with Stilton

SPICY KOREAN CUCUMBER SALAD

Serves 4

1 large English cucumber, halved, seeded
   and thinly sliced on the diagonal
1 tsp salt
½ brown onion, thinly sliced
1 spring onion, thinly sliced
1 large carrot, julienned
2 cloves garlic, minced
2 thumbs ginger, grated on
   a microplane
1 tbsp fish sauce
1 tbsp gochugaru (Korean hot
   pepper flakes)

1   Sprinkle the cucumber slices with salt and leave them to sweat for about 30 minutes.
2   Rinse them with water, pat them dry and add them to a mixing bowl with the onion,
     spring onion, carrot, garlic, ginger, fish sauce and gochugaru and mix well.
3   Leave the mix in the fridge for 24 hours and serve.

GOES WELL WITH: Dak Galbi Korean Chicken Stir Fry, Dark Salty Pork Ribs.

CUCUMBER RIBBONS WITH MINT YOGHURT

Serves 4

2 medium English cucumbers, peeled
   and shaved into ribbons
1 tsp salt
250ml double thick Greek yoghurt
Juice and zest of 1 lemon
1 handful fresh mint, finely chopped
2 tbsp toasted black
   sesame seeds
Salt and black pepper

1   Sprinkle the cucumber ribbons with salt and leave them in a bowl for 30 minutes.
2   Meanwhile, mix the yoghurt with the lemon juice, zest and mint, and season it with
     salt and pepper. (You can dilute it with a little water if you like a thinner consistency.)
3   Rinse the ribbons and spin or pat them dry, then lay them out on a platter.
4   Cover them liberally with the yoghurt dressing and the sesame seeds, and serve.

GOES WELL WITH: Greek Kale Salad with Tahini Dressing, Tarragon Roasted Chicken,
Persian-style Stuffed Fish Bake.

STIR-FRIED CUCUMBER WITH SESAME SEEDS

Serves 4

1 tbsp sesame oil
2 large Japanese cucumbers or 1 large
   English cucumber, cut into quarters
   lengthways, then into 3cm chunks
½ tsp salt
1 spring onion, thinly sliced
2 tbsp toasted sesame seeds

1   Get the sesame oil nice and hot in a large pan.
2   Add the cucumber and sauté for about 5 minutes until tender.
3   Chuck in the salt, spring onion and sesame seeds. Serve immediately.

GOES WELL WITH: Beef Tataki, Stir-fried Spring Onions and Pak Choi.

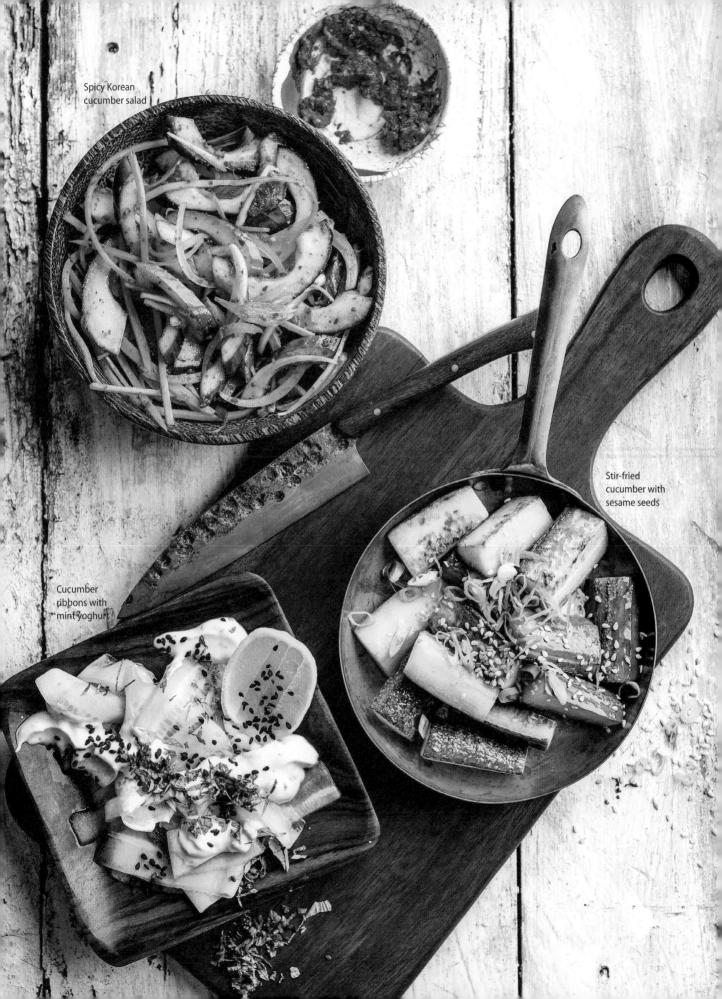

Spicy Korean cucumber salad

Stir-fried cucumber with sesame seeds

Cucumber ribbons with mint yoghurt

MARINATED ENDIVES WITH PECORINO, WALNUTS AND EPIC BLUE CHEESE DIP

See page 76

Serves 4

45g blue cheese like Stilton,
Gorgonzola, Roquefort, etc
50ml buttermilk
40g cream cheese
½ handful flat-leaf parsley, chopped
½ handful chives, finely chopped
2 large endives
3 tbsp olive oil
1 tbsp white wine vinegar
Juice and zest of 1 lemon
40g pecorino shavings
60g toasted walnuts
Salt and pepper

1 Place the blue cheese, buttermilk, cream cheese, parsley and chives in a small jug and blitz them with a stick blender. Pop the mix in the fridge to firm up and for the flavours to infuse.
2 Cut the endives into quarters, lengthways, before removing the core and slicing the quarters into quarters again, horizontally.
3 Toss the leaves in a large bowl with the olive oil, vinegar, lemon juice, zest and seasoning and leave overnight.
4 Arrange the endives on a serving platter and top them with the pecorino shavings, toasted walnuts and lashings of blue cheese dip.

For the full recipe for Epic Blue Cheese Dip, see page 274.

ENDIVE GRATIN

See page 76

Serves 4

750ml water

½ tbsp salt

2 large yellow endives, trimmed
  and cut in half lengthways

250g streaky bacon

4 tbsp butter

250ml cream

1 pinch ground nutmeg

100g grated Gruyère or other good
  grilling cheese

Salt and pepper

1 Preheat your oven to 200°C.

2 Bring the water and salt to a steady simmer in a medium-sized pot.

3 Add the endives to the pot, pop the lid on and leave them to simmer for 5 minutes until they are tender.

4 While the endives are simmering, fry the bacon in the butter until it is cooked, then add the cream, nutmeg and some seasoning and bring it to the boil.

5 Remove the endives from the water, draining all excess liquid back into the pot. Once they're cool, squeeze them and add the excess liquid to the pot.

6 Add half of the cooking liquid to the bacon cream and reduce it by half.

7 Pack the endives into a small baking dish or deep roasting tray and cover them with the bacon cream.

8 Pop the dish, uncovered, into the oven for 20 minutes to get the creamy sauce bubbling and thick.

9 Remember that everyone's oven is different, so this recipe might vary. If it's too runny, you may need it to stay in the oven longer to reduce more. If you see it getting too thick and starting to burn, skip to the next step before 20 minutes is up.

10 Remove the dish from the oven, top it with the cheese and put it back in the oven for another 10 minutes to gratinate before serving.

GRILLED ENDIVES WITH PECAN GREMOLATA

See page 77

Serves 4

4 tbsp olive oil

2 large endives, quartered lengthways

1 garlic clove, minced

Juice and zest of 1 lemon

40g toasted pecan nuts,
    roughly chopped

1 handful flat-leaf parsley,
    roughly chopped

Salt and black pepper

1 Heat a medium-sized pan up to medium heat and add 2 tablespoons of olive oil.

2 Add the endives and sauté them for about 6 minutes, turning them occasionally until they are wilted and lightly coloured.

3 While the endives are sizzling away, mix the garlic, lemon juice, zest, pecan nuts and parsley with the remaining olive oil in a medium-sized mixing bowl.

4 Once the endives look caramelised, add the garlic mixture and toss them quickly before tipping them out of the pan into a mixing bowl to infuse for 10 minutes.

5 Season to taste and serve hot or cold.

GOES WELL WITH: Roasted Baby Gems, 'Beeten' Salmon, Köttbular.

FENNEL AND SOUR CREAM SALAD

See page 77

Serves 4

2 fennel bulbs, shaved on a mandolin
    or with a peeler, or sliced super-thinly

½ red onion, thinly sliced

2 sticks celery, thinly sliced

1 tsp Dijon mustard

2 tbsp sour cream

1 pinch cayenne pepper

½ tsp smoked paprika

2 tbsp olive oil

Juice and zest of 1 lemon

1 small bunch chives, finely chopped

1 Combine all the ingredients in a large mixing bowl and serve immediately.

GOES WELL WITH: Carciofi alla Romana, Eisbein.

BRAISED FENNEL

See page 76

Serves 4

3 tbsp butter

8 baby fennel bulbs, trimmed
and halved

1 garlic clove, thinly sliced

250ml vegetable or chicken broth

½ small handful fresh oregano,
destemmed and chopped

Salt and pepper

1 Heat the butter in a large pot over a medium heat and add the fennel.
2 Cook the fennel for about 3 minutes on each side until golden-brown, then add the garlic and cook for another minute.
3 Add the broth and bring to the boil, then reduce it to a gentle simmer and pop the lid on. Leave it to tick away for about 10 or 12 minutes.
4 Remove the fennel from the pot and reduce the broth until it's thick and rich.
5 Return the fennel to the pot with the oregano and give it a good coating of the sauce.
6 Season with salt and pepper before serving.

GOES WELL WITH: Eisbein, Tarragon Roasted Chicken or any fish dish.

CARAMELISED GARLIC FENNEL

See page 76

Serves 4

4 tbsp olive oil

8 baby fennel bulbs, cut into
3cm chunks

6 garlic cloves, roughly chopped

80ml water

1 lemon, cut into wedges

Salt and black pepper

1 Get the olive oil nice and hot in a medium-sized pan and add the fennel chunks.
2 Sauté for about 5 minutes, until they begin to colour.
3 Add the garlic and sauté for another 5 minutes.
4 Add the water, pop the lid on and cook for 10 minutes until the fennel is tender.
5 Take the lid off, pump up the heat and let it boil aggressively until all the excess moisture has evaporated.
6 Season to taste and serve with lemon wedges and some fresh fennel fronds if you have them.

GOES WELL WITH: Sole Meunière, Greek Pork Chops.

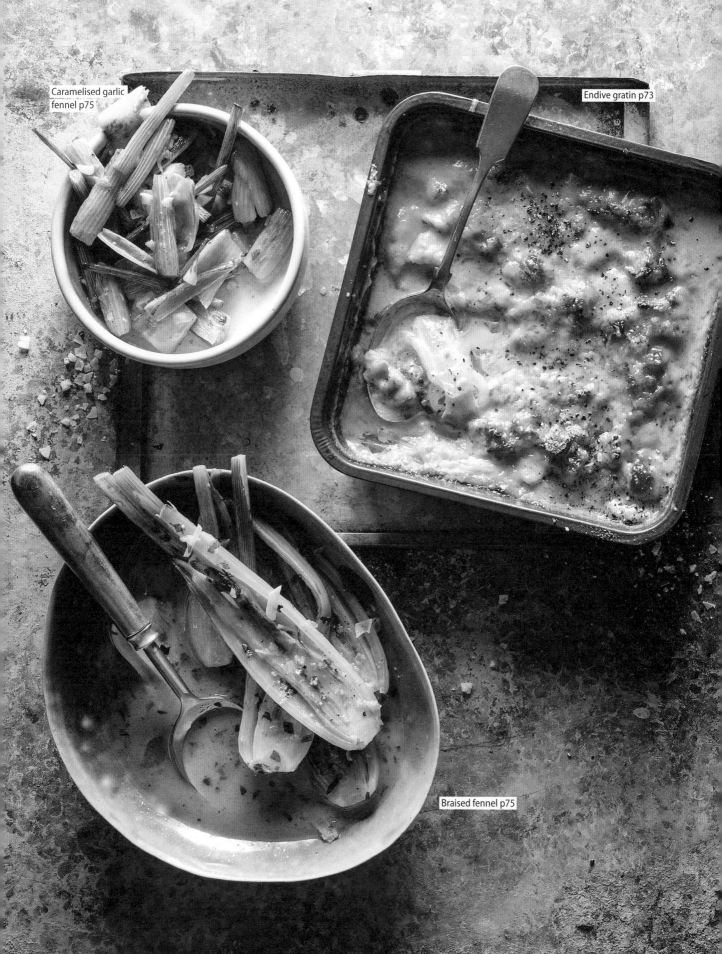

Caramelised garlic
fennel p75

Endive gratin p73

Braised fennel p75

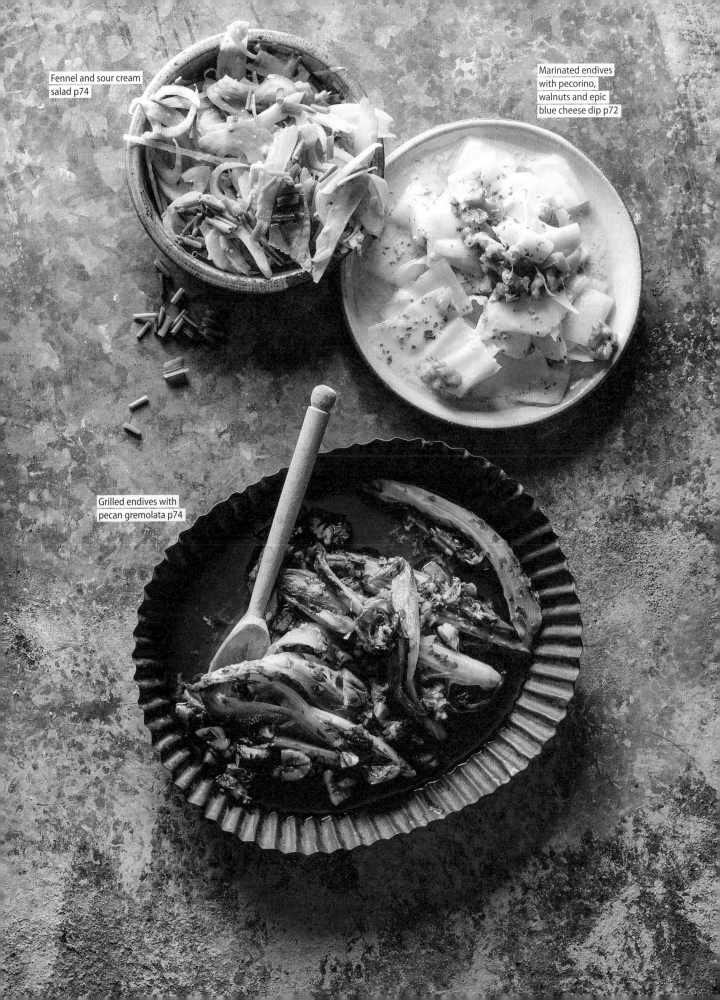

Fennel and sour cream
salad p74

Marinated endives
with pecorino,
walnuts and epic
blue cheese dip p72

Grilled endives with
pecan gremolata p74

SPAGHETTI SQUASH FRITTERS

Serves 4

350g cooked and shredded spaghetti
   squash (or gem squash)
1 egg yolk
2 tbsp olive oil
1 tsp salt

1   Drain the squash by wringing it out in a muslin cloth, then mix it with the egg yolk in a mixing bowl.
2   Heat the oil to a medium heat in a large frying pan.
3   To make the fritters, use your fingers and palms to shape and compress the squash (about 2 heaped tablespoons per fritter) into little cakes. Now drop them into the pan.
4   Cook them for about 5 minutes on each side, then drain them on a paper towel.
5   Give them a sprinkling of salt and serve with garlic mayo or a squeeze of lemon.

GOES WELL WITH: Walnut and Sage Courgettes with Stilton, 'Beeten' Salmon, Aioli.

ROASTED BABY SQUASH

Serves 4

400g baby gem squash, cut into
   quarters
2 tbsp olive oil
Salt and pepper

1   Line a baking tray with foil and heat your oven to 200°C.
2   In a mixing bowl, toss the baby gems in olive oil and season, then tip them out onto the baking tray.
3   Pop them in the oven for 20 minutes and serve immediately.

GOES WELL WITH: Grilled Endive with Pecan Gremolata, Cod au Gratin.

NUTTY SAGEY GEM SQUASH PURÉE
This is a great way to use any leftover squash.

Serves 4

3 tbsp butter
10 big sage leaves, shredded
125ml cream
Flesh of 4 gem squash, steamed
   and seeded
Salt and black pepper

1   Melt the butter in a medium pot and heat it until it goes nutty-brown.
2   The moment it turns brown, add the sage and stir it in as it crackles and spits.
3   Quickly add the cream and bring it to the boil, then simmer it gently until it reduces by half.
4   Now add the flesh of the squash, crushing and stirring it gently with a wooden spoon over the heat until the cream is incorporated and the moisture has evaporated so that the purée is thick and holding its shape.
5   Season with salt and pepper to taste and serve immediately.

GOES WELL WITH: Roasted Kale, Winter Salad of Radicchio with Parsley and Sweet Sautéed Onion, Slow-Roasted Lamb Shoulder with Lemon and Capers.

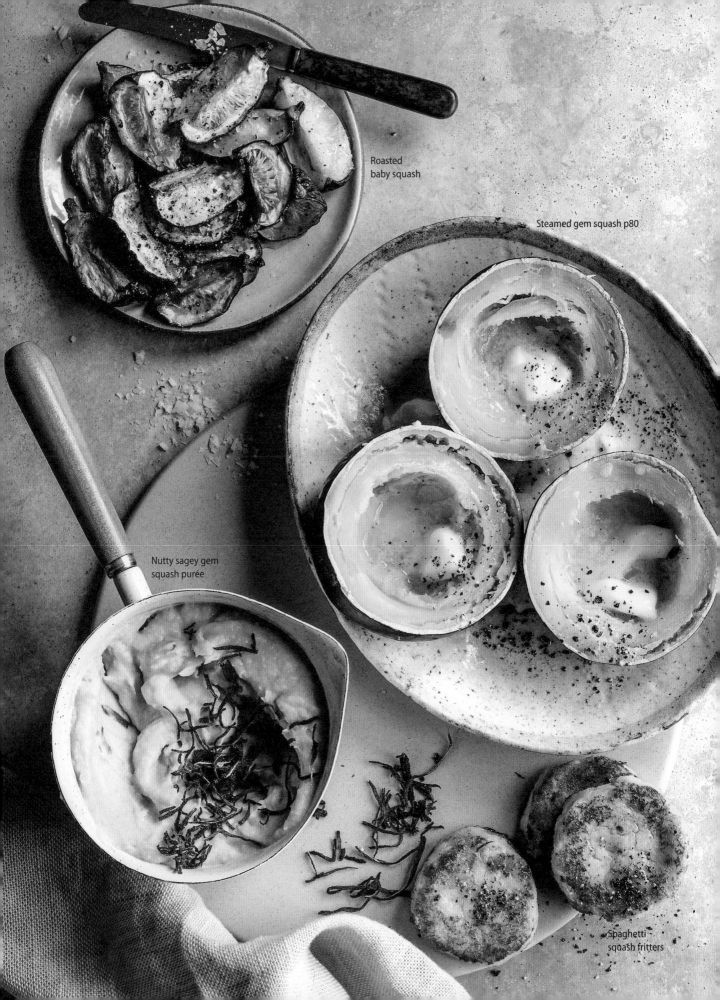

Roasted
baby squash

Steamed gem squash p80

Nutty sagey gem
squash purée

Spaghetti
squash fritters

STEAMED GEM SQUASH

See page 79

Serves 4

4 gem squash, halved
8 tsp butter
Salt and black pepper

1 Add 750ml of water to a large pot and heat it up to a rolling boil.
2 Tightly pack the squash into the pot, pop the lid on and let them steam away.
3 After 15 minutes, turn off the heat, take the lid off and remove the squash.
4 Scoop out the seeds of each squash with a spoon, if necessary.
5 Dot the squash with butter, 1 teaspoon per half, and season liberally with salt and pepper.

GOES WELL WITH: Walnut and Sage Courgettes with Stilton, Red Wine-Braised Radishes with Bacon.

IF YOU ARE WHAT YOU EAT, WHERE DOES THAT LEAVE YOU IF ALL YOU EAT IS JUNK?

EDAMAME BEAN AND RADISH SALAD

See page 85

Serves 4

1kg edamame beans in their pods
10 baby red radishes, thinly sliced or
  shaved (the latter is always better)
1 red onion, finely chopped
2 tbsp apple cider vinegar
6 tbsp olive oil
1 handful flat-leaf parsley,
  roughly chopped
Salt and black pepper

1 Blanch the beans for about 3 minutes, then refresh them in iced water – see lesson on blanching on page 38.
2 Squeeze the beans out of the pods into a large mixing bowl and discard the shells.
3 Add the remaining ingredients and mix well before serving.

GOES WELL WITH: Roasted Broccoli, Stir-fried Cucumber with Sesame Seeds, Salt and Pepper Calamari.

FRIED GARLIC GREEN BEANS

See page 84

Serves 4

4 tbsp butter
6 garlic cloves, thinly sliced
1 big pinch dried chilli flakes
300g green beans, trimmed and cut
  in half
2 tbsp soy sauce
2 tsp paprika

1 Heat the butter to a medium heat in a large pan and drop in the garlic and chilli flakes.
2 After a minute of stirring them quickly, add the beans and stir-fry them for about 10 minutes.
3 Now toss in the soy sauce and paprika, and keep cooking for another 5 minutes until all of the moisture has evaporated.
4 Serve the beans with an extra dusting of chilli flakes, depending on your liking.

GOES WELL WITH: Spicy Aubergine, Penny's Durban Curry, Xinjiang Cumin Spiced Lamb Skewers.

SAUTÉED MANGE TOUT WITH MINT, LEMON AND RICOTTA

See page 84

Serves 4

2 tbsp olive oil
300g mange tout
2 spring onions, thinly sliced
Juice and zest of 1 lemon
100g ricotta
1 small bunch mint, leaves picked and
  roughly chopped
Salt and black pepper

1 Heat the olive oil to a medium heat in a large pan and add the mange tout.
2 After about 2 minutes of sautéing and stirring constantly, add the spring onions and lemon zest and sauté for another minute.
3 Tip the beans out onto a serving platter and cover them with crumbles of ricotta, shredded mint and a squeeze of lemon juice before serving.

GOES WELL WITH: Roasted Cherry Tomato Caprese, Baked Fish with Almond and Peppers.

BEANS WITH CAPER DRESSING

See page 85

Serves 4

300g fine French green beans
50ml basic vinaigrette
4 tbsp capers, roughly chopped
Zest and juice of 1 lemon
1 handful flat-leaf parsley, chopped

For the full recipe for Basic Vinaigrette, see page 272.

1 Blanch the beans for about 3 minutes, then refresh them in iced water – see lesson on blanching on page 38.
2 Whisk together the vinaigrette with the capers, lemon zest, juice and parsley and season to taste with salt and pepper. (If you want to be brave, you can add anchovies instead of salt.)
3 Lay the beans out on a platter and douse them liberally with the dressing.

GOES WELL WITH: Drunken Lamb Ribs, Oxtail Stew.

FASOLAKIA LADERA – GREEN BEANS COOKED IN TOMATO

See page 85

Serves 4

80ml olive oil
1 red onion, finely diced
3 garlic cloves, minced
400g green beans, ends trimmed
6 plum tomatoes, peeled and chopped (or a tin of whole peeled tomatoes, chopped)
80ml water
1 handful flat-leaf parsley, roughly chopped
Salt and black pepper

1 Heat the olive oil in a large pot, add the onion and sauté for 2 minutes.
2 Chuck in the garlic and mix it around until fragrant, then add the beans and stir until they are well coated.
3 Now, add the tomatoes, water and a pinch of salt and cover with a lid. Then simmer for 1 hour.
4 Remove the lid and season to taste with salt and pepper.
5 Pump up the heat to a fast simmer and stir through the parsley, then remove from the heat and serve.

GOES WELL WITH: Greek Kale Salad with Tahini Dressing, Greek Pork Chops.

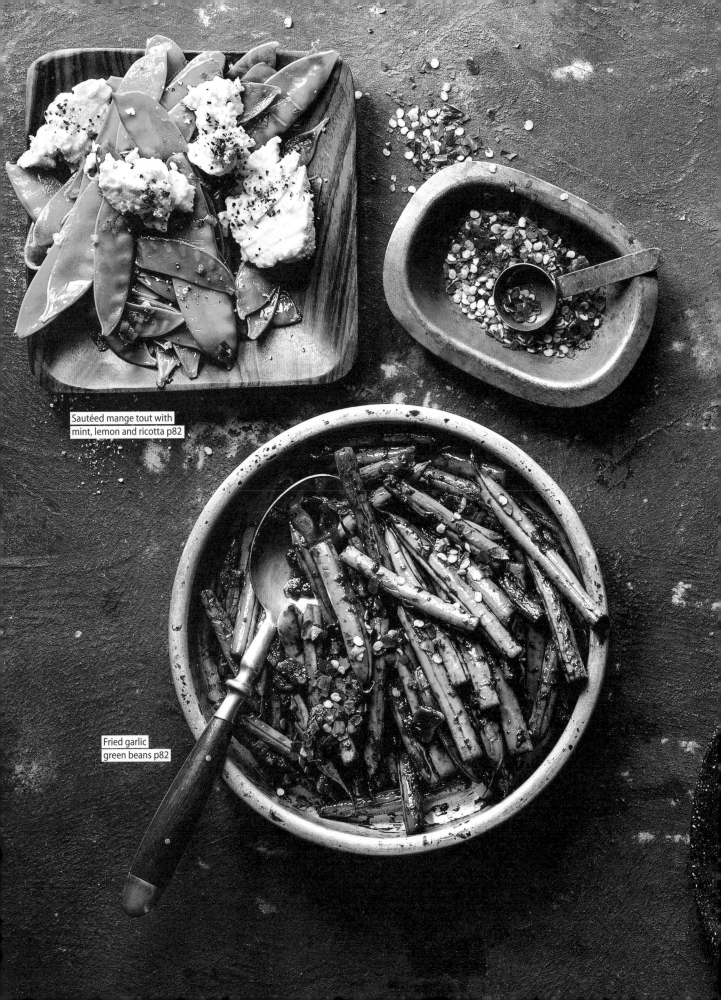

Sautéed mange tout with mint, lemon and ricotta p82

Fried garlic green beans p82

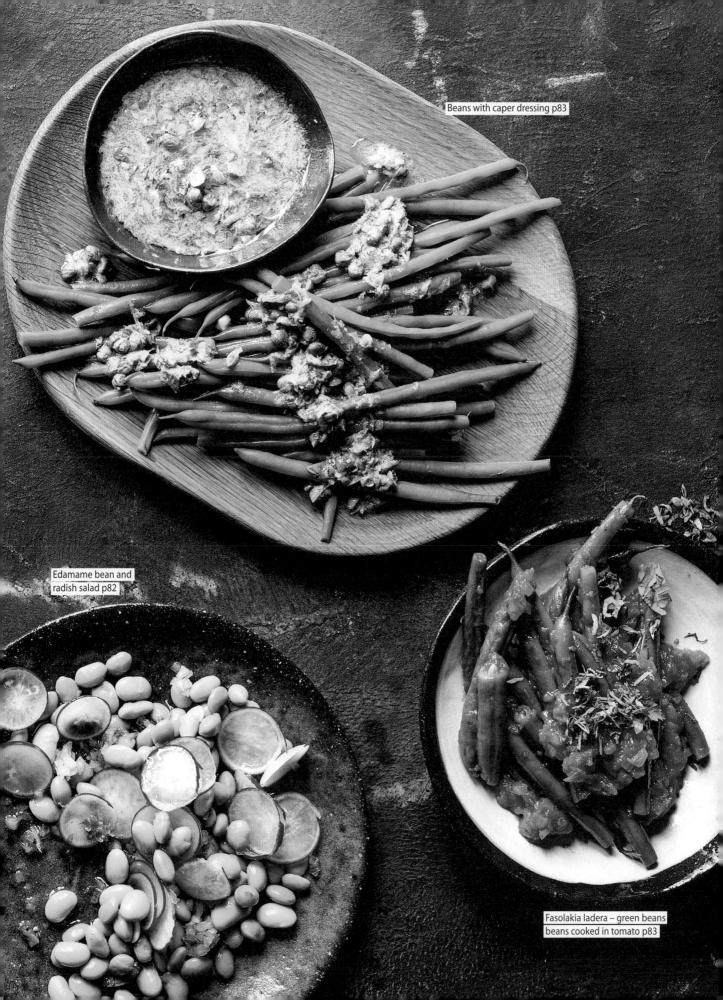

Beans with caper dressing p83

Edamame bean and
radish salad p82

Fasolakia ladera – green beans
beans cooked in tomato p83

KALE AND CABBAGE SALAD

See page 88

Serves 4

Juice of 1 lemon
125ml olive oil
1 tbsp apple cider vinegar
½ handful basil, torn
200g kale, destemmed and
   roughly chopped
¼ red cabbage, shredded
1 large carrot, grated
40g walnuts, toasted
1 avocado, cut into chunks
Salt and black pepper

1 Make the dressing by whisking the lemon juice, olive oil, vinegar and basil in a medium mixing bowl. Season with salt and pepper.
2 Massage the kale leaves with half a teaspoon of fine salt to soften them.
3 Toss the kale, cabbage and carrots in the mixing bowl with the dressing, then tip them onto a platter.
4 Top the salad with walnuts and avocado and serve immediately.

GOES WELL WITH: Wet Jerk Spiced Chicken, Whole Roasted Jerk Cauliflower.

ROASTED KALE

See page 89

Serves 4

400g kale, rinsed and thick stems
   removed
1 garlic clove, minced
3 tbsp olive oil
2 tbsp pine nuts, toasted
Salt and black pepper

1 Preheat your oven to 180°C and line a large baking tray with foil.
2 Mix the kale, garlic, olive oil with some salt and pepper with your hands in the baking tray, making sure the leaves are well coated with all of the seasonings.
3 Roast the kale in the oven for 20 minutes until the leaves are crunchy at the edges.
4 Serve them on the tray or place on a platter with a scattering of pine nuts.

GOES WELL WITH: Nutty Sagey Gem Squash Purée, Caprese Salad, Sardines with Warm Chorizo and Tomato Dressing.

BUTTERED KALE

See page 88

Serves 4

300g kale, destemmed and cut
   into big pieces
2 tbsp butter
Salt and black pepper

1 Blanch the kale in a medium-sized pot for 3 minutes, then refresh in iced water – see lesson on blanching on page 38.
2 Once cooled, remove from the water and wring out with your hands.
3 Melt the butter over a high heat until it is sizzling, then add the kale and toss it until it is heated through.
4 Season with salt and pepper and serve hot.

GOES WELL WITH: Pan-fried Sweetbreads Piccata, Pan-fried Haddock with Olives and Tomatoes.

GREEK KALE SALAD WITH TAHINI DRESSING

See page 89

Serves 4

200g kale, destemmed and cut into
   large strips
½ tsp fine salt
90g pitted kalamata olives,
   thinly sliced
20g sun-dried tomatoes in olive
   oil, rinsed and drained
60g Parmigiano Reggiano, grated
35g sunflower seeds, toasted
1 tbsp olive oil
4 tbsp tahini
Juice of 2 lemons
1 garlic clove, minced
½ tsp Dijon mustard
2 tbsp water
Salt and black pepper

1 Place the kale in a bowl and massage the leaves with 1 teaspoon of fine salt until the leaves go darker in colour and look bruised.
2 Make the dressing by adding the tahini, lemon juice, garlic, mustard and water to a small bowl. While whisking continuously, slowly add more water, 2 tablespoons at a time, until the dressing reaches the consistency of drinking yoghurt.
3 Now, add the remaining salad ingredients to the kale, along with some dressing, and mix gently until all of the ingredients are well coated.
4 Serve immediately.

GOES WELL WITH: Greek Pork Chops, Charred Okra with Coriander and Lemon Dressing, Spanakopita Filling.

KALE, BACON AND SWEET ONIONS WITH ROASTED GARLIC

See page 89

Serves 4

1 head roasted garlic, as per recipe on
   page 286
250ml olive oil
1 sprig thyme
2 tbsp butter
120g streaky bacon, cut into lardons
1 large onion, cut into thick slices
6 sprigs thyme
200g kale, rinsed and
   thick stems removed
Salt and black pepper

1 For the salad, get the butter nice and hot in a medium-sized pan and cook the bacon for about 10 minutes. Take it out once it's caramelised but leave the fat in the pan.
2 Add the onions and the thyme sprigs and sauté them, stirring only every couple of minutes, so that the onions get nice and dark on the sides but keep their crunch in some parts. In South Africa we would make these onions for a boerie roll.
3 While this is going on, blanch the kale for 3 minutes and refresh it in some iced water before wringing it out with your hands.
4 To finish it off, drop the kale back into the onion, followed by the bacon bits, the roast garlic and a dusting of salt and pepper and get it nice and hot.
5 Once the bits of roasted garlic catch on the pan and start to caramelise, you're in business. Serve immediately.

GOES WELL WITH: Tarragon Roasted Chicken, Creamy Brussels Sprouts.
For the full recipe for Roasted Garlic, see page 286.

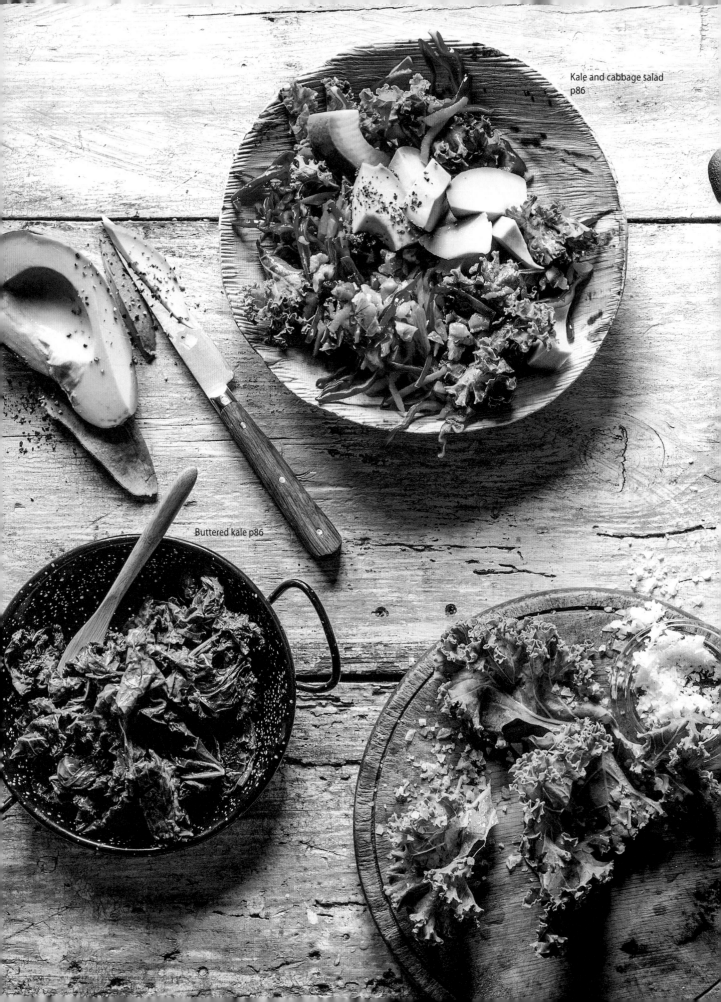

Kale and cabbage salad
p86

Buttered kale p86

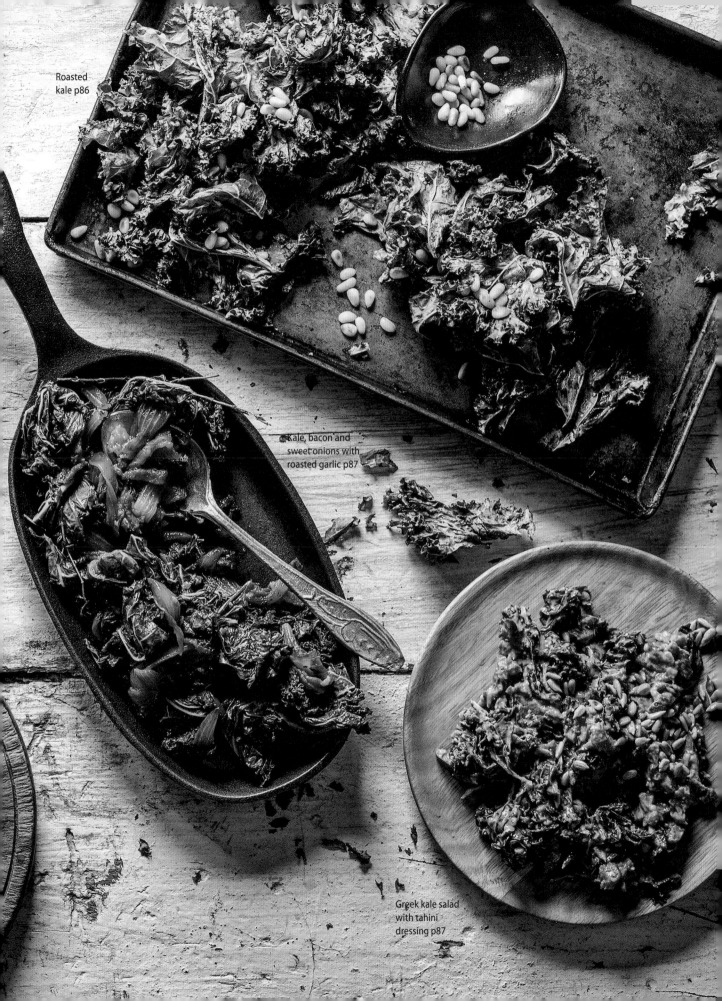

Roasted
kale p86

Kale, bacon and
sweet onions with
roasted garlic p87

Greek kale salad
with tahini
dressing p87

CHARRED LEEKS WITH ALMOND NOISETTE DRESSING AND CRÈME FRAÎCHE

See page 93

Serves 4

4 leeks, washed and halved lengthways

4 tbsp butter

35g almonds, toasted and roughly chopped

2 tbsp apple cider vinegar

125ml crème fraîche

Black pepper

1 Fire up the barbecue to a high heat and place the leeks directly over the hottest coals (not over the flames).

2 Char them on all sides then push them to one side of the coals to continue to cook gently. Or you can wrap them tightly in foil after they have been charred, so that they continue to steam in their own heat – up to you.

3 Melt the butter in a pan over a medium heat until it turns brown, then add the nuts and vinegar and simmer for 2 minutes. Remove the mix from the heat.

4 Once the leeks are cooked, lay them out on a platter and spoon over the almond dressing, finishing it off with lashings of crème fraîche and a crack of black pepper.

GOES WELL WITH: Tarragon Roasted Chicken, Creamy Brussels Sprouts.

HOBOCHOKES

See page 92

Serves 4

Leeks done in the style of artichokes, aka poor man's artichoke, or Hobochokes. Hint – get leeks with the longest white stem you can find.

4 tbsp olive oil

4 giant leeks, washed and cut into 3cm cylinders

1 garlic clove, roughly chopped

1 small bunch thyme sprigs

2 bay leaves

500ml white wine

1 large handful flat-leaf parsley, roughly chopped

Salt and black pepper

1 Heat the olive oil in a large pot and add the leeks, cut-side down, and the garlic. Fry the leeks for about 2 minutes on each side until lightly brown.

2 Add the thyme, bay leaves and white wine, reducing the heat to a simmer and leaving it to tick away with the lid on for about 40 minutes.

3 After 40 minutes, remove the lid and turn up the heat to reduce the sauce by half (with the leeks still in the pot).

4 Finally, season with salt and pepper and stir through the parsley before serving.

5 If you're going to bottle them, make sure both the jars and the leeks are steaming hot when the lid goes on, to create a sterile vacuum.

GOES WELL WITH: Sardines with Warm Chorizo and Tomato Dressing, Baked Fish with Almond and Peppers, Slow-roasted Lamb Shoulder with Lemon and Capers.

CARAMELISED ENDIVE AND LEEKS

See page 93

Serves 4

2 tbsp butter

3 tbsp olive oil

3 leeks, trimmed and halved
   lengthways and washed

3 endives, halved lengthways

2 tbsp red wine vinegar

50g Gorgonzola

Salt and black pepper

1   Heat the butter and olive oil to a medium heat in a large frying pan. Add the leeks and endives.
2   Let them tick away, turning them occasionally, for about 15 minutes, until they are dark on all sides and soft in the middle.
3   Add the vinegar and season with salt and pepper, and stir it all around to make sure the steam from the vinegar penetrates the leeks and endives.
4   Tip them out, juice and all, onto a platter and crumble the Gorgonzola over them before serving.

GOES WELL WITH: Nutty Sagey Gem Squash Purée, Creamy Bacon Onions, Winter Salad of Radicchio with Parsley and Sweet Sautéed Onion.

CONFIT LEEKS

See page 92

Serves 4

4 large leeks, halved lengthways and
   washed

3 garlic cloves, sliced in half

1 small sprig rosemary

½ tsp fennel seeds

¼ tsp black peppercorns

1 tsp salt

3 tbsp red wine vinegar

500ml olive oil

1   Preheat your oven to 140°C and line a small baking tray with foil.
2   Tightly pack the leeks, garlic, rosemary, fennel seeds, peppercorns and salt in the tray, then cover them with the vinegar and oil. If the leeks are covered without using all the oil, there's no need to add the rest.
3   Pop the tray in the oven for one-and-a-half hours, then turn off the oven and leave the tray in there until it's cool.
4   Take the tray out and tip the leeks into a bowl for a salad or reserve to stir through your next batch of roast vegetables.

GOES WELL WITH: Provençal Mushrooms, Tarragon Roasted Chicken, Casablanca Chicken Casserole.

TURNIP SKORDALIA

See page 92

Serves 4

400g turnips, peeled and diced

8 garlic cloves, peeled

4 tbsp olive oil

375ml veg or chicken broth/stock

1 tsp of lemon juice

1 tbsp butter

Salt and black pepper

1   Preheat your oven to 180°C. Place all of the ingredients in a baking tray, cover with foil, then bake in the oven for 50 minutes.
2   Tip the contents into a medium pot and bring to the boil, stirring regularly, until the juices have evaporated.
3   Blitz with a stick blender, spoon into a serving dish and top with a generous glug of olive oil before serving.

GOES WELL WITH: Greek Pork Chops, Flash-fried Mange Tout, Olives and Tomato.

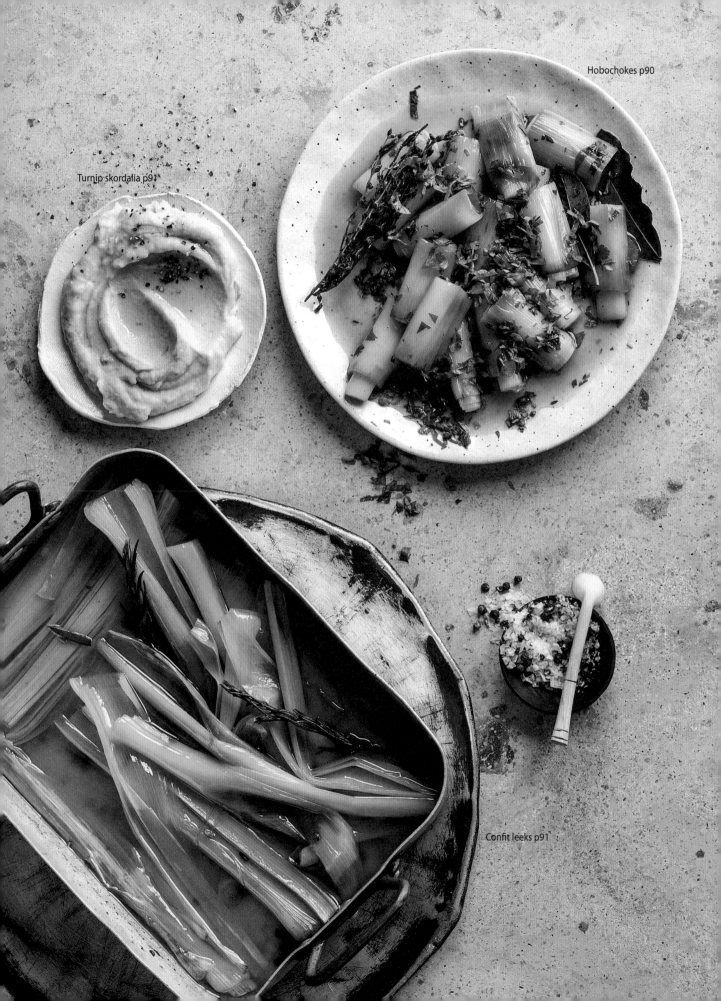

Turnip skordalia p91

Hobochokes p90

Confit leeks p91

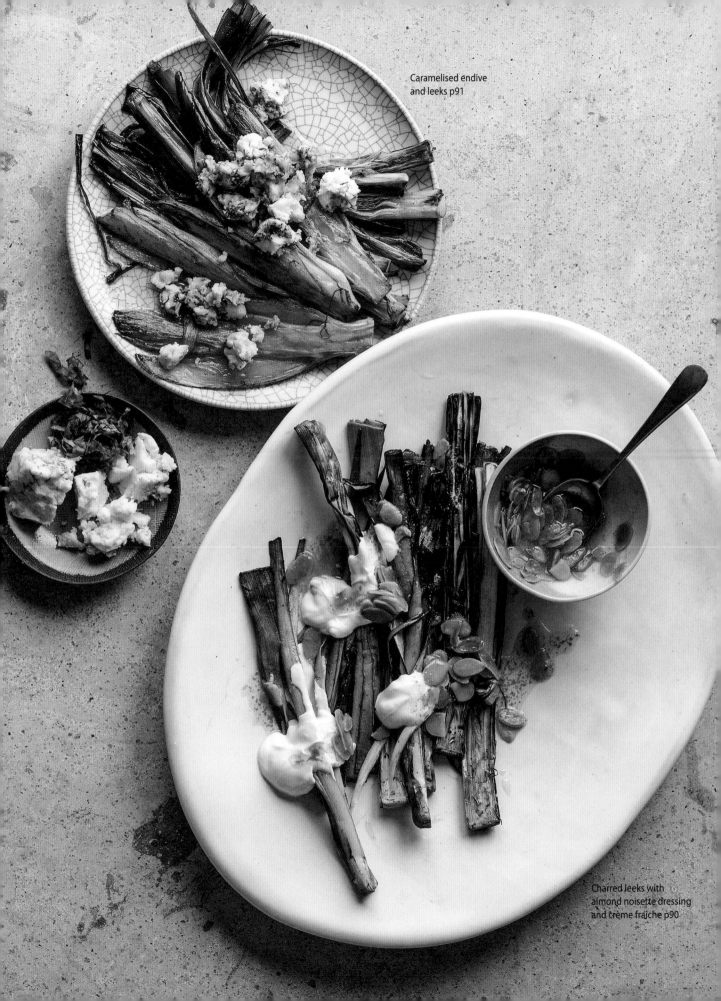

Caramelised endive
and leeks p91

Charred leeks with
almond noisette dressing
and crème fraîche p90

LIME, CHILLI AND SESAME STIR-FRIED MANGE TOUT

Serves 4

400g mange tout

2 tbsp coconut oil

1 red onion, finely chopped

1 red chilli, deseeded and thinly sliced

2 tbsp toasted sesame seeds

1 tbsp sesame oil

Juice of 1 lime

1 tbsp fish sauce

½ handful fresh coriander,
   roughly chopped

1   Blanch the mange tout as per the blanching lesson on page 38.

2   Heat the coconut oil in a large pan, add the onion and chilli and sauté until they're soft and about to caramelise.

3   Add the mange tout, sesame seeds, sesame oil, lime juice, fish sauce and fresh coriander and toss until they're heated through and the flavours are well combined.

4   Serve immediately with an extra sprinkle of sesame seeds.

GOES WELL WITH: Pork Bulgogi, Spicy Aubergine, Stir-fried Spring Onions and Pak Choi.

MANGE TOUT WITH HAZELNUT NOISETTE

Serves 4

400g mange tout

4 tbsp butter

50g hazelnuts, roughly chopped

Salt and black pepper

1   Blanch the mange tout as per the blanching lesson on page 38.

2   Heat the butter to sizzling hot in a medium-sized frying pan.

3   As it turns nutty brown, throw in the hazelnuts and stir them around for a minute.

4   Add the mange tout and toss to coat them evenly with the butter and nuts.

5   Season them to taste with salt and pepper and serve immediately.

GOES WELL WITH: Greek Pork Chops, Provençal Mushrooms, Tarragon Roasted Chicken.

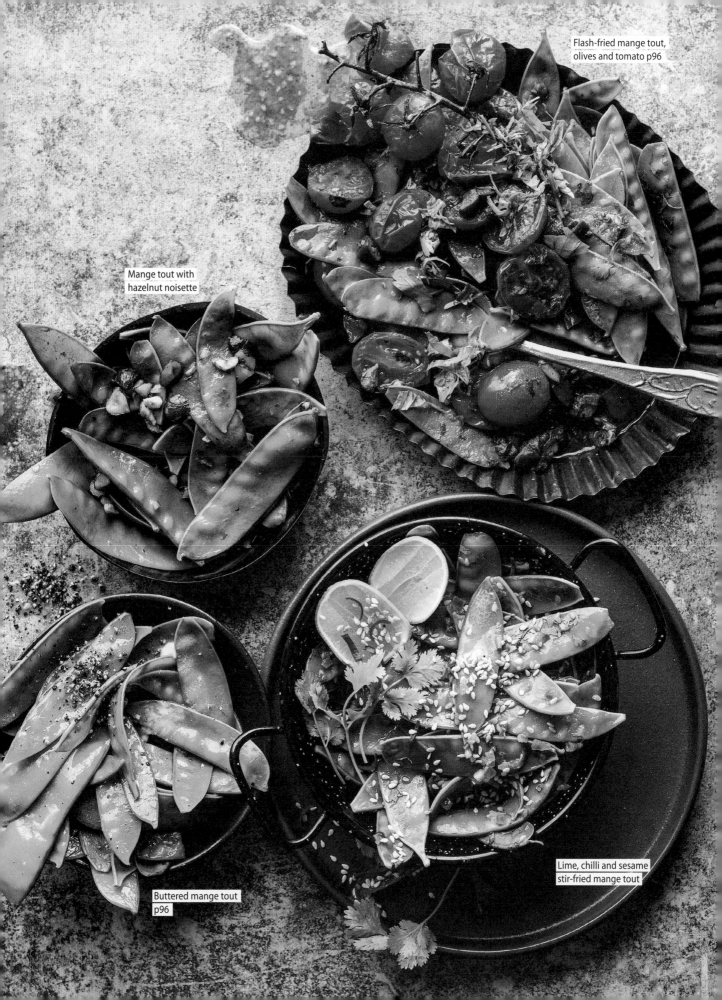

Flash-fried mange tout, olives and tomato p96

Mange tout with hazelnut noisette

Buttered mange tout p96

Lime, chilli and sesame stir-fried mange tout

FLASH-FRIED MANGE TOUT, OLIVES AND TOMATO

See page 95

Serves 4

400g mange tout, ends trimmed

2 tbsp olive oil

200g baby plum tomatoes, halved

3 garlic cloves, halved

90g good-quality black olives, chopped

1 tbsp brine/oil from olives

1 handful flat-leaf parsley, chopped

Salt and black pepper

1 Blanch the mange tout as per the lesson on blanching on page 38.

2 Add the oil to a large pan and get it outrageously hot.

3 As the oil begins to smoke, add the tomatoes and garlic and pop the lid on, shaking the pan once every minute for 5 minutes. The tomatoes should be slightly charred and very soft.

4 Take the lid off and add the mange tout, olives and olive brine or oil, and toss together until they are hot.

5 Finally, toss in the parsley, add salt and pepper and give it a final mix before serving.

GOES WELL WITH: Greek Pork Chops, Greek Kale Salad with Tahini Dressing, Spanakopita Filling.

BUTTERED MANGE TOUT

See page 95

Serves 4

400g mange tout

2 tbsp butter

Salt and black pepper

1 Blanch the mange tout for about 2 minutes, then drop them straight into a medium-sized pan on a medium heat with the butter.

2 Season them with salt and pepper and toss them in the pan for 3 or 4 minutes, then serve immediately.

GOES WELL WITH: Chermoula Fish BBQ, Prosciutto-wrapped Radicchio, Shaved Radish Salad.

GARLIC, THYME & TRUFFLE MUSHROOM SOSATIES

See page 99

Serves 4

You won't often find sosatie recipes from South Africa that feature truffle oil and fresh herbs. I love this recipe because you get that bittersweet caramel flavour from the garlic and lemon zest over the flames, as well as the raw potent garlic from the final basting of marinade. The truffle oil just elevates everything to the next level.

250ml olive oil

1 handful thyme, destemmed

3 garlic cloves, peeled

Juice and zest of 1 lemon

600g button mushrooms, halved

8 bamboo skewers, soaked in water

2 tbsp truffle oil

Salt and black pepper

1 Heat a barbecue or griddle pan up to a high heat.

2 Using a stick blender, blitz the olive oil, thyme, garlic, lemon zest, juice as well as salt and pepper in a narrow jar.

3 Place the mushrooms in a large mixing bowl and cover them with three-quarters of the marinade. Toss until well coated. Once they have soaked up the marinade, thread them onto the bamboo skewers.

4 Mix the remaining marinade with the truffle oil. Keep a basting brush handy.

5 Grill the skewers over direct heat on the BBQ or on the griddle pan. Aim for 3 minutes on each side, so they end up tender with good caramelisation.

6 Give them one final basting with the remaining marinade and another minute on the heat, then transfer them to a serving dish.

7 Splash them with whatever marinade is left and add plenty of salt. Serve immediately.

GOES WELL WITH: Tarragon Roasted Chicken, Courgetti with Mint, Basil and Pine Nuts, or just eat them on their own.

STIR-FRIED MUSHROOMS WITH BAMBOO SHOOTS

See page 99

Serves 4

12 dried black mushrooms

125ml chicken stock or broth
  (see page 232)

1 tbsp rice wine vinegar

1 tbsp oyster sauce

2 tbsp soy sauce

3 tbsp coconut oil

1 garlic clove, minced

200g bamboo shoots, rinsed

1 tbsp sesame oil

1 Soak the mushrooms in a bowl of hot water for 20 minutes. Drain the water and squeeze out any excess liquid from the mushrooms. Slice thickly.

2 In a small bowl, whisk together the chicken broth, vinegar, oyster sauce and soy sauce.

3 Heat the coconut oil in a wok over a medium-high heat. Add the garlic and sauté for a minute. Add the mushrooms and bamboo shoots. Stir-fry for 2 minutes.

4 Add the sauce and cook it until it is reduced to a thick consistency. Remove from the heat.

5 Transfer to a serving bowl and drizzle with sesame oil.

GOES WELL WITH: Fried Garlic Green Beans, Stir-fried Spring Onions and Pak Choi, Confit Duck.

PROVENÇAL MUSHROOMS

Serves 4

3 tbsp olive oil
1 garlic clove, roughly chopped
½ tsp fresh rosemary, finely chopped
½ tsp fresh thyme, finely chopped
1 tsp fresh oregano, finely chopped
½ tsp dried marjoram (or fresh,
   if you are lucky enough to find it)
400g portobello mushrooms
Salt and black pepper
Lemon

1 Heat the olive oil to very hot in a large frying pan.
2 Add the garlic, rosemary, thyme, oregano and marjoram and let them sizzle in the oil for a minute.
3 Add the mushrooms and stir them until their juices are released and have evaporated.
4 Once the mushrooms are caramelised all over, give them a liberal seasoning of salt and pepper. Serve with a twist of lemon.

GOES WELL WITH: Steamed and Buttered Courgettes, Tarragon Roasted Chicken, Confit Duck.

SAUTÉED MUSHROOMS WITH SOY BUTTER SAUCE

Serves 4

3 tbsp butter
400g assorted mushrooms (enoki,
   shiitake, maitake, shimeji, porcini, etc)
1 garlic clove, finely chopped
1 tbsp soy sauce
2 spring onions, finely sliced

1 Melt half the butter in a large pan and wait for it to get hot (on the verge of nutty).
2 Add the mushrooms and sauté them for about 5 minutes. Try to stir them only once in this time – you'll get better caramelisation.
3 Once they are caramelised, add the garlic and toss them for a minute until the garlic becomes fragrant.
4 Add the soy sauce and the remaining butter. Toss to melt the butter, then coat the mushrooms with the sauce.
5 Finally, add the spring onions and give it one last toss before serving.

GOES WELL WITH: Dark Salty Pork Ribs.

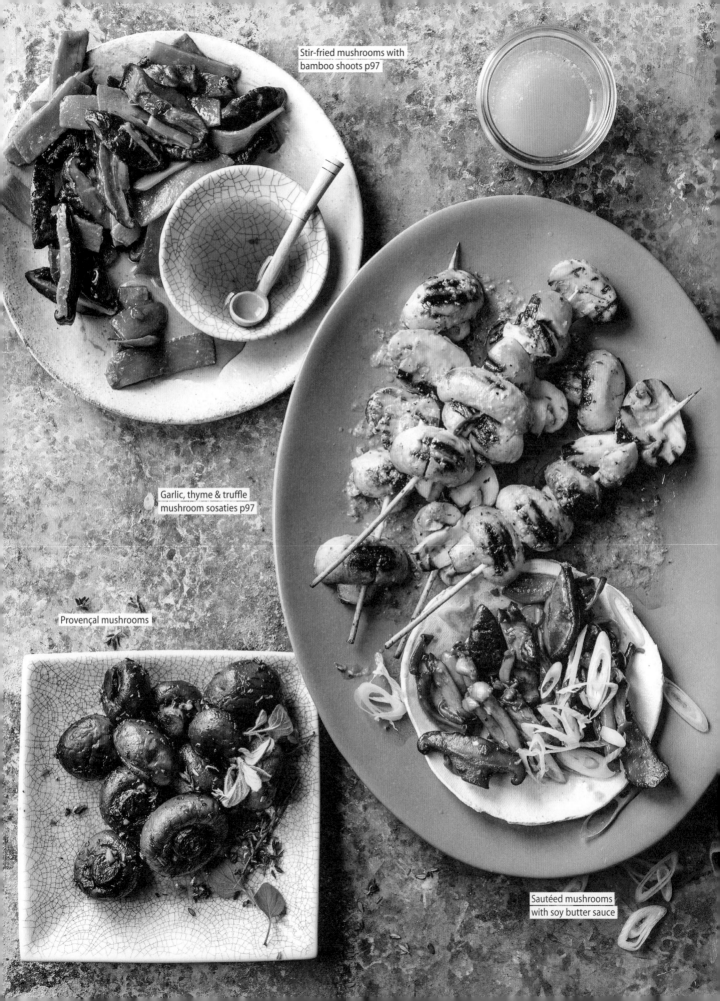

Stir-fried mushrooms with bamboo shoots p97

Garlic, thyme & truffle mushroom sosaties p97

Provençal mushrooms

Sautéed mushrooms with soy butter sauce

GRIDDLED OKRA AND TOMATO RAGOUT

See page 102

Serves 4

300g okra
4 tbsp white wine vinegar
500ml water
3 tbsp olive oil
1 red onion, finely chopped
1 garlic clove, minced
400g plum tomatoes, halved (or
    canned whole peeled tomatoes)
1 tsp smoked paprika
1 pinch cayenne pepper
2 tbsp finely chopped mint leaves
30g toasted pine nuts
Salt and black pepper

1   Place the okra in a large bowl, cover it with vinegar and water, and leave it to soak for 40 minutes.
2   Get a griddle pan really hot and rinse the okra before tossing it in a bowl with 1 tablespoon of the olive oil and a little salt.
3   Grill the okra for 1-2 minutes on each side on the griddle pan until it is nicely charred on all sides.
4   While you're doing this, or while the okra is soaking, heat the remaining olive oil in a medium-sized pan. Add the red onion and garlic, and sauté until they are softened.
5   Add the tomatoes, paprika and cayenne pepper, and pop the lid on for 10 minutes, stirring every 2 or 3 minutes.
6   Remove the sauce from the heat, add the mint and season with salt and pepper. Use a potato masher (if you still have one) to mash the tomatoes into a chunky sauce, and set aside.
7   Add the okra and stir it occasionally for 10 minutes while the sauce thickens and the okra gets cooked through.
8   Transfer to a serving dish and sprinkle with toasted pine nuts.

GOES WELL WITH: Blackened Swordfish with Guacamole, Roasted Artichokes with Lemon and Dill Vinaigrette.

CHARRED OKRA WITH CORIANDER AND LEMON DRESSING

See page 102

Serves 4

If you're not keen on firing up the BBQ for this, you can char the okra over a gas flame, much like you would do a pepper (see page 108). But don't overdo the charring – remember you can't remove the skin.

4 tbsp olive oil
Juice and zest of 1 large lemon
¼ red onion, super-finely chopped
1 garlic clove, minced
½ red chilli, finely chopped
½ handful coriander, roughly chopped
300g okra
Salt and black pepper

1   Get your barbecue up to a medium heat.
2   To make the dressing, whisk the olive oil, lemon juice, zest, onion, garlic, chilli and coriander together in a large mixing bowl, and season with salt and pepper.
3   Place the okra on the grill or flame for 3 minutes on each side until evenly charred.
4   While still hot, toss the okra in the dressing.
5   Tip the okra onto a platter and serve hot or cold.

GOES WELL WITH: Greek Pork Chops, Greek Kale Salad with Tahini Dressing, Turnip Skordalia, Persian-style Stuffed Fish Bake.

BHINDI MASALA

See page 103

Serves 4

3 tbsp coconut oil

300g okra, ends trimmed and cut in half

1 tsp cumin seeds

2 onions, roughly chopped

1 tsp ground coriander

1 tsp ground turmeric

1 tsp red chilli powder

1 tsp garam masala

1 green chilli, finely chopped

1 tsp garlic, minced

1 tsp ginger, grated on a microplane

3 tomatoes, chopped

1 tbsp fenugreek

2 tsp salt

1 small handful fresh coriander, roughly chopped, stems and all

1 Heat a large pan and add 1 tablespoon of the coconut oil and the okra, and stir-fry it until it is golden and soft.

2 Remove the okra from the pan and set aside. Add the remaining oil along with the cumin seeds, onion, ground coriander, turmeric, chilli powder, garam masala, green chilli, garlic and ginger and cook until the onion becomes soft and golden.

3 When the onions are soft, add the tomatoes and the fenugreek and cook, stirring constantly, over a gentle heat until the tomatoes are mushy and properly cooked.

4 Now add the okra, pop the lid on and leave it to cook on a gentle heat for 15 minutes.

5 Just before serving, pump up the heat, season to taste, and stir through the fresh coriander.

GOES WELL WITH: Saag Paneer, Cumin Carrot Kraut, Tzatziki.

SPICY ROASTED OKRA

See page 103

Serves 4

300g okra, halved lengthways

2 tbsp olive oil

½ tsp ground cumin

1 pinch ground coriander

½ tsp smoked paprika

1 pinch cayenne pepper

1 tsp salt

Lemon wedges

1 Heat your oven up to 200°C.

2 Toss all the ingredients (except the lemon wedges) together in a large mixing bowl, tip them onto a baking tray, and spread them out evenly in one layer only. Then roast for 15 minutes.

3 Arrange on a platter and serve with lemon wedges.

GOES WELL WITH: Pulled Shawarma-style Lamb, Roasted Spring Onions, Tomatoes on the Grill.

BUTTERED OKRA

See page 103

Serves 4

300g okra, halved lengthways

2 tbsp butter

Salt and black pepper

1 Blanch the okra for about 4 minutes as per the blanching lesson on page 38.

2 Melt the butter in a large pan over a medium heat and add the okra to warm through, then season with salt and pepper.

3 Serve immediately.

GOES WELL WITH: Romesco Chicken Tray Bake, Sardines with Warm Chorizo and Tomato Dressing.

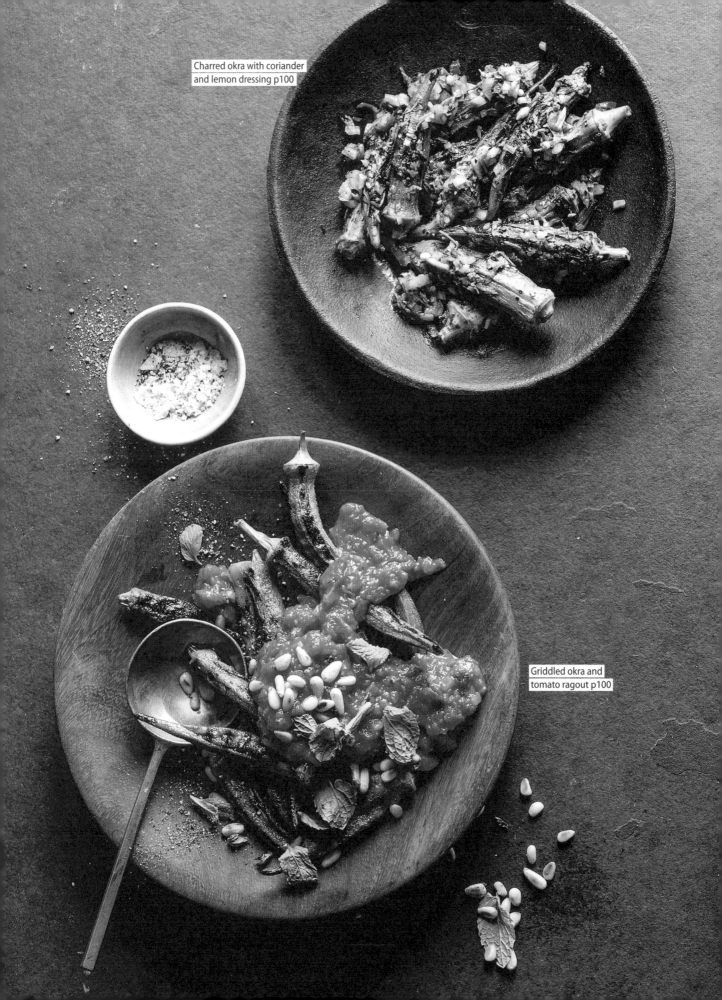

Charred okra with coriander and lemon dressing p100

Griddled okra and tomato ragout p100

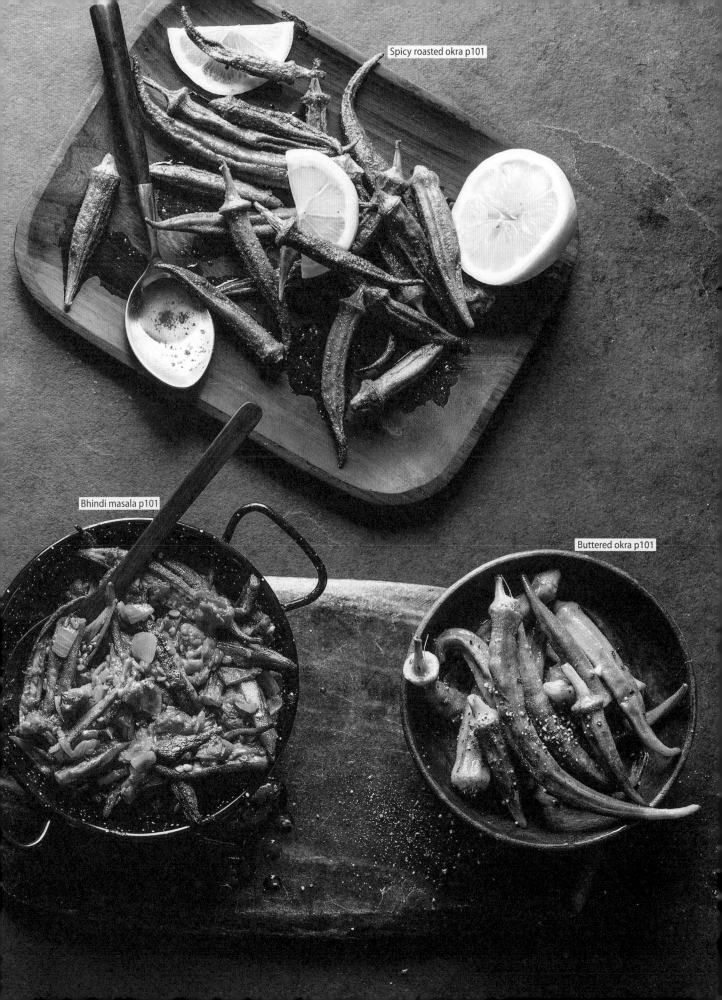

Spicy roasted okra p101

Bhindi masala p101

Buttered okra p101

STIR-FRIED SPRING ONIONS AND PAK CHOI

See page 106

Serves 4

1 tbsp coconut oil

2 bunches spring onions, trimmed and cut into 10cm lengths

2 bunches pak choi, ends trimmed and quartered lengthways

2 garlic cloves, thinly sliced

1 tbsp grated ginger

½ tsp chilli flakes

Juice of 1 lime

1   Heat the oil in a pan over a medium-high heat, add the spring onions and stir-fry for 1 minute.

2   Add the pak choi, garlic and ginger and sauté for another minute until the leaves start to wilt.

3   To finish it off, sprinkle the chilli flakes over the mix and drizzle with lime juice. Serve immediately.

GOES WELL WITH: Broccolini in Oyster Sauce, Shanghainese Poached Chicken, Xinjiang Cumin-spiced Lamb Skewers.

BUTTER-BRAISED SPRING ONIONS WITH LOTS OF CHIVES

See page 106

Serves 4

300g spring onions, root ends trimmed

125ml of water

4 tbsp butter

1 small handful chives, snipped

Salt and black pepper

1   Place the spring onions, water and butter in a small pot, bring to a simmer, then pop the lid on and leave it to cook for 5 minutes.

2   Take the lid off and fire up the pan to reduce the mix until it starts bubbling and spitting, so that, basically, only the butter is left.

3   Throw in the chives, some salt and pepper, give it all a stir and serve.

GOES WELL WITH: Provençal Mushrooms, Deconstructed Ratatouille, Tarragon Roasted Chicken.

ROASTED SPRING ONIONS

See page 106

Serves 4

125ml olive oil

2 bunches spring onions, washed and roots trimmed

4 whole garlic cloves, peeled

Salt and black pepper

1   Heat your oven to 200°C.

2   Put the olive oil, spring onions and garlic in a roasting tray with some salt and pepper and roast them for 30 minutes until golden-brown.

3   Pour the oil off into something for later use – perhaps a roast-garlic dressing – then serve the onions as they are or in a salad.

GOES WELL WITH: Caprese Salad, Drunken Lamb Ribs, Prosciutto-wrapped Radicchio.

CREAMY BACON ONIONS

See page 107

Serves 4

4 tbsp olive oil

2 onions, topped, tailed, peeled
  and halved

250ml beef stock or broth
  (see page 232)

125ml cream

8 rashers streaky bacon

2 tsp thyme leaves, chopped

90g Parmigiano Reggiano, grated

Salt and black pepper

1 Preheat your oven to 180°C.

2 Heat the oil in a large pan and add the onions. Leave them to go dark brown on one side before turning them. Once they are brown, remove them from the heat.

3 In a bowl, whisk together the beef broth and cream.

4 Wrap the bacon rashers around the onions, pinning them with cocktail sticks to stay in place, and pack them tightly in a baking dish.

5 Pour the cream mixture around them and give the onions a drizzle of olive oil, a sprinkling of thyme, and some salt and pepper.

6 Roast them, uncovered, for 40 minutes.

7 Before serving, top each onion with some grated Parmigiano Reggiano and pop them back in the oven either under the grill or at a high heat to get that cheese golden and gooey.

GOES WELL WITH: Steamed and Buttered Courgettes, Caramelised Endive and Leeks.

KOREAN SPRING ONION SALAD

See page 107

Serves 4

For extra crunch, pop the onions in the fridge for an hour after they've been washed.

2 bunches spring onions, thinly sliced
  or, even better, julienned

2 tbsp soy sauce

2 tbsp sesame oil

3 tsp rice wine vinegar

1 garlic clove, minced

1 tsp Korean chilli flakes (gochugaru)

2 tsp toasted sesame seeds

1 Wash the spring onions in fresh running water, then leave them in a colander to drain for 10 minutes.

2 In the meantime, whisk together everything apart from the sesame seeds and the spring onions.

3 Add the spring onions to the dressing and toss them until they are well coated. Tip them out onto a platter.

4 Scatter them with sesame seeds and serve immediately.

GOES WELL WITH: Crispy Asian Pork Belly, Kimchi Jjigae.

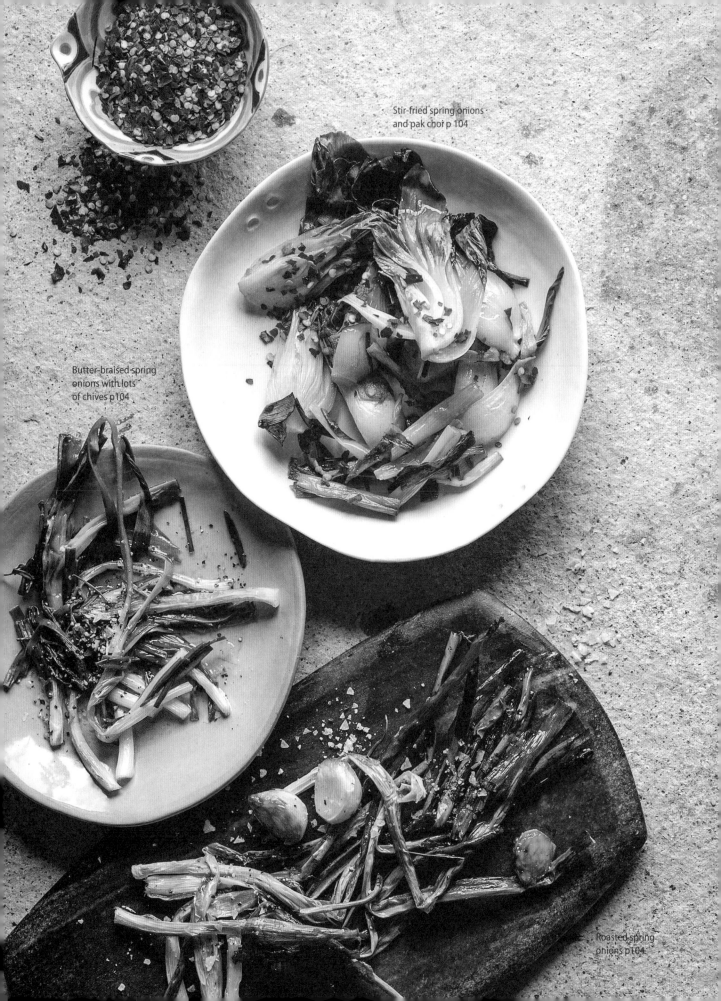

Stir-fried spring onions
and pak choi p 104

Butter-braised spring
onions with lots
of chives p104

Roasted spring
onions p104

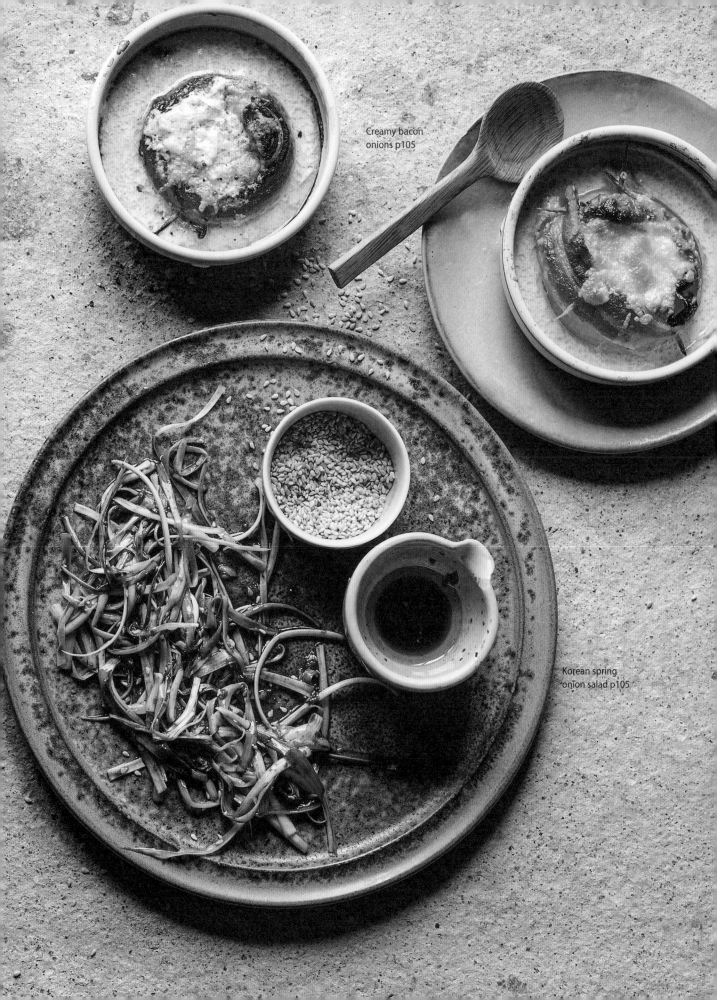

Creamy bacon
onions p105

Korean spring
onion salad p105

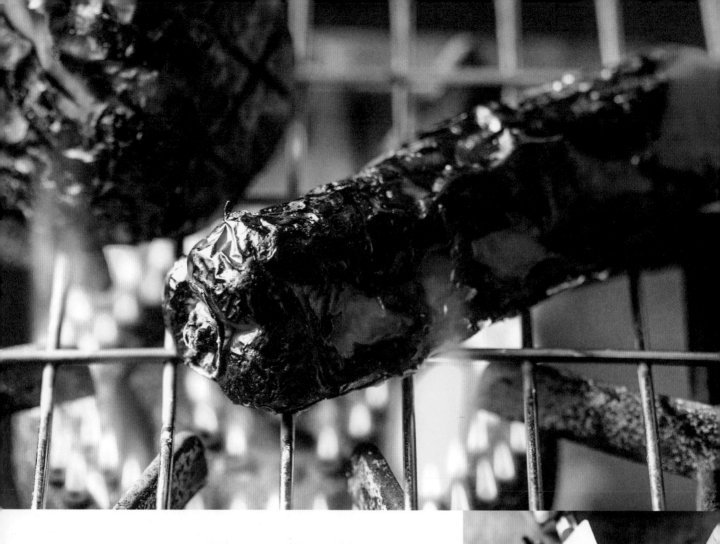

CHARRING PEPPERS

Some of the pepper recipes call for charred peppers. Tomatoes, chillies, peppers and other nightshades all have the amazing ability to endure being burnt to a crisp and, under all that char, still harbour the most delicious complex smoky flavours in generally undamaged 'meat'.

To char any of them, peppers in particular, place them directly over a flame (on a small grid if you like) and turn them until they are black all over.

Once they are blackened, place them in an airtight container until they cool to room temperature.

At this point, use your fingers or a knife to scrape the charred skin from the veg.

Then continue as per the recipe.

CARMEN'S CHARRED RED PEPPER SOUP

See page 111

Serves 4

1 tbsp olive oil

2 tbsp butter

1 red onion, finely chopped

1 tbsp chopped thyme leaves

½ handful basil, chopped

3 charred red peppers, seeded and
cut into strips (see charring lesson
opposite)

150g plum tomatoes, halved

500ml tomato purée

250ml chicken broth

125ml cream

Salt and black pepper

1 Heat the olive oil and butter to a high heat in a medium-sized pot; throw in the onion and let it become slightly caramelised.

2 Add the thyme and half the basil and sauté until they become fragrant.

3 Add the red peppers and tomatoes and cook them until slightly caramelised.

4 Stir in the tomato purée and chicken broth and bring to the boil, stirring occasionally, then reduce the heat and simmer, covered, for 15 minutes.

5 Remove the soup from the heat, add the cream and blitz the mix with a stick blender until smooth, then place it back on the heat to simmer for 3 minutes.

6 Season to taste, then add the remaining basil seconds before serving (whether it is served hot or cold).

Thanks to Carmen Roux, my legendary assistant on this book, for this recipe.
It stands on its own as amazing starter.

SAUTÉED PEPPERS WITH SPICY VINAIGRETTE

See page 111

Serves 4

3 tbsp red wine vinegar

6 tbsp olive oil

1 jalapeño chilli, cored, seeded
and thinly sliced

2 tbsp finely chopped marjoram leaves

1 red onion, thinly sliced

1 garlic clove, thinly sliced

2 red bell peppers, cored, seeded and
jullienned

2 yellow peppers, cored, seeded and
jullienned

Salt and black pepper

1 In a small mixing bowl, whisk together 3 tablespoons of olive oil, the vinegar, chilli and marjoram, and season with salt and pepper.

2 Heat the remaining oil to medium heat in a large pan and add in the onion and garlic, and sauté until softened.

3 Add the peppers and sauté for another 10 minutes.

4 Once the peppers are cooked, pour in the dressing. Immediately remove from the heat and leave to cool.

GOES WELL WITH: Classic Slaw, Vaca Frita.

RATATOUILLE

Serves 8

4 tbsp olive oil

2 medium aubergines, cut into cubes

1 red onion, sliced

2 red peppers, sliced

1 bay leaf

1 tbsp tomato paste

4 tbsp chicken broth

3 baby marrows, sliced

2 garlic cloves, minced

300g plum tomatoes, halved

1 tsp fresh oregano, chopped

½ handful basil, roughly chopped

Salt and black pepper

1 Heat half the olive oil to a medium heat in a large saucepan and add the aubergine cubes to sauté for 5 minutes until golden, then remove them from the pan and set aside.
2 In the same pan, add the rest of the oil and heat it.
3 Add the onion, peppers and bay leaf and sauté until softened.
4 Add the tomato paste and stir until well combined, then pour in the chicken broth and cook until thick and saucy.
5 Add the baby marrows and cook them until tender, stirring occasionally.
6 Finally, add the garlic, tomatoes and oregano, and cook until the tomatoes start to become mushy.
7 Add the aubergines to the saucepan and stir them through until they're hot.
8 Just before serving, stir through the basil and season to taste with salt and pepper.

GOES WELL WITH: Chicken Parmigiana.

DECONSTRUCTED RATATOUILLE

Serves 6

1 medium aubergine, halved lengthways, then sliced in half-disks

2 red bell peppers, sides cut off and halved

1 red onion, thickly sliced

2 large courgettes, sliced into small disks

3 large tomatoes, halved and sliced into small half-disks

125ml olive oil

2 garlic cloves, roughly chopped

2 tbsp chopped fresh oregano

1 tbsp chopped fresh thyme leaves

500ml passata

Salt and black pepper

1 Preheat your oven to 180°C.
2 Toss the aubergine, peppers, onion, courgettes and tomatoes in olive oil in a mixing bowl.
3 Mix the garlic, oregano and thyme into the passata, then spoon a third of the mix evenly over the base of a baking dish.
4 Layer the aubergine, peppers, onion, courgettes and tomatoes in the dish, making sure they are tightly packed (as pictured opposite).
5 Give the bake a liberal seasoning of salt and pepper, then top with the remaining passata mix and drizzle with a little extra olive oil.
6 Place in the oven to roast for 35 minutes until all the vegetables are tender, then serve.

GOES WELL WITH: Butter Braised Spring Onions with Lots of Chives, Tarragon Roasted Chicken.

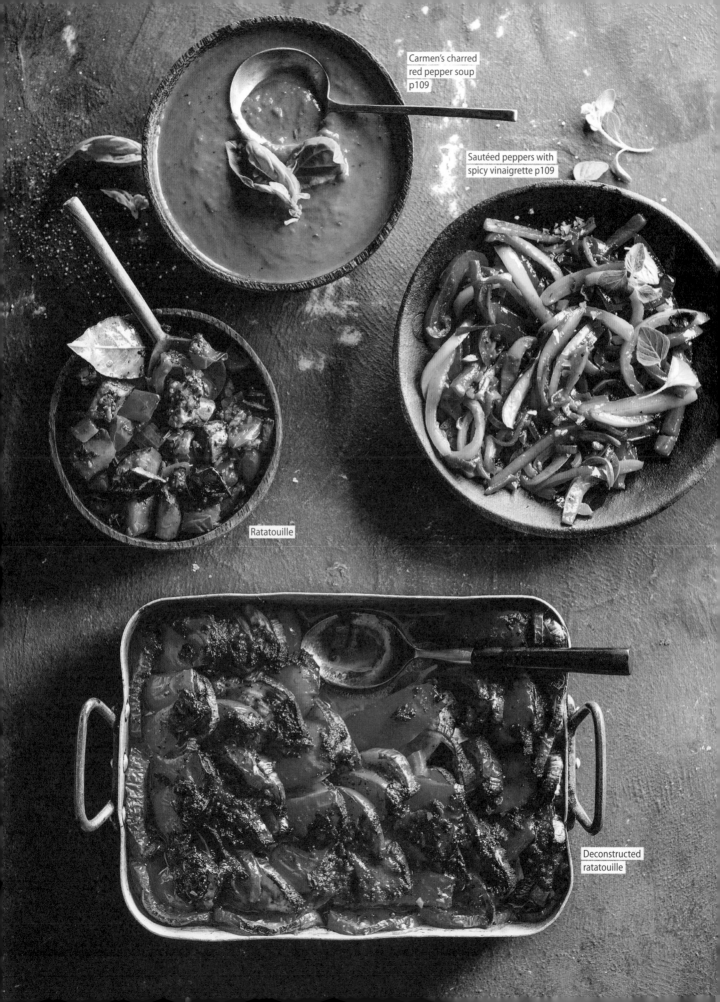

Carmen's charred red pepper soup p109

Sautéed peppers with spicy vinaigrette p109

Ratatouille

Deconstructed ratatouille

PROSCIUTTO-WRAPPED RADICCHIO

See page 115

Serves 4

2 heads radicchio, outer leaves
  discarded, quartered
8 big slices of Parma ham (prosciutto)
2 tsp olive oil
125ml white wine
3 tbsp butter
Salt and black pepper

1 Preheat your oven to 180℃.
2 Wrap each radicchio quarter in prosciutto and give them a brush of olive oil and a sprinkling of salt and pepper.
2 Place the wraps in a small baking dish, add the wine and butter, and roast them for 15 minutes.
3 Baste them with sauce from the dish and serve immediately.

GOES WELL WITH: Buttered Mange Tout, Roasted Spring Onions, Caprese Salad.

SHAVED RADISH SALAD

See page 114

Serves 4

100g mixed radishes, thinly sliced,
  preferably on a mandolin
100g fennel, thinly sliced, preferably
  on a mandolin
100g cucumber, thinly sliced,
  preferably on a mandolin
1 large handful mint leaves
4 tbsp basic vinaigrette (page 272)
60g toasted walnuts, lightly crushed
Salt and black pepper

1 Toss the radish, fennel, cucumber and half the mint in a mixing bowl with salt, pepper and vinaigrette. Spoon onto a serving platter.
2 Scatter with the toasted walnuts and the remaining mint leaves.

GOES WELL WITH: Confit Duck, 'Beeten' Salmon.

RED WINE-BRAISED RADISHES WITH BACON

See page 114

Serves 4

1 tbsp butter
120g diced bacon (streaky is best)
2 shallots, sliced to medium thickness
300g radishes, topped, tailed
  and halved
80ml water
80ml red wine
2 sprigs thyme
1 handful flat-leaf parsley, chopped
Salt and black pepper

1 Melt the butter in a medium-sized pan over a medium heat. Add the bacon, shallots and radishes, and sauté them for 10 minutes. The mix should caramelise and catch a little on the bottom.
2 Add the water, wine and thyme, and bring to the boil. Then reduce to a simmer and pop the lid on for it to tick away for 10 minutes.
3 Remove the lid and reduce the liquid to a sticky-glaze consistency. Season to taste.
4 Stir through three-quarters of the parsley. Place in a serving dish, scatter the rest of the parsley over the top and serve.

GOES WELL WITH: Buttered Chard, Spaghetti Squash Fritters, Roasted Kale.

STEAMED RADISH RÉMOULADE WITH CHIVES

See page 115

Serves 4

180ml mayonnaise

1 tsp sherry vinegar
  (or tarragon vinegar)

½ celery stalk, finely chopped

1 tbsp Dijon mustard

1 tbsp wholegrain mustard

1tbsp grated horseradish (creamed if
  you can't get fresh)

2 tsp capers, minced

1½ tsp sweet paprika

1 tsp Tabasco

400g radishes, ends trimmed

2 tbsp finely chopped chives

4 hard-boiled eggs, roughly grated

Salt and black pepper

1 Make the rémoulade in advance by mixing the mayonnaise, sherry vinegar, celery, mustards, horseradish, capers, paprika and Tabasco together. Leave in the fridge for an hour or so to infuse.

2 Bring a pot of water to the boil, place the radishes in a colander over the pot, cover with a lid and and steam them for 8 minutes.

3 Remove from the heat and allow the radishes to cool down before slicing them as thinly as possible, or shaving them on a mandolin.

4 Mix the radishes, chives, eggs and rémoulade together well in a medium mixing bowl. Season well and serve with another scattering of chives.

GOES WELL WITH: Buttered Asparagus.
For the full recipe for Rémoulade, see page 294.

WINTER SALAD OF RADICCHIO WITH PARSLEY AND SWEET SAUTÉED ONION

We've gone easy on the bacon in this book, but some crispy bacon bits really would take this to the next level.
See page 114

Serves 4

3 tbsp butter

2 onions, thickly sliced

250ml water

2 heads radicchio, shredded

1 large handful flat-leaf parsley,
  roughly chopped

1 splash basic vinaigrette
  (see page 272)

Salt and black pepper

Optional: 250g streaky bacon, chopped
  and fried until crispy

1 Melt the butter in a large pan over a medium heat and add the onions.

2 Sauté the onions until they start to go brown – about 10 minutes.

3 Add a quarter of the water. As it bubbles, use a wooden spoon to scrape the sediment off the bottom of the pan.

4 Leave the water to evaporate completely, and repeat the process about three times. Let the onions get darker each time, then stop the caramelisation by adding in a little water, letting it lift the flavour off the pan and back into the onions.

5 Once the onions are dark and sticky (after the third or fourth round), remove them from the heat and let them cool.

6 Place the onions with the radicchio, parsley and vinaigrette in a bowl, season with salt and pepper and toss gently together until the salad is mixed well. Add the bacon if you like, then serve.

GOES WELL WITH: Caramelised Endive and Leeks, Chocolate Braised Short Ribs, Caribbean-spiced Lamb Shanks.

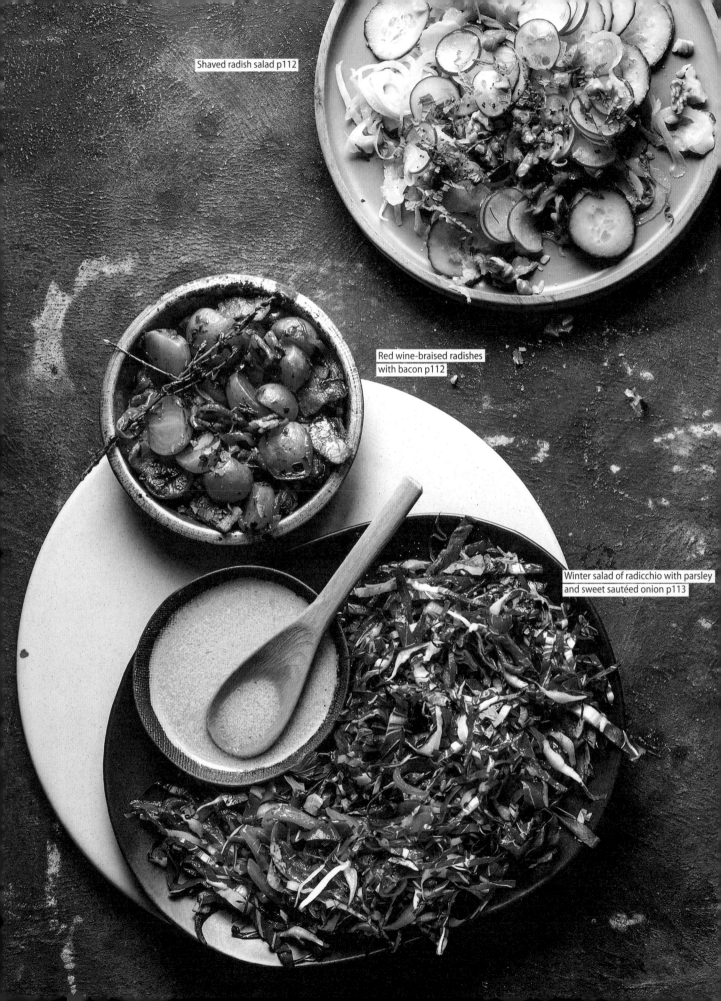

Shaved radish salad p112

Red wine-braised radishes with bacon p112

Winter salad of radicchio with parsley and sweet sautéed onion p113

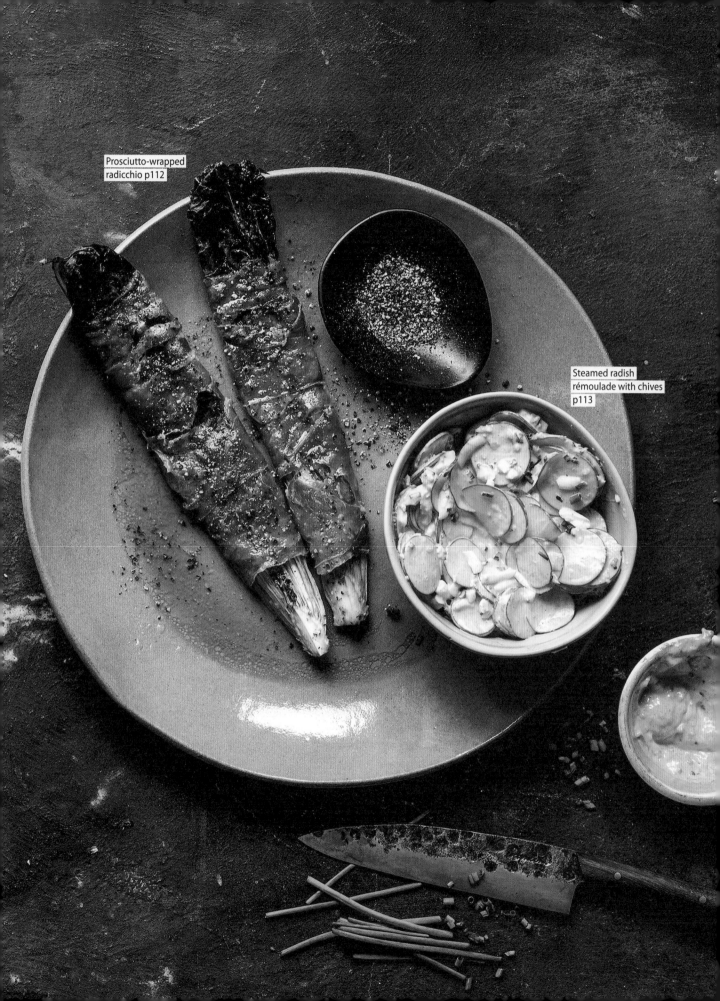

Prosciutto-wrapped radicchio p112

Steamed radish rémoulade with chives p113

GOMEN WAT

Serves 4

1 tbsp coconut oil
1 onion, chopped
¼ tsp ground allspice
½ tsp ground turmeric
3 garlic cloves, finely chopped
300g spinach, rinsed, trimmed
  and chopped
375ml water
1 red pepper, roughly chopped
1 yellow pepper, roughly chopped
1 green pepper, roughly chopped
1 tbsp fresh lemon juice
1 tbsp ginger, minced
1 tsp paprika
Salt and pepper

1   Heat the oil in a large pan over a medium heat and add the onions, allspice and turmeric to cook until the onions are tender and golden-brown.
2   Add the garlic and sauté for a minute, then add the spinach and water and simmer gently for 15 minutes until the water has almost completely evaporated.
3   Add the red, yellow and green peppers, lemon juice, ginger and paprika and cook for 5 minutes until peppers are soft.
4   Check the seasoning, remove from the heat and serve immediately.

GOES WELL WITH: Harissa Chicken Wings, Berbere Cauliflower with Tarator.

SPANAKOPITA FILLING

Serves 4

1 tbsp olive oil
1 onion, finely chopped
1 garlic clove, minced
300g spinach, rinsed and spun dry
1 handful flat-leaf parsley
  leaves, chopped
4 eggs, beaten
4 tbsp crumbled feta
2 tsp chopped dill
Salt and pepper

1   Preheat your oven to 160°C and oil a small baking dish.
2   Heat the oil to a medium heat in a large frying pan, add the onions and sauté them until they are softened.
3   Add the garlic and stir until it becomes fragrant, then add the spinach.
4   Cook the spinach until it has wilted and the pan juices have dried up. This takes up to 10 minutes on a medium heat.
5   Once the spinach has cooled, combine all the ingredients in a large bowl, place in a baking dish and spread them out evenly.
6   Bake in the oven for 40 minutes until cooked and set, then serve with any Greek dish.

GOES WELL WITH: Turnip Skordalia, Greek Pork Chops, Pulled Shawarma-style Lamb.

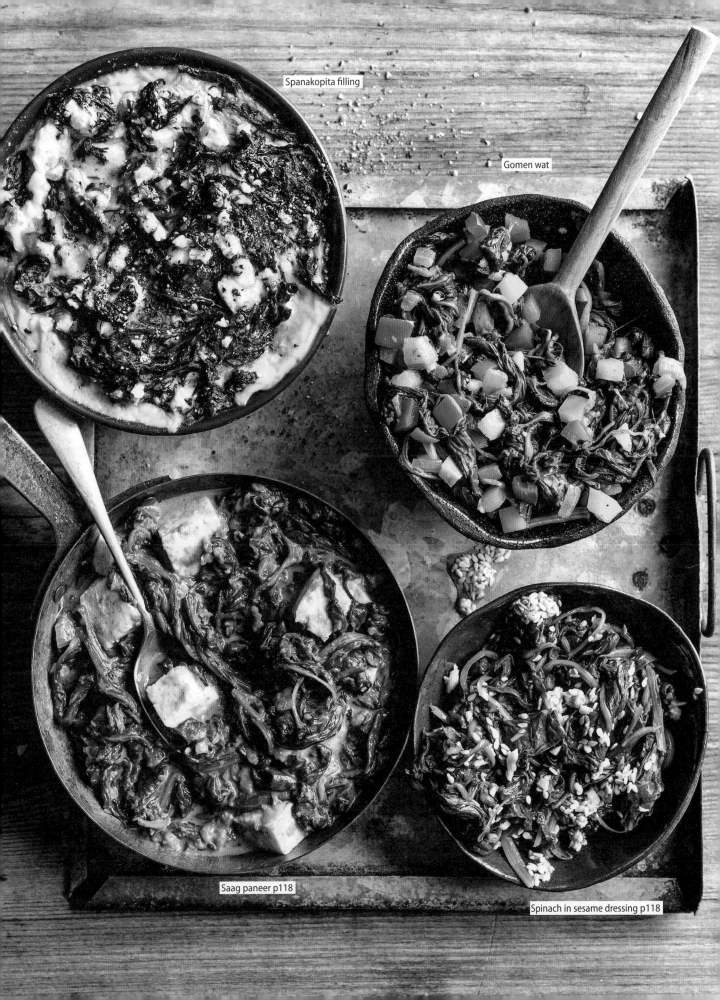

Spanakopita filling

Gomen wat

Saag paneer p118

Spinach in sesame dressing p118

SPINACH IN SESAME DRESSING

See page 117

Serves 4

1 tbsp sesame oil

1 tbsp toasted sesame seeds

2 garlic cloves, minced

1 tsp lime juice

1 tsp soy sauce

Water

400g baby spinach

1 Whisk together the sesame oil, sesame seeds, garlic, lime juice and soy sauce in a small mixing bowl.

2 Quarter-fill a medium-sized pot with water and bring to a boil over a high heat.

3 Blanch the spinach as per the lesson on blanching on page 38.

4 Squeeze out excess water, then toss the spinach in the dressing and serve. This dish can be served hot or cold.

GOES WELL WITH: Sautéed Mushrooms with Soy Butter Sauce, Dark Salty Pork Ribs.

SAAG PANEER

See page 117

Serves 4

5 tbsp olive oil

1 onion, finely chopped

1 tbsp ginger, minced

4 garlic cloves, minced

1 green chilli, finely chopped

½ tsp garam masala

2 tsp ground coriander

1 tsp ground cumin

1 tsp turmeric

300g spinach, chopped

125ml plain yoghurt

120g paneer, cut into 1.5cm cubes

½ tsp cayenne pepper

½ tsp salt

1 In a large pan, heat the olive oil to a medium heat. Add the onion, ginger, garlic and chilli, and sauté for 10 minutes until well caramelised.

2 Add the garam masala, coriander, cumin and turmeric and cook for about 5 minutes.

3 Add the spinach and stir well, tossing to coat it in the spices.

4 Once mixed, add 125ml water and cook uncovered until the water has completely reduced.

5 Remove the mix from the heat and stir in the yoghurt, 1 tablespoon at a time.

6 Finally, add the paneer, season to taste with cayenne pepper and salt. Mix gently on a low heat until ready to serve. (Be careful: if it gets too hot, the yoghurt will split.).

A DISH ON ITS OWN.

MOJO-ISH MARINATED TOMATOES

See page 121

Serves 4

Traditional mojo sauce usually contains orange, lime, grapefruit or some other kind of citrus juice. We've made this with just lime juice, which gives it a slightly more savoury flavour.

1 garlic clove

4 tbsp fresh lime juice

4 tbsp olive oil

1 small handful fresh oregano leaves

1 tsp ground cumin

1 pinch salt

½ tsp black pepper

8 plum tomatoes, cored and quartered

1   Use a stick blender to blitz the garlic, lime juice, olive oil, oregano, cumin, salt and pepper together to make the dressing.

2   Add the tomatoes to a small bowl, smother them in the mojo sauce and leave them to marinate for 2 hours before serving.

3   You could serve these as a side dish, or add them to a salad for a punch.

GOES WELL WITH: Cuban Ropa Vieja, Sautéed Peppers with Spicy Vinaigrette.

ROASTED CHERRY TOMATO CAPRESE

See page 121

Serves 4

200g cherry tomatoes

3 tbsp olive oil

2 garlic cloves, cut into quarters

4 sprigs thyme

1 ball buffalo mozzarella, torn

½ handful fresh basil leaves

Salt and black pepper

1   Preheat your oven to 180°C and line a baking tray with foil.

2   Place the tomatoes, olive oil, garlic and thyme in a roasting tray and season with salt and pepper.

3   Roast them in the oven for 35 minutes until lightly browned.

4   Arrange the tomatoes on a serving platter with the buffalo mozzarella and the basil.

5   Before serving, drizzle everything with the juices from the roasting tray and give it a sprinkle of salt and a crack of black pepper.

GOES WELL WITH: Roasted Artichokes with Lemon and Dill Vinaigrette, Sautéed Mange Tout with Mint, Lemon and Ricotta, Slow-roasted Lamb Shoulder with Lemon and Capers.

CAPRESE SALAD

Serves 4

Unlike the roasted variation, where you can add flavour by cooking, this variation relies solely on the quality and ripeness of the tomatoes. You want them on the edge of turning: soft, blood-red and juicy as hell, otherwise don't bother. Also, we would traditionally drizzle a caprese with balsamic vinegar, but it is very syrupy and sugary. We've substituted vinaigrette here. This is not an Italian way to deal with the problem.

4 ultra-ripe plum tomatoes, cut into
    2cm slices
2 balls buffalo mozzarella, cut into
    2cm slices
1 handful basil leaves
4 tbsp basic vinaigrette (see page 272)
Salt and black pepper

1 On a large serving platter, arrange the tomato slices, mozzarella slices and basil leaves by alternating and overlapping them.
2 Season with salt and pepper, splash with the vinaigrette and serve.

GOES WELL WITH: Pan-fried Haddock with Olives and Tomatoes, Prosciutto-wrapped Radicchio, Roasted Spring Onions.

TOMATOES ON THE GRILL

Serves 4

4 plum tomatoes, halved lengthways
2 tbsp olive oil
Salt and black pepper

1 Prepare the barbecue or a griddle pan for a high heat.
2 Once the coals or the griddle are ready, season the tomatoes with salt and pepper and place them cut-side down directly on the grill. Grill each side for 5 minutes until nicely charred.
3 Remove from the heat and arrange on a serving dish and drizzle with olive oil.
4 You could eat them just like this with other vegetables or add them to your next soup, sauce, salad or stew for a deliciously charred flavour.

GOES WELL WITH: Courgetti with Basil, Mint and Pine Nuts, Spicy Roasted Okra, Takeaway Chicken.

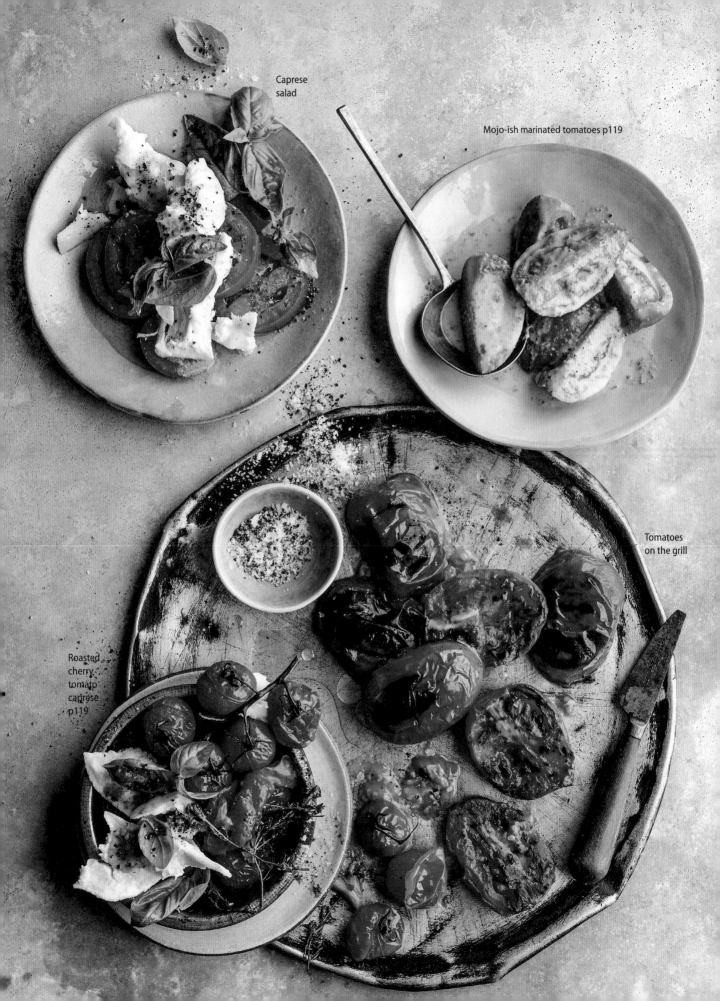

Caprese salad

Mojo-ish marinated tomatoes p119

Tomatoes on the grill

Roasted cherry tomato caprese p119

DRINK?

'What can I drink?' – a question I'm often asked.

I get it. This is a serious consideration for someone who's quitting sodas and cordials.

When I'm asked this question, I often see the serial dieters anxiously waiting for me to unveil my collection of 'low-carb' cordials and products that allow them to change nothing about their behaviour. Unfortunately, that's not my style.

I don't believe in the 'Don't drink that sweet drink, drink *my* sweet drink' model, and I think you'll benefit more if you prepare your drinks yourself. (On a related note, I take a dim view on powdered shakes, special supplements and protein bars.)

So, my usual answer to the question, 'What can I drink?' is as follows.

We were designed to drink water. And that's what you should drink.

If you're new to drinking water, here are some tips and info to soften the belly-flop into the world of basic hydration.

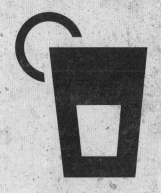

★ The idea that you need to stay hydrated or you will die comes from marketers and compromised scientists out to sell more of the brand-drinks that sponsored their research. (That is, I believe, about as accurate a short summary of *Waterlogged* by Professor Tim Noakes as you will get.)

★ It's totally okay to drink water before, after and while you're exercising, instead of Gatorade, Powerade, colas, powdered magic potions, etc. You won't bonk (run out of fuel). I swam 459km in 23 days once and drank water and tea. To be honest, I also had coffee. But I'd hardly call coffee with milk an extreme performance-enhancer.

★ You do not need to drink 2/4/8 glasses, or any fixed amount, of water per day. Drink when you're thirsty.

★ If your pee is yellow that does not mean you are dehydrated. It might mean you're urinating out all the money you've spent on multivitamins.

There's a steamy double-page spread of fruits and herbs over the page, which was laid out as inspiration for you to flavour your waters and teas, and throughout this short section I've offered a range of specific suggestions.

HOT (AND COLD) TIPS

★ Use any fruit to flavour your drinks, but not necessarily to eat – unless you're happy to eat fruit.

★ Bubbles make it better. I have a SodaStream at home and I always have at least three bottles of cold water in the fridge. It may sound strange, but bubbles make it seem more like a soda, which, if that's what you're trying to give up, is good.

★ Acidity also helps. Low-carb diehards often talk about putting apple cider vinegar in the water. It does help lower your blood sugar after a meal, and vinegar does have other health benefits, so there's that. Alternatively, add a squeeze of lemon to your water. It will taste like nothing for your first soda-free week, but eventually, as your palate adjusts, you'll take pleasure in being a discerning lemon buyer (choose the plump ones with the thick waxy skin).

★ Tea can also be a cold drink. In fact, tea teams up very well with a number of fruits, herbs and spices. The best iced teas are those that have been left to infuse overnight. There are also loads of infused teas that you can buy off the shelf. Just brew them in volume, refrigerate, then mix with ice, sparkling water and some fruit – and you'll be laughing.

HOT DRINKS

These are my favourite recipes. Each one is designed to use 1½ litres of water and the exact same method.

Add the tea bags/herbs/spices/fruit to a pot with the water. Bring it all to the boil then strain the mixture into a cup. Drink immediately as is, or with extra fruit if required.

ROOIBOS CARDAMOM TEA

4 rooibos tea bags, 5 cardamom pods

HIBISCUS TEA

1 small handful hibiscus flowers, 1 stick cinnamon, lime slices

RUG SHOP TEA

4 tbsp dried Moroccan mint, slices of apple

SPICED EARL GREY

4 Earl Grey tea bags, 4 sticks of cassia,
10 pieces allspice, half a nutmeg

LEMON AND BAY

4 Earl Grey tea bags, 2 bay leaves,
4 thick slices of lemon

GINGER AND LAVENDER

4 tbsp dried lavender, 2 thumbs thickly sliced ginger

TURKISH CHOCOLATE

4 tbsp cocoa nib husks, 5 tbsp rose water

STRAIGHT UP GINGER

3 thumbs grated ginger, juice pressed into the water

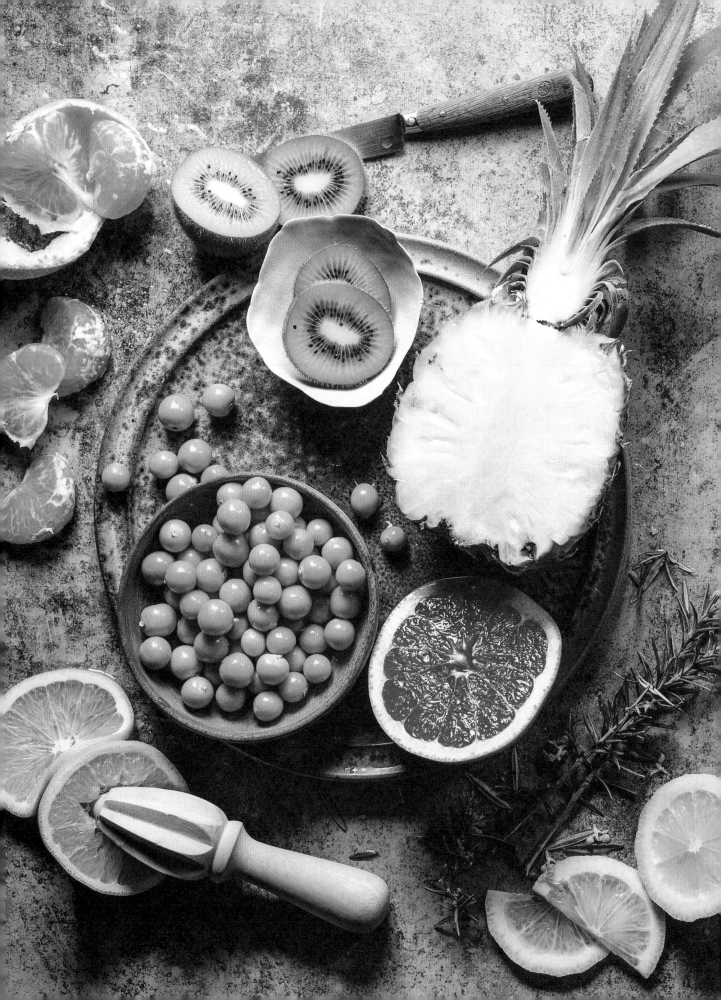

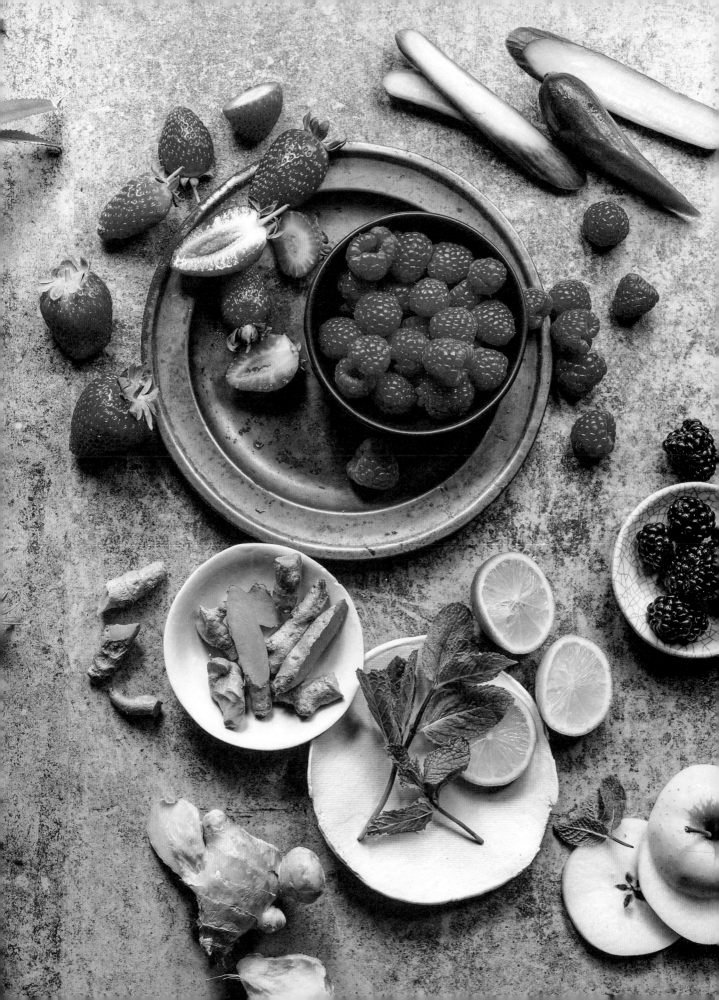

COLD DRINKS AND 'FIZZES'

There are three ways to go about getting cold drinks down.

The first is to just drink cold water, with a twist of lemon if you like.

The second is to add sliced fruit to a glass, and top it up with ice and sparkling water.

The third, which may seem worth it to those who are really struggling to quit sodas, is to let one of the hot infusions here cool in the fridge, and enjoy them on the rocks mixed 50/50 with sparkling water.

That said, there are some ideal fruits to add to your drinks. Here are a few things I throw into water or iced tea when I have guests coming over: slices of fresh ginger, slices of apple, lemon, orange, grapefruit, lime, cucumber, kiwi, pineapple or mandarin. Alternatively, you can drop in whole or macerated strawberries, raspberries, blackberries or any other berries, for that matter. And, of course, fresh mint leaves – even muddled slightly – will give a lift to your glass of anything.

If you're looking for specific ideas, you may find inspiration from the recipes over the next four pages.

CHAMOMILE AND VANILLA TEA

Serves 4

1¼ litres water
4 chamomile tea bags
1 vanilla pod, halved lengthways
750ml ice

1 In a medium saucepan, bring the water, tea bags and vanilla pod to a boil over a medium heat, then leave them to cool to room temperature.
2 Remove the tea bags and vanilla pod.
3 Serve on ice once the drink has cooled.

ROOIBOS, HONEYBUSH AND ORANGE ICED TEA

Serves 4

1¼ litres water
3 rooibos tea bags
2 honeybush tea bags
6 slices orange peel
750ml ice
4 strips orange peel

1 In a medium saucepan, bring the water to a boil over a medium heat.
2 Add the tea bags and orange peel. Remove the saucepan from the heat and let it cool to room temperature.
3 Remove the tea bags and orange peel.
4 Place the ice in a water jug and fill it up with the tea.
5 Garnish with fresh orange peel.

ELDERFLOWER AND PEPPERMINT WATER

Serves 4

1 litre water
1 handful elderflowers
4 sprigs mint
500ml ice
250ml sparkling water
2 sprigs mint

1 In a medium saucepan, bring the water to a boil over a medium heat.
2 Remove the saucepan from the heat, and add the elderflowers and mint to the water. Let it cool to room temperature.
3 Remove the flowers and mint from the water.
4 Place the ice in a water jug and fill it up with the infused water. Top it up with the sparkling water and garnish with fresh mint.

ICED GREEN TEA WITH ROSE WATER

Serves 4

1¼ litres water

3 decaffeinated green tea bags

2 tbsp rose water

750ml ice

8 pink rose petals (optional)

1 In a medium saucepan, bring 1 litre of the water to a boil over a medium heat.

2 Add the tea bags. Remove the saucepan from the heat and let it steep for 5 minutes.

3 Remove the tea bags. Add the remaining cold water and the rose water. Let it cool to room temperature.

4 Place the ice in a water jug and fill it up with the tea.

5 Garnish with rose petals.

LEMON AND GINGER WATER

Serves 4

1 litre water

6 slices lemon

thumb-sized piece ginger, peeled
   and thinly sliced

500ml ice

250ml sparkling water

4 slices lemon

1 In a medium saucepan, bring the water to a boil over a medium heat.

2 Remove the saucepan from the heat and add the lemon and ginger to the water. Let it cool to room temperature.

3 Remove the lemon and ginger from the water.

4 Place the ice in a water jug and fill it up with the infused water. Top it up with the sparkling water and garnish with slices of lemon.

APPLE, MINT AND GREEN TEA INFUSION

Serves 4

2 decaffeinated green tea bags

250ml boiling water

750ml cold water

1 tbsp chopped mint leaves

1 green apple, thinly sliced

750ml ice

250ml sparkling water

4 mint sprigs

1 Place the green tea bags in a cup of boiling water and brew for 2 minutes. Remove the tea bags. Let the tea cool to room temperature.

2 Place the tea, cold water, mint leaves and apple slices in a glass water jug and place it in the fridge for 30 minutes.

3 Top up the jug with the ice and sparkling water.

4 Garnish with the mint sprigs.

ROOIBOS, ORANGE AND CLOVE TEA

Serves 4

1¼ litres water
4 rooibos tea bags
6 slices orange peel
6 cloves
4 slices orange peel

1 In a medium saucepan, bring the water to a boil over a medium heat.
2 Add the tea bags, orange peel and cloves. Reduce the heat to low and let the mix steep for 3 minutes.
3 Remove the tea bags, orange peel and cloves.
4 Place a slice of fresh orange peel in each cup and fill each one with the tea. Serve hot or cold.

STRAWBERRY AND LEMON INFUSION

Serves 4

1 lemon
8 strawberries, sliced
1 litre cold water
750ml ice
250ml sparkling water

1 Remove the peel of the lemon, slice it into thin strips and juice the lemon.
2 Place half of the strawberries, half of the lemon peel and all of the lemon juice in a glass water jug.
3 Add the water to the jug and place in the fridge for 30 minutes.
4 Top up the jug with the ice and sparkling water.
5 Garnish with the remaining strawberries and the remaining lemon peel.

BERRY INFUSION

Serves 4

60g frozen raspberries
60g frozen blueberries
750ml cold water
500ml ice
250ml sparkling water
4 sprigs thyme

1. Place the frozen berries in a blender and blend until smooth. Add the water and blend until thoroughly mixed.
2. Pour the berry water into a glass water jug.
3. Top up the jug with the ice and sparkling water.
4. Garnish with the thyme sprigs.

ORANGE AND CINNAMON INFUSION

Serves 4

4 cinnamon sticks
250ml boiling water
2 oranges
500ml cold water
750ml ice
250ml sparkling water
Orange peel

1. Fill a cup with boiling water and add cinnamon sticks.
2. Remove the peel of the oranges and cut into thick slices. Discard the rest of the orange.
3. Place half of the orange peel in the cup of water with the cinnamon sticks. Let it cool to room temperature.
4. Place the cooled infusion in a glass water jug. Top up the jug with the cold water, ice and sparkling water.
5. Garnish with the remaining orange peel.

FIZZ OF CUCUMBER, LIME AND BASIL

Serves 4

12 slices cucumber
2 limes, thinly sliced
2 basil sprigs
750ml cold water
750ml ice
250ml sparkling water
4 basil sprigs

1. Place the cucumber slices, lime slices and basil sprigs in a glass water jug.
2. Add the water to the jug and place in the fridge for 30 minutes.
3. Top up the jug with the ice and sparkling water.
4. Garnish with the basil sprigs.

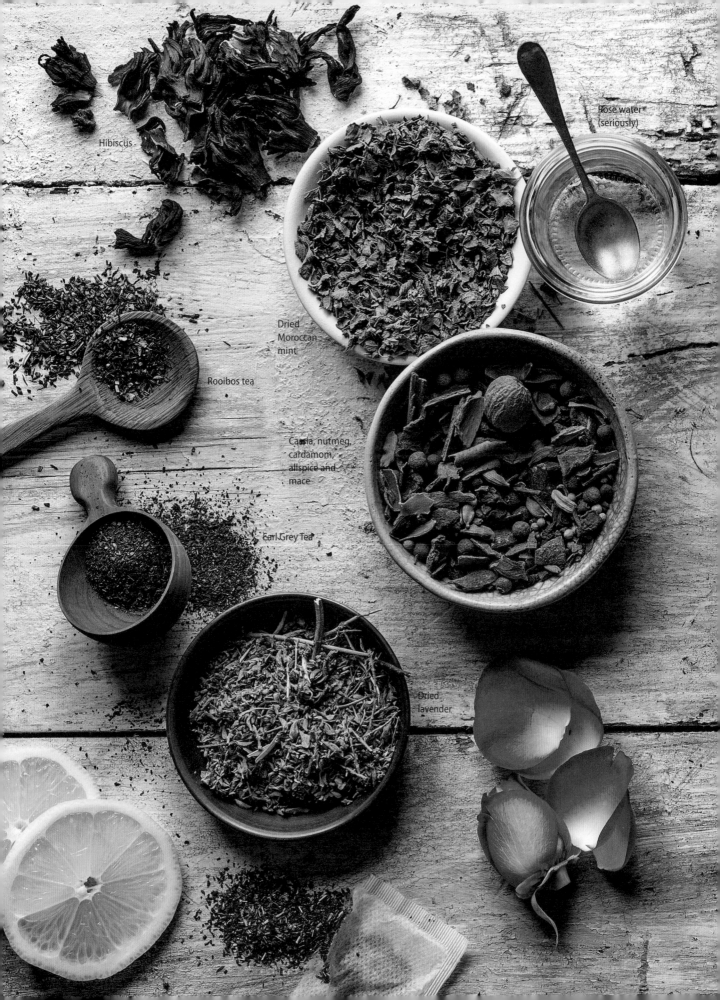

Hibiscus

Rose water*
(seriously)

Dried
Moroccan
mint

Rooibos tea

Cassia, nutmeg,
cardamom,
allspice and
mace

Earl Grey Tea

Dried
lavender

MEAT & POULTRY

Team these meat dishes with any of the sauces in the Sauces, Seasonings and Condiments section, and two or more of the dishes in the Vegetables section.

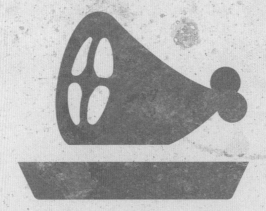

SZECHUAN BOILED BEEF

See page 135

Serves 4

2 tbsp coconut oil

1 thumb ginger, grated

1 tsp ground Szechuan peppercorns

2 garlic cloves, roughly chopped

1 heaped tbsp fermented chilli
    bean paste

500ml broth or stock (preferably beef,
    but chicken will do)

400g Chinese greens (pak choi, tatsoi,
    asparagus lettuce, etc), chopped into
    bite-sized pieces

400g sirloin, sliced into thin finger-
    length strips

1 handful fresh coriander,
    roughly chopped

Juice of 1 lime

150g mung bean sprouts

1 tsp dried ground chilli flakes

1 Get the coconut oil very hot in a medium pot and add the ginger, peppercorns and garlic, and stir quickly.

2 When the garlic becomes fragrant, add the bean paste and keep stirring.

3 When the aroma of the bean paste is released, pour in the stock and bring to the boil.

4 Add the greens and allow them to wilt.

5 Add the beef and stir to separate the strips. Leave the beef to boil for about a minute.

6 Add the coriander and a splash of lime, then divide the sprouts among four serving bowls. Divide the beef among the four bowls.

7 Sprinkle each portion with chilli flakes and serve.

GOES WELL WITH: Broccolini in Oyster Sauce, Lime, Chilli and Sesame Stir-fried Mange Tout, Stir-fried Mushrooms with Bamboo Shoots.

CHOCOLATE BRAISED SHORT RIBS

See page 135

Serves 4

4 tbsp olive oil

1.8kg (6 bone-in pieces) beef short ribs

1 tsp ground coriander

1 tsp ground cumin

1 tsp cinnamon

1 big pinch ground cloves

1 onion, roughly chopped

3 celery stalks, roughly chopped

1 large carrot, roughly chopped

1 x 400g tin chopped tomatoes

1 litre beef stock or broth (see
    page 232)

1 pinch cayenne pepper

2 tbsp cocoa powder

Salt and black pepper

1 Preheat your oven to 160°C.

2 Get half the olive oil nice and hot in a large pot and sear the short ribs. Turn them every few minutes until they are dark brown all over, then remove them and set aside.

3 Place the remaining olive oil, coriander, cumin, cinnamon, cloves, onion, celery and carrot in the pot and sauté them on a medium heat until they are well caramelised.

4 Add the tomatoes, broth, cayenne pepper and cocoa powder. Bring to a gentle simmer, pop the lid on, and leave for 3 hours to braise.

5 Either stir in the excess fat or skim it off – it's up to you.

GOES WELL WITH: Guacamole, Classic Slaw, Sautéed Peppers with Spicy Vinaigrette.

BAKED CHILLI

Serves 4

600g stewing beef (chuck), cut into 3cm cubes
2 tbsp chilli powder
½ tsp cayenne pepper
1 tbsp cumin seeds
¼ tsp ground cinnamon
1 tsp dried oregano
½ tsp black pepper
2 tsp salt
1 tbsp olive oil
1 onion, chopped
2 celery stalks, chopped
2 garlic cloves, chopped

1 jalapeño chilli, seeded and chopped
1 tsp tomato paste
250ml beef stock or broth (page 232)
1 x 400g tin tomatoes
2 bay leaves
½ handful fresh coriander, chopped
½ handful flat-leaf parsley, chopped
2 spring onions, chopped
Sour cream, to serve
Limes, to serve

You could do your baked chilli in a slow cooker or a pot, but in my experience wrapping it in foil, putting it in a baking dish and letting it do its thing in the oven offers the least risk of the sauce catching and blackening the stew. If you don't have time to watch a pot for two hours, I recommend this route.

1 Preheat your oven to 160°C.
2 In a large mixing bowl, mix the beef with the chilli powder, cayenne pepper, cumin, cinnamon, oregano, pepper and salt.
3 Heat the olive oil in a large pan and add the beef cubes. Only add enough cubes to cover three-quarters of the base of the pan, otherwise they won't brown nicely.
4 Cook the meat cubes on each side until they are dark brown, then repeat with the remaining cubes and set them aside.
5 In the same pan, add the onion and celery and sauté them until soft. Add the garlic and jalapeño, and cook until fragrant.
6 Finally, return the beef to the pan and add the tomato paste, stock or broth, chopped tomatoes and bay leaves, and bring to the boil.
7 Spoon everything into a baking dish and cover it in foil (or just put the lid on if the pot is ovenproof) and put it in the oven for 2 hours.
8 After 2 hours, remove the cover, stir through the herbs and scatter with spring onions before serving. Serve it with a dollop of sour cream and a twist of fresh lime.

CUBAN ROPA VIEJA

Serves 4

500g whole chuck steak
4 tbsp olive oil
1 onion, sliced
2 red peppers, thinly sliced
2 cloves garlic, minced
1 tsp ground cumin
1 pinch ground allspice
1 pinch ground clove
375ml chicken stock or broth (page 232)
1 x 400g tin chopped tomatoes

3 tbsp tomato paste
1 tsp sweet paprika
½ tsp smoked paprika
1 tsp dried oregano
250ml pitted green olives
2 tbsp chopped capers
1 bay leaf
1 big handful flat-leaf parsley, roughly chopped

This is brilliant with pork too. You could replace the chuck with pork rump in the same quantities.

See page 137

1 Preheat your oven to 160°C.
2 Season the meat liberally with salt and pepper and sear it in the olive oil at a medium-high heat in an ovenproof pot.
3 When the meat is dark brown all over, remove it from the pot and add the onions and peppers to cook until they are caramelised.
4 Add the garlic, cumin, allspice and cloves and cook for another minute.
5 Add the stock and bring to the boil, using a wooden spoon to scrape the sediment off the bottom of the pot.
6 Add the chopped tomatoes, tomato paste, paprika, smoked paprika, oregano, olives, capers and the bay leaf and return the meat to the pot. Pop the lid on and put it in the oven for 4 hours.
7 Remove the pot from the oven. Remove the meat and shred it before adding it back to the sauce.
8 Place the sauce back on the heat and reduce it gently until it gets thick and stewy.
9 Just before serving, check the seasoning for salt and pepper and stir through the parsley.

GOES WELL WITH: Guacomole, Cauliflower Colcannon.

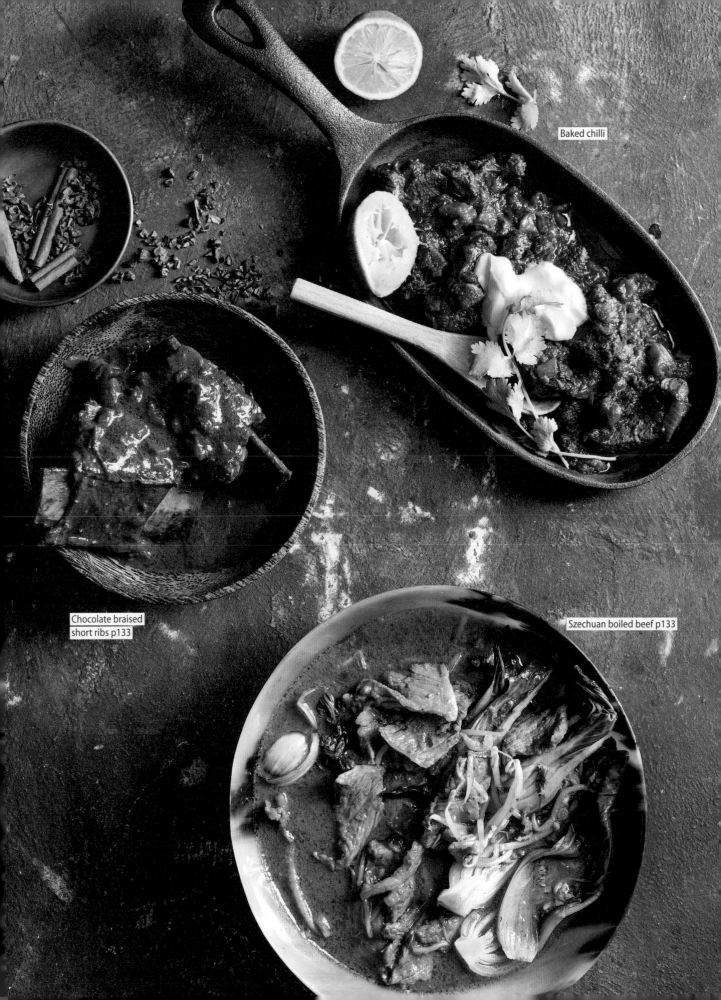

Baked chilli

Chocolate braised
short ribs p133

Szechuan boiled beef p133

BEEF RENDANG

Serves 4

4 tbsp coconut oil

10 dried red chillies, plumped in
    boiling water, then drained

1 onion, finely chopped

4 garlic cloves

2 lemongrass stalks, white part, sliced

1 tbsp fresh galangal, grated

1 tbsp ginger, grated

600g chuck steak, cut into
    4cm x 2cm cubes

2 tsp tamarind paste

1 cinnamon stick

¼ tsp ground cloves

2 star anise

¼ tsp ground cardamom

1 lemongrass stick, cut into 4 pieces

400ml coconut milk

3 large kaffir lime leaves, finely sliced

20g desiccated coconut

Salt

1   Blitz 2 tablespoons coconut oil, chillies, onion, garlic, sliced lemongrass, galangal and ginger in a food processor until smooth and set aside.

2   Heat another 2 tablespoons of coconut oil in a large saucepan over a medium heat and sear the beef, stirring until brown all over.

3   Remove the beef from the pot and add the tamarind paste to cook, stirring until it starts to darken.

4   Return the beef to the pot, add all the other ingredients and stir to combine.

5   Bring the curry up to a very gentle simmer, pop the lid on and let it tick away for about 3 hours, until the beef is tender. You will have to top it up with water every 30 minutes or so, giving it a good stir each time, to prevent it drying out.

6   Once the meat is falling apart, remove the lid, turn the heat up a bit and let it reduce until the sauce is thick and gooey.

7   Season with salt and serve immediately.

GOES WELL WITH: Fried Garlic Green Beans.

FILIPINO BISTEK WITH BAY LEAVES

I've changed the method in this bistek from the traditional way so that you can enjoy your steak medium rare.

Serves 4

See page 137

2 tbsp coconut oil

8 fresh bay leaves

1 onion, sliced into thick rings

3 cloves garlic, roughly chopped

4 tbsp soy sauce

4 tbsp calamondin (or lemon) juice

400g rib-eye, cut into four steaks (small
    and thick, rather than large and thin)

Salt and black pepper

1   Heat half the oil to a medium-high heat in a large pan and add the bay leaves to crisp up.

2   Add the onion rings and let them caramelise well. Avoid stirring them too much.

3   Once they're the right colour, add the garlic and sauté for another 2 minutes.

4   Pour in the soy sauce and juice and bring to the boil.

5   Use a slotted spoon to remove the onion rings and bay leaves, then reduce the sauce to a quarter of its original volume.

6   Return the onion and bay leaves to the pot. Remove from the heat.

7   Season the meat. Heat the remaining oil to really hot in a medium-sized pan.

8   Sear the meat aggressively for about 2 minutes on each side, for medium-rare steaks.

9   Add the onions and bay leaves to the pan and boil everything together, basting the meat in the sauce, for about two minutes.

10 Serve this immediately or the meat will overcook in the sauce.

GOES WELL WITH: Sautéed Mushrooms with Soy Butter Sauce, Korean Spring Onion Salad, Spinach in Sesame Dressing.

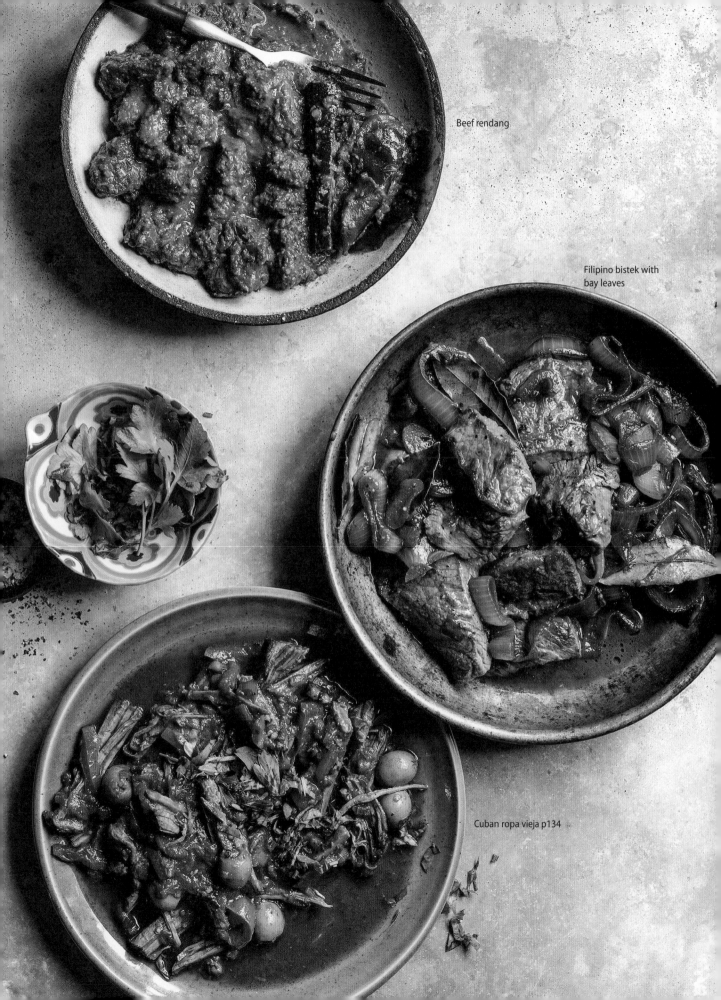

Beef rendang

Filipino bistek with
bay leaves

Cuban ropa vieja p134

BEST DRY-RUBBED BRISKET

Serves 4 to 6

This requires 24 hours of cooking, but it's very easy to reheat. Best to cook it far in advance so there's space in the oven for other stuff.

1 tbsp chilli powder
1 tbsp paprika
1 tbsp salt
1 tsp garlic powder
1 tsp onion powder

1 tsp black pepper
1 tsp cayenne
1 tsp mustard powder
1 tsp ground cumin
600g brisket

1 Mix the spices together, rub them on the meat and leave it, covered, overnight in the fridge.
2 When you're ready to cook, preheat your oven to 90°C.
3 Place the meat in a deep roasting pan, cover with foil and pop it into the oven for 24 hours.
4 Remove it from the oven and let it rest for 30 minutes.
5 Slice it up and serve with homemade dill pickles, gravy, vegetables – and whatever else tickles your fancy.

GOES WELL WITH: Dill Pickle, Classic Slaw.

BEEF TATAKI

Makes 4 starter portions

6 tbsp soy sauce
4 tbsp mirin
2 tbsp lime juice
2 tbsp grated ginger
2 garlic cloves, minced
400g beef fillet

100g daikon, grated and drained of excess moisture
2 spring onions, finely sliced
½ tsp good Japanese chilli sauce
1 handful watercress

1 In a small mixing bowl, combine the soy sauce, mirin, lime juice, ginger and garlic, and mix well.
2 Cover the fillet with half of this mixture and leave it to marinate.
3 After 2 hours, pat the fillet dry. Get a small pan very, very hot and seal the fillet until brown on all sides. Leave it to cool.
4 In a small bowl, mix together the daikon, spring onions and chilli sauce.
5 Slice the meat into very thin strips and arrange them on a serving platter or plates, then drizzle with the remaining marinade.
6 Cover the meat evenly with the daikon salad and top with watercress.

STEAK TARTARE

Makes 4 starter portions

400g beef tenderloin, finely diced or minced
4 tbsp olive oil
2 tbsp Dijon mustard
1 tbsp red wine vinegar
2 tsp capers, chopped
½ red onion, finely chopped

3 medium anchovy fillets, minced
1 egg yolk
1 small handful flat-leaf parsley, finely chopped
Salt and black pepper
Tabasco sauce to taste

1 Mix everything together in a bowl and leave it in the fridge for an hour before serving.

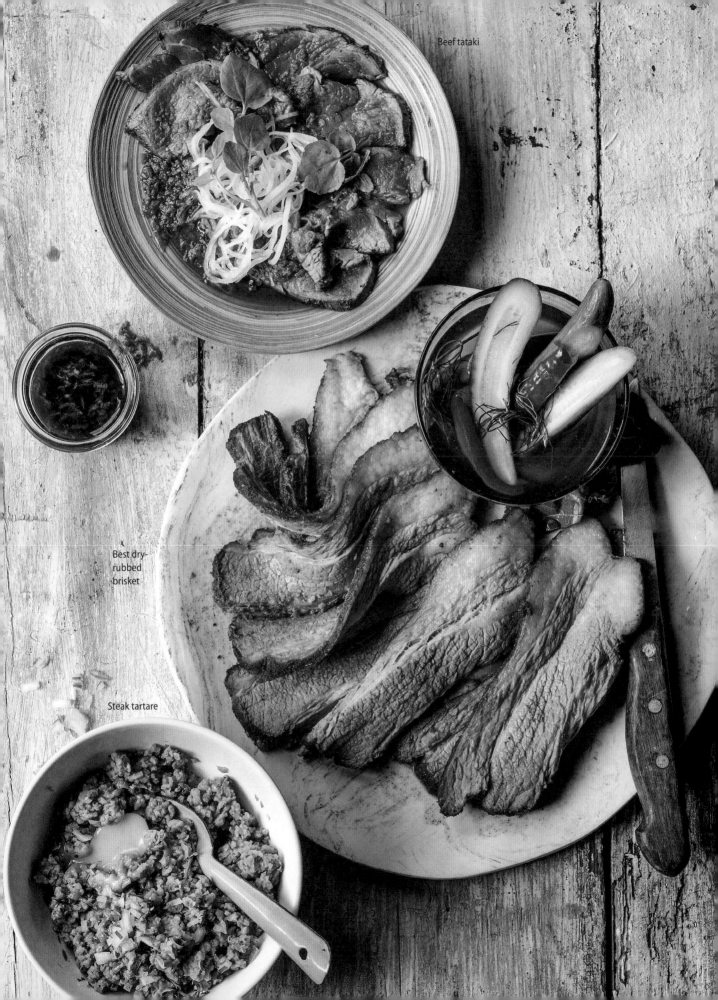

Beef tataki

Best dry-rubbed brisket

Steak tartare

MEATBALL BAKE

See page 142

Serves 4

600g lamb mince

1 small red onion, finely chopped

3 cloves garlic, minced

4 tbsp olive oil

2½ tsp ground cinnamon

250ml white wine

1½ tsp dried chilli flakes

2 x 400g tin chopped tomatoes

1 handful flat-leaf parsley,
   roughly chopped

1 small handful fresh oregano,
   roughly chopped

Salt and pepper

1 Preheat your oven to 150°C.

2 Combine the lamb, red onion, garlic in a mixing bowl and season with salt and pepper. Use your hands to roll 16 meatballs.

3 Heat the olive oil in a large ovenproof casserole or dish with a lid. Fry the meatballs in small batches at a time, so they don't crowd the pot, until dark brown all over. Set them aside but keep the casserole hot.

4 Add the cinnamon. If the pan is a bit dry, pour in a little more oil and sizzle the cinnamon for a minute or two until it is fragrant.

5 Add the wine and chilli flakes, and reduce the wine by half.

6 Add the tomatoes and bring the sauce to a gentle simmer.

7 Add the meatballs, pop the lid on and pop the dish in the oven for an hour.

8 Remove the lid, then pop the dish back in the oven for another 30 minutes.

9 Before serving, gently stir in the parsley and oregano. Season to taste.

GOES WELL WITH: Charred Okra with Coriander and Lemon Dressing, Greek Kale Salad with Tahini Dressing, Turnip Skordalia.

QUICK STICKS DONER

See page 143

Serves 4

1 tbsp fresh oregano, chopped

1 tbsp fresh thyme, chopped

1 tbsp sumac

½ red onion, peeled and
   cut into chunks

125ml double thick yoghurt

4 tbsp olive oil

1 tsp salt

½ tsp pepper

600g deboned lamb shoulder, sliced
   into strips

2 large, thick bamboo skewers, soaked
   in water, or metal skewers

1 Place the oregano, thyme, sumac, onion, yoghurt, oil, salt and pepper in a food processor and whizz them into a smooth paste.

2 Cover the lamb slices thoroughly with the paste. Place them in the fridge for 1 to 2 hours to infuse.

3 While the lamb is marinating, fire up the barbecue (you can do this on a griddle pan or hot pan too).

4 Thread the lamb onto the skewers, packing each piece as tightly as possible.

5 Place the skewers on the hottest part of the fire to get as much charring as possible. Five minutes a side should do it.

6 If you want them cooked all the way through, pop them in the oven at 200°C for another 5 to 10 minutes, or place them to one side of the hot coals and leave them in the Weber with the lid on for 10 minutes.

7 To check how pink the skewers are, use your fingers or a pair of tongs to pull the meat slices apart. You should be able to see all the way through to the skewer.

8 When they've reached the desired 'doneness', remove them from the heat. With one hand, stand the skewers upright. With the other hand, use a knife to carve the skewers like a Turkish pro. You guests will dig it.

GOES WELL WITH: Tzatziki, Tomatoes on the Grill.

PULLED SHAWARMA-STYLE LAMB

See page 143

Serves 4

600g deboned leg of lamb

6 tbsp olive oil

2 tsp dried oregano

250ml white wine

500ml water

2 tbsp ground cumin

1 large onion, thickly sliced

2 green peppers, thickly sliced

3 garlic cloves, roughly chopped

2 tbsp sweet paprika

1 big handful flat-leaf parsley, roughly chopped

Salt and black pepper

1　Preheat your oven to 150°C.

2　Rub the lamb with 2 tablespoons of the oil, oregano and salt and pepper.

3　Pop it into a deep tray, pour in the wine and half the water, then cover the tray tightly in two layers of foil. Place in the oven for 4 hours.

4　After 4 hours remove from the oven and leave to cool. Then use your hands to shred it into strips, mixing it with any leftover juices and bits of fat.

5　Heat the remaining oil to a medium heat in a large frying pan, and add the cumin, onion and peppers, and sauté for about 10 minutes.

6　When the vegetables are caramelised (and slightly darker than golden-brown), add the garlic and stir until it becomes fragrant.

7　Add the lamb and paprika and keep it cooking, turning it every minute or so until there are some 'burnt ends' or dark brown bits of lamb, and the paprika is well incorporated.

8　Season liberally with salt and pepper. Add the parsley and the water.

9　While the water is bubbling away, use a wooden spoon to scrape any bits off the bottom of the pan and mix it into the meat.

10 Once all the water has evaporated and the mix starts crackling and spitting in the pan, the dish is ready to serve.

GOES WELL WITH: Greek Kale Salad with Tahini Dressing, Tzatziki, Flash-fried Mange Tout, Olives and Tomato.

DRUNKEN LAMB RIBS

See page 143

Serves 4

12 free-range lamb ribs

250ml dry white wine

Zest and juice of 2 lemons

180ml olive oil

2 large sprigs rosemary, destemmed

2 garlic cloves, peeled

Sea salt and black pepper

1　Preheat your oven to 180°C.

2　Pack the lamb ribs tightly in a medium-sized baking dish.

3　In a small jug, blitz the remaining ingredients with a stick blender and pour the mixture over the lamb, using a spoon to spread it evenly.

4　Cover the tray in foil and pop it in the oven for 90 minutes.

5　After 90 minutes, uncover the meat, drain off most of the liquid into a bowl or jug and pop the dish back in the oven for a further 15 to 20 minutes to brown.

6　Meanwhile, scoop most of the fat off the roasting juices and pour what is left into a small pot. Reduce it by two-thirds.

7　When the ribs are ready, transfer them to a platter and drizzle them with the fatty pan-juice reduction.

GOES WELL WITH: Cucumber Ribbons with Mint Yoghurt, Greek Kale Salad with Tahini Dressing, Turnip Skordalia.

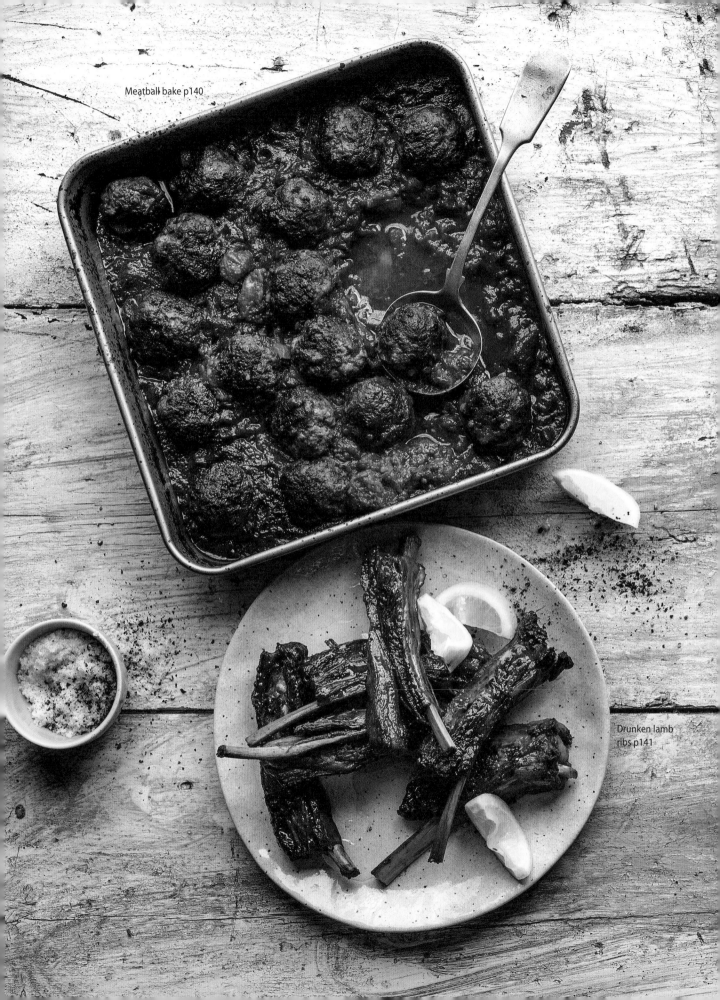

Meatball bake p140

Drunken lamb ribs p141

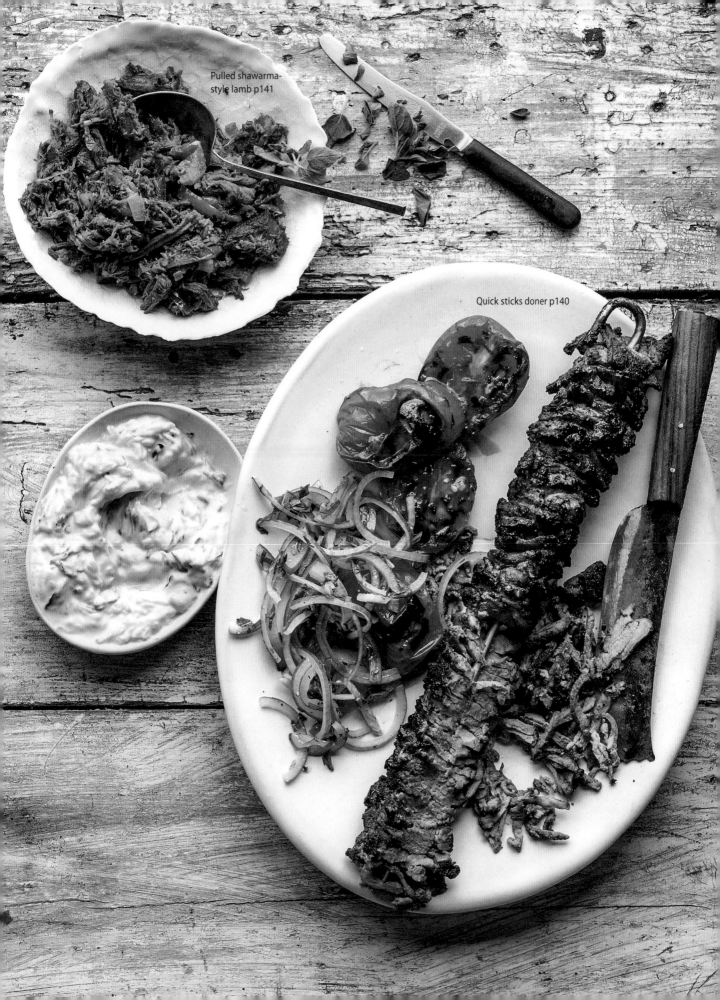

Pulled shawarma-style lamb p141

Quick sticks doner p140

XINJIANG CUMIN SPICED LAMB SKEWERS

Serves 4

400g lamb leg or shoulder, cut
   into bite-sized pieces
200g lamb belly fat, cut into pieces
   half the size of the meat pieces
3 tbsp avocado oil
3 tbsp ground cumin
1 tsp white pepper
2 tsp salt
1 tbsp dried chilli flakes
3 large cloves of garlic, minced
8 bamboo skewers, soaked in water
Lemon wedges

1 Prepare a barbecue to a medium-high heat.
2 In a large mixing bowl, combine the lamb, fat, avocado oil, spices and garlic. Mix well, then leave to marinate for at least an hour.
3 Make the skewers by alternating a piece of fat with a piece of lamb on all the skewers until the meat is used up.
4 Grill the skewers for about 3 minutes on each side, making sure the fat is crisp and juicy and the meat is well charred.
5 Serve immediately with wedges of lemon.

GOES WELL WITH: Spicy Aubergine, Stir-fried Spring Onions and Pak Choi.

LAMB-STUFFED AUBERGINES

Serves 2

2 medium aubergines, halved
   lengthways, flesh scored in
   a diamond pattern
4 tbsp olive oil
½ tsp ground cumin
2 tsp ground cinnamon
1 onion, roughly chopped
250g lamb mince
2 tbsp pine nuts
1 small handful flat-leaf parsley,
   roughly chopped
1 small handful mint,
   roughly chopped
2 tsp tomato paste
2 tsp sweet paprika
125ml chicken stock
Juice of ½ lime
1 tsp tamarind paste
Salt and black pepper

1 Preheat your oven to 200°C.
2 Brush the flesh of the aubergines with half of the olive oil, sprinkle with salt and roast them flesh-side up for 20 minutes.
3 Heat the remaining oil up to a medium heat in a medium-sized pan and add the cumin, cinnamon and onion to caramelise.
4 Once the onion is brown, add the lamb, pine nuts, parsley, mint, tomato paste and paprika and stir over a medium heat until most of the moisture has evaporated and the lamb is cooked.
5 Reduce the oven to 175°C. In a separate bowl, mix the stock, lime juice, tamarind paste and seasoning together.
6 Pack the aubergine halves into a baking dish and spoon some lamb mixture into each aubergine half.
7 Pour the tamarind stock around the aubergines, cover with foil and pop the dish back in the oven for 90 minutes.
8 Check the aubergines after 45 minutes to make sure they haven't dried out. Baste them with the tray juices. If they are drying out, top up the juices with a little water.
9 After 90 minutes, they are ready to serve, hot or cold.

A MEAL ON ITS OWN.

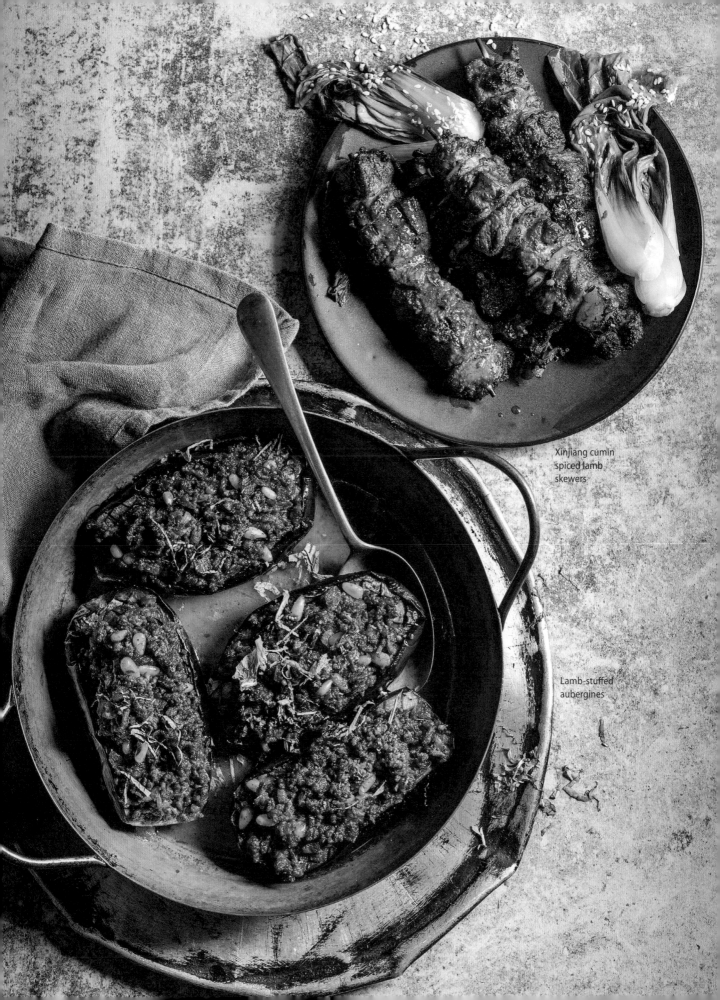

Xinjiang cumin
spiced lamb
skewers

Lamb-stuffed
aubergines

SLOW-ROASTED LAMB SHOULDER WITH LEMON AND CAPERS

Serves 6

1 handful rosemary sprigs, leaves
    removed and finely chopped
4 tbsp olive oil
4 garlic cloves, finely chopped
4 tbsp capers, finely chopped
6 anchovy fillets, finely chopped
Zest and juice of 1 lemon
1½ kg lamb shoulder, on the bone
2 white onions, cut into thick disks
250ml dry white wine

1   Preheat your oven to 160°C.
2   Using a stick blender, blitz the rosemary, olive oil, garlic, 2 tablespoons of the capers, 3 of the anchovies and half of the lemon juice together.
3   Pour the marinade over the lamb shoulder and massage it into every nook and cranny.
4   Lay the onion disks down to create a nest in the middle of a medium roasting pan, then place the lamb on top of the onion and roast for an hour in the oven.
5   Pour the wine and the remaining lemon juice into the tray, reduce the heat to 140°C, cover with foil, and roast for a further 3 hours.
6   Remove the lamb from the oven and allow to rest for 20 minutes.
7   While it's resting, make the drizzle. Pour all the liquid from the tray through a sieve and pop it into a small pot.
8   Bring to the boil, and add the lemon zest and remaining capers and anchovies. If the consistency is too thin, reduce it; otherwise just keep it hot until the meat is ready to be carved.
9   Slice the meat and serve on a platter, smothered with the drizzle.

GOES WELL WITH: Fasolakia Ladera, Hobochokes, Roasted Cherry Tomato Caprese.

PENNY'S DURBAN CURRY

Serves 6

Durban, South Africa, is home to one of the largest Indian communities outside of India, and every Durbanite reckons no-one knows how to make curry like they do. My good friend Penny is no different. Penny is our bookkeeper, team-spirit sergeant and general hero of everything at RMR – and this is her Durban Curry recipe.

250ml coconut oil
1kg lamb knuckles
3 tbsp curry powder
1 tbsp cumin seeds
1 tbsp black and yellow
    mustard seeds
1 onion, sliced
2 heaped tsp garlic, minced
1 thumb fresh ginger, grated
1 tbsp curry leaves (fresh or dried)
500ml beef stock or broth (see page 232)
2 tomatoes, diced
Salt and black pepper

1   Heat the coconut oil in a heavy-bottomed pot.
2   Season the lamb knuckles with salt and pepper and fry them in the oil until brown all over. This should take about 15 minutes.
3   Remove the knuckles and set aside. Add the curry powder, cumin and mustard seeds and toast until the mustard seeds begin to pop.
4   Add the onion slices and sauté until they are golden-brown.
5   Add the garlic, ginger and curry leaves, and stir until they become fragrant.
6   Put the knuckles back in the pot with the stock and the tomatoes, and top with water to cover. Pop the lid on and simmer gently for 2 hours.
7   Remove the lid, season to taste and serve.

GOES WELL WITH: Saag Paneer, Spicy Roasted Cabbage Wedges, Spicy Roasted Okra.

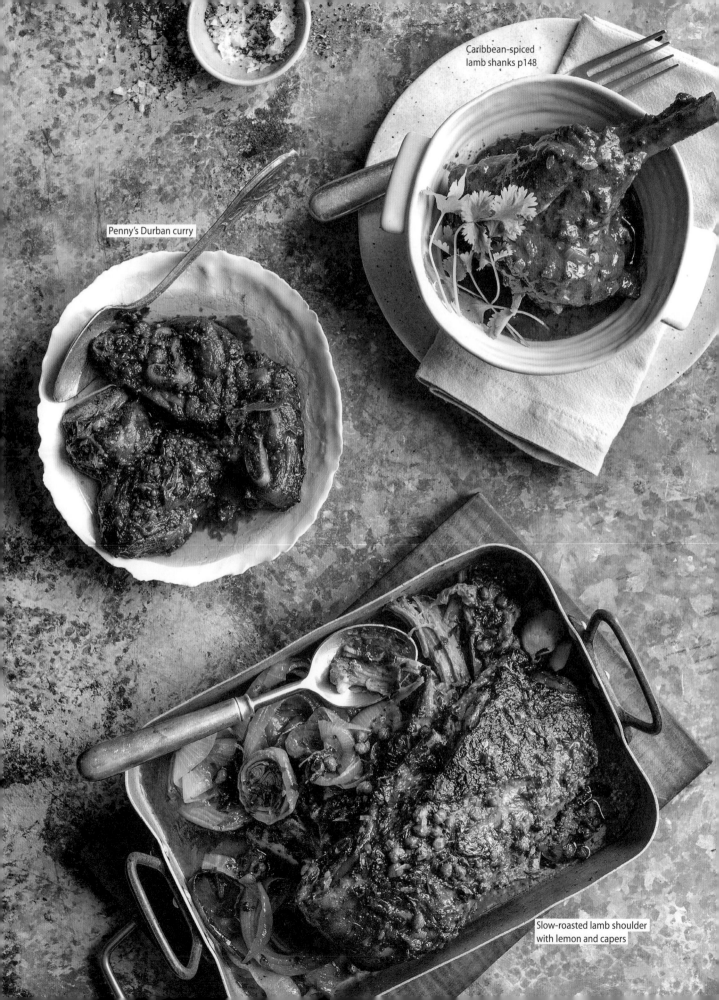

Caribbean-spiced
lamb shanks p148

Penny's Durban curry

Slow-roasted lamb shoulder
with lemon and capers

CARIBBEAN-SPICED LAMB SHANKS

See page 147

Serves 6

6 medium-sized lamb shanks

3 tbsp coconut oil

2 tbsp curry powder

1 tbsp cinnamon

1½ tsp ground allspice

1½ tsp ground coriander

1½ tsp ground cumin

1½ tsp ground ginger

5 medium carrots, cut into chunks

2 onions, thinly sliced

5 garlic cloves, minced

2 tsp salt

1 x 50g can tomato paste

1¼ litres beef stock or broth

1 tbsp chilli powder

1 large handful fresh coriander, roughly chopped

Salt and black pepper

1. Preheat your oven to 160°C and season the shanks liberally with salt and pepper.

2. Get the oil nice and hot in a large pan and drop in the shanks (as many as will fit in the pan without being squashed). Cook them, turning sometimes, until they are completely brown all over. Be patient: it will be worth it.

3. Leaving the fat in the pan, remove the shanks and pack them tightly into a deep roasting pan. There should be only enough space for the liquid (below) to fit.

4. Add the curry powder, cinnamon, allspice, ground coriander, cumin and ginger to the pan and sauté the spices in the lamb fat for a few minutes until well toasted.

5. Add the carrots and onions and sauté them until they are caramelised. Add the garlic.

6. When the garlic becomes fragrant, add the salt and tomato paste and sweat the garlic for 3 or 4 minutes.

7. Add the stock and chilli powder, using a wooden spoon to scrape any sediment off the bottom of the pan.

8. Once the sauce comes to the boil, pour it over the shanks, cover the dish with a double layer of foil and pop it in the oven for 2 to 3 hours.

9. Remove the dish from the oven and remove the foil. The shanks should be falling off the bone and the sauce should be dark.

10. Serve them just like this, with fresh coriander stirred through the sauce, or drain off the sauce and reduce it by half for a slightly more potent flavour. Up to you.

GOES WELL WITH: Spicy Roasted Cabbage Wedges, Whole Roasted Jerk Cauliflower, Kale and Cabbage Salad.

PORK BULGOGI

See page 151

Serves 4

The direct translation of Korean Bulgogi is 'fire meat'. If your palate is sensitive, adjust the pepper flakes and paste to your liking. Bulgogi goes really well with pickled daikon. If you can't get hold of that, serve it with any pickle from your collection of fertilisers.

600g pork loin, thinly sliced,
  skin removed

2 tbsp soy sauce

6 garlic cloves, minced

3 spring onions, finely chopped

1 onion, thinly sliced

2 tbsp toasted sesame seeds

2 tbsp gochujang (Korean red
  pepper paste)

3 tbsp gochugaru (Korean red
  pepper flakes)

2 tbsp coconut oil

1 lime, cut into quarters

1 Mix all the ingredients, except the coconut oil and lime, in a bowl and place it in the fridge for 1 hour to marinate.

2 Get a large, heavy-based pan very hot and pour in a splash of coconut oil.

3 Just before the oil begins to smoke, add half the pork mixture and stir-fry it until it has developed a bit of colour and is cooked through. This should take no more than a couple of minutes.

4 Repeat with the remaining mixture. Serve with lime.

GOES WELL WITH: Spicy Korean Cucumber Salad, Mad's Kimchi and any other pickles.

COCOA AND FENNEL PORK FILLET WITH COLOMBIAN HOT SAUCE

See page 151

Serves 4

1 habanero chilli (if you're soft like me,
  use a less aggressive chilli)

1 big handful fresh coriander, chopped

8 spring onions, chopped

2 big, ripe and juicy tomatoes

Juice of 2 big limes

2 tbsp apple cider vinegar

1 large pork fillet, cleaned and sinew
  removed

¼ tsp ground cinnamon

2 tbsp dark cocoa powder

2 tbsp cocoa nibs

1 tsp fennel seeds

1 pinch cayenne pepper

2 tbsp olive oil

Salt and pepper

1 To make the Colombian hot sauce, blitz the chilli, coriander, spring onions, tomatoes, lime juice and vinegar with some salt and pepper in a small jug and leave it in the fridge to infuse for up to 24 hours (or at least 1 hour).

2 Preheat your oven to 200°C and line a roasting tin with foil.

3 Dust the fillet with the cinnamon and cocoa powder. Season it with salt and pepper.

4 Using a pestle and mortar or spice grinder, grind the cocoa nibs and fennel seeds together until coarse, then mix in the cayenne pepper.

5 Heat 1 tablespoon of the olive oil in a medium-sized pan and add the fillet, turning until it is brown all over. Remove from the heat.

6 Tip the fennel-spice mix onto a small baking tray, then transfer the meat to the tray and roll it in the spices until the fillet is nicely encrusted in the rub. Place the fillet in the foil-lined roasting dish, drizzle with the remaining olive oil and pop it in the oven for 15 minutes.

7 Remove the fillet from the oven and let it rest for 10 minutes. Slice it thinly and serve with the Colombian hot sauce.

GOES WELL WITH: Classic Slaw, Caramelised Garlic Fennel, Fennel Kraut.

For the full recipe for Colombian Hot Sauce, see page 287.

PORK BELLY FROM SOMEWHERE IN ASIA

Serves 4

I don't know where this recipe comes from, but I used to make it back in my restaurant days – and it's delicious.

800g–1kg pork belly, deboned,
   skin on
1 tbsp coconut oil
2 tbsp fine salt
1 litre water
4 tbsp dark soy sauce
4 tbsp fish sauce
4 tbsp rice vinegar
4 tbsp dry sherry
2 whole cloves garlic
1 thumb of ginger, grated
½ tsp white pepper
1 big handful fresh coriander,
   roughly chopped
1 red chilli, finely sliced
1 fresh lime

1. Preheat your oven to 160°C.
2. Use paper towels to pat the pork belly dry and massage in the coconut oil and salt. Don't bother scoring it.
3. Place the water, soy, fish sauce, vinegar, sherry, garlic, ginger and white pepper in a medium roasting pan and mix well.
4. Rest a cooling rack on top of the pan and place the pork on the rack, skin-side up.
5. Pop the pan on the bottom rack in the oven, leaving it to roast for between 1½ to 2 hours.
6. After 1½ hours, check to see how crispy the crackling is. If it isn't super-crispy yet, pour half or a full cup of water into the tray, and let the pork cook for another 30 minutes.
7. Check again after 30 minutes. If it isn't crackly all over, crank the heat up to 200°C and leave it for a further 20 minutes. You will achieve crackling success (but do keep an eye on it – you don't want it to burn).
8. Once it's done, drain all the juices from the tray into a small saucepan and bring to the boil, then start reducing.
9. Once it has reduced to about a cup (about 250ml), remove it from the heat and add the coriander, chilli and juice of the lime. For extra flavour, you can add the lime shells.
10. Cut the pork into four large chunks and serve with generous lashings of sauce.

GOES WELL WITH: Classic Slaw, Stir-fried Spring Onions and Pak Choi.

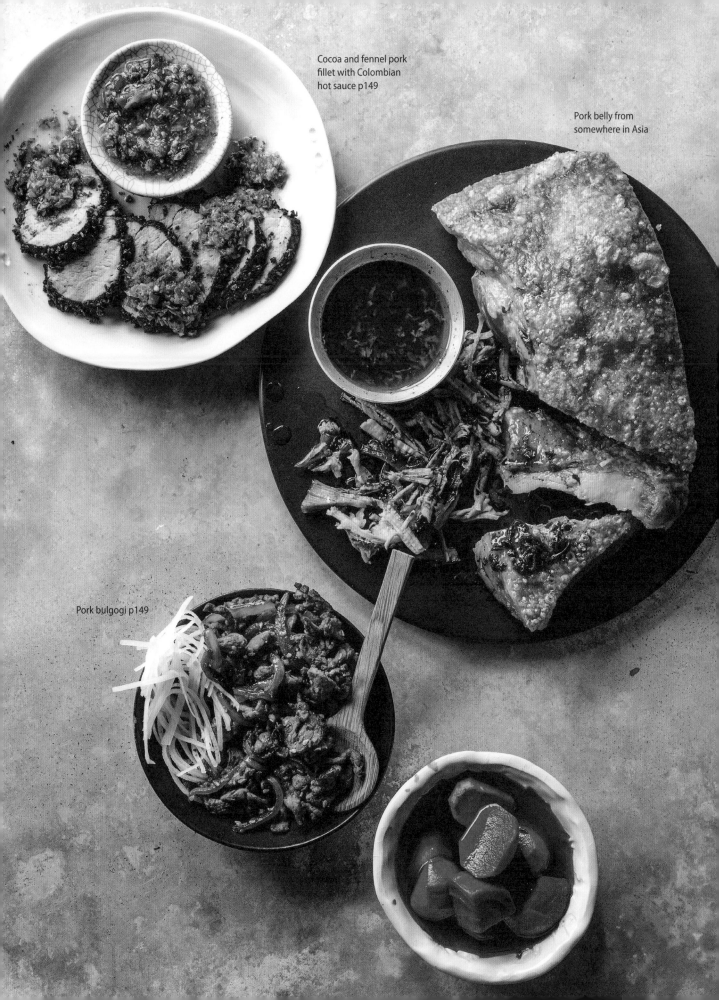

Cocoa and fennel pork
fillet with Colombian
hot sauce p149

Pork belly from
somewhere in Asia

Pork bulgogi p149

DARK SALTY PORK RIBS

Serves 4

2kg pork ribs, cut into individual ribs

4 tbsp white vinegar

4 tbsp oyster sauce

4 tbsp soy sauce

1 tbsp tomato paste

4 tbsp lemon juice

2 apples, peeled, cored and chopped

2 tbsp ginger, diced

1 tbsp minced garlic

1 litre water or chicken stock

2 tbsp toasted sesame seeds

4 spring onions, chopped

1   Preheat your oven to 180°C.
2   Place all the ingredients (except the sesame seeds and spring onions) in a deep roasting pan, cover it with foil and pop it into the oven for 2 hours.
3   Remove the ribs and leave them to cool, covered, then pour the tray juices into a pot and reduce the sauce until it is thick. Blitz it with a stick blender.
4   While the sauce reduces, prepare a barbecue for a medium-high heat.
5   When the coals are ready and the sauce is reduced, put the ribs on the grill. Let them caramelise nicely on each side before giving them the first basting of the sauce.
6   Keep turning and basting them every 2 minutes or so until the sauce is nearly finished and you have some good charring on each rib.
7   Transfer the ribs to a serving platter and drizzle them with the final drops of marinade, sesame seeds and spring onions.

GOES WELL WITH: Stir-fried Cucumber with Sesame Seeds, Spinach in Sesame Dressing.

EISBEIN

Serves 4 very hungry people

The direct translation of the German word Eisbein is 'ice bone'. Back in the day, they used the pork hock bone for the blades of ice skates. It doesn't affect this recipe at all, but I thought you'd like to know.

4 cured, smoked ham hocks

2 onions, quartered

2 carrots, chopped

3 bay leaves

1 tbsp salt

1   Place all the ingredients in a medium or large pot and cover with water.
2   Bring the water to the boil, then reduce it to a simmer and let it tick away for a good 1½ hours.
3   Remove the hocks and leave them to chill in the fridge, uncovered, to dry out overnight.
4   Reserve the stock for broth or a soup, or discard it.
5   About an hour before you're ready to eat, heat the oven to 240°C.
6   Place the hocks in a roasting pan and pop them in the oven until the skins are crisp. This should take 30 minutes. But keep an eye on it – it could be less than that or it could take up to an hour.
7   Once you have good crackling, serve.

GOES WELL WITH: Fennel and Sour Cream Salad, Sauerkraut.

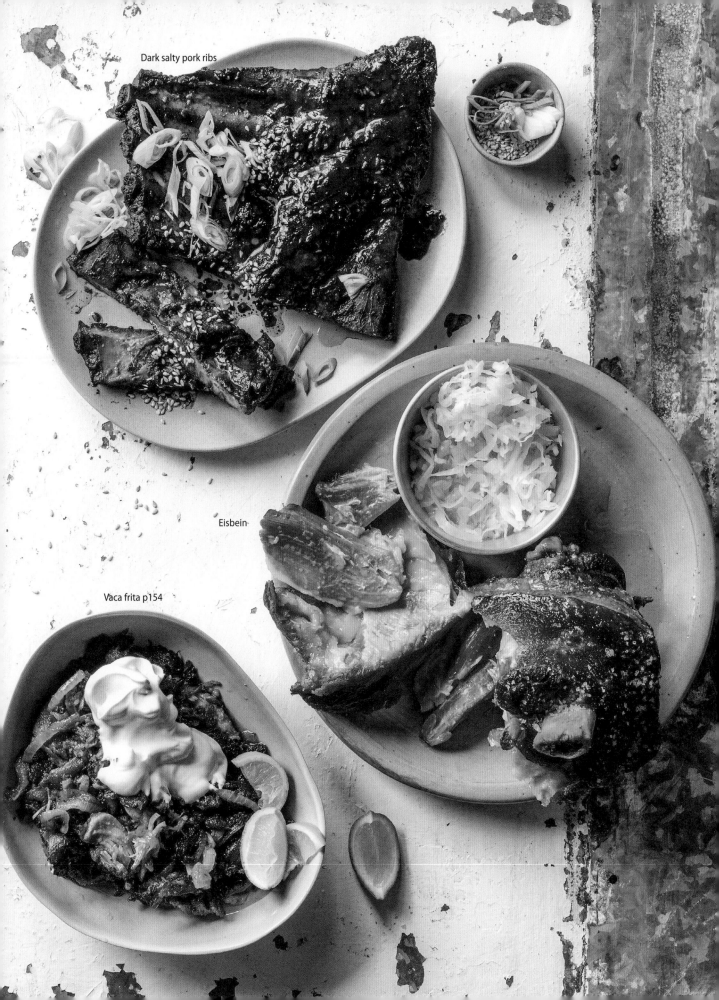

Dark salty pork ribs

Eisbein

Vaca frita p154

VACA FRITA

See page 153

Serves 6 if you're using it for lettuce tacos; 4 for a meat-and-two-veg type of meal

This is a Cuban take on pulled pork. The second cooking stint creates glorious burnt ends that will take your lettuce leaf – because you won't eat the taco, will you? – to the next level. You can use a slow cooker for the first part if you like.

800g deboned pork shoulder

4 plum tomatoes, chopped

1 onion, chopped

2 red bell peppers, chopped

3 bay leaves

½ tsp ground coriander

½ tsp paprika

½ tsp ground cumin

¼ tsp salt

1 onion, sliced

2 garlic cloves, minced

2 or 3 limes, cut into quarters

1   Place the pork, tomatoes, onion, peppers, bay leaves, coriander, paprika, cumin and salt in a medium-sized pot. Add enough water to cover the meat.

2   Pop the lid on and leave it to simmer at a very low heat for 8 hours (or cook it in the oven at 110°C for 8 hours). A slow cooker will also take about 8 hours.

3   Remove the pork and set aside. Strain the vegetables, then discard them. Reserve the broth.

4   Once the pork has cooled, shred the meat with your hands, separating the cooked fat.

5   Heat the fat in a large pan over a medium heat until it starts spitting.

6   Add the meat pieces and let them cook, without stirring, for about 10 minutes. They should crisp up and be well caramelised. Then gently flip the pieces over and repeat the process.

7   Add the sliced onion and sauté until the pork is crispy and the onion soft, then add the garlic and give it all a final stir for about 3 or 4 minutes.

8   Add the reserved broth and reduce until it is thick and sticky.

9   Serve with lime wedges, and anything else that goes well with a (lettuce) taco.

GOES WELL WITH: Classic Slaw, Sautéed Peppers with Spicy Vinaigrette, Mojo-ish Marinated Tomatoes.

KÖTTBULLAR – SWEDISH PORK MEATBALLS

See page 157

Serves 4

500g pork mince
¼ tsp ground allspice
¼ tsp ground nutmeg
½ tsp garlic powder
¼ tsp black pepper
½ tsp salt
1 tbsp olive oil
2 tbsp butter
½ white onion, finely chopped
1 clove garlic, minced
1 tsp Dijon mustard
250ml beef stock or broth (see page 232)
250ml double (heavy) cream
½ handful flat-leaf parsley, chopped
2 tbsp sour cream
Salt and black pepper

1. In a medium bowl, mix the pork, allspice, nutmeg, garlic powder, pepper and salt until well combined, then roll the mixture into 20 meatballs.
2. Heat olive oil and butter in a large pan to a medium heat and seal the meatballs, turning them until they are brown on each side.
3. Transfer them to a plate, but keep the pan going.
4. Add the onion and a little extra oil or butter if needed, and sauté until golden. Add the garlic.
5. As the garlic becomes fragrant, add the mustard and stir it around for a minute.
6. Pour in the broth or stock and bring to the boil, then add the cream. Keep it simmering gently until the sauce begins to thicken.
7. Finally, add the meatballs and simmer them until they are cooked through (no more than 5 minutes).
8. Remove from the heat. Stir through the parsley, the sour cream and salt and pepper to taste and serve.

GOES WELL WITH: Buttered Brussels Sprouts, Buttered Chard, Braised Fennel.

MOREISH PORK FILLET

Serves 4

1 tsp sweet smoked paprika
1 tsp sweet paprika
1 tsp ground cumin
1 tsp dried oregano
1 tbsp fresh thyme leaves
2 garlic cloves
1 red chilli, destemmed
3 tbsp old sherry vinegar
125ml olive oil
2 small pork fillets, cut in half
4 thick bamboo skewers,
   soaked in water
Lemon
Salt and black pepper
Romesco Sauce, optional
   (see page 296)

1 Prepare a barbecue for a medium-high heat, or get a griddle pan smoking-hot.
2 To make the marinade, use a stick blender to blitz all of the ingredients, except the pork and lemon (and skewers!), with some salt and pepper in a small jug.
3 Mix the pork with the marinade. Place the fillets, tightly packed, flat on a cutting board. Run the skewers, 4cm apart, through all of the fillets, creating a 'mat' of pork.
4 Grill the pork mat for 3 or 4 minutes on each side, then continue turning every minute until they are cooked (test by slicing down to the skewers to see how pink the meat is).
5 Once they're cooked to your liking, get stuck in with a twist of lemon and some Romesco Sauce if desired.

GOES WELL WITH: Sautéed Peppers with Spicy Vinaigrette, Romesco Sauce.

GREEK PORK CHOPS

Serves 4

4 pork loin chops, skin on
1 handful fresh oregano
1 handful fresh mint
1 sprig rosemary, destemmed
1 garlic clove
125ml olive oil
Zest and juice of 1 lemon
½ tsp salt
¼ tsp black pepper

1 Lay the chops down on a cutting board and use a knife (and your body weight) to cut through the fat and rind at 2cm intervals. Place in a small dish.
2 Blitz all the other ingredients in a small jug with a stick blender and pour over the chops, then leave them to marinate for an hour or so.
3 Heat a large ovenproof frying pan to a medium-high heat.
4 Scrape any marinade off the chops, then stack them together to make a reconstructed loin.
5 Hold the 'loin' together with tongs and place it fat-side down in a pan to crisp up the fat. This should take about 5 minutes.
6 Spread the chops out and fry them for 4 minutes on each side, turning them only once.
7 Turn your oven up to the highest temperature, and put on the grill setting.
8 Pour the leftover marinade over the chops and pop them under the grill for another 3 or 4 minutes.

GOES WELL WITH: Fasolakia Ladera, Greek Kale Salad with Tahini Dressing, Turnip Skordalia.

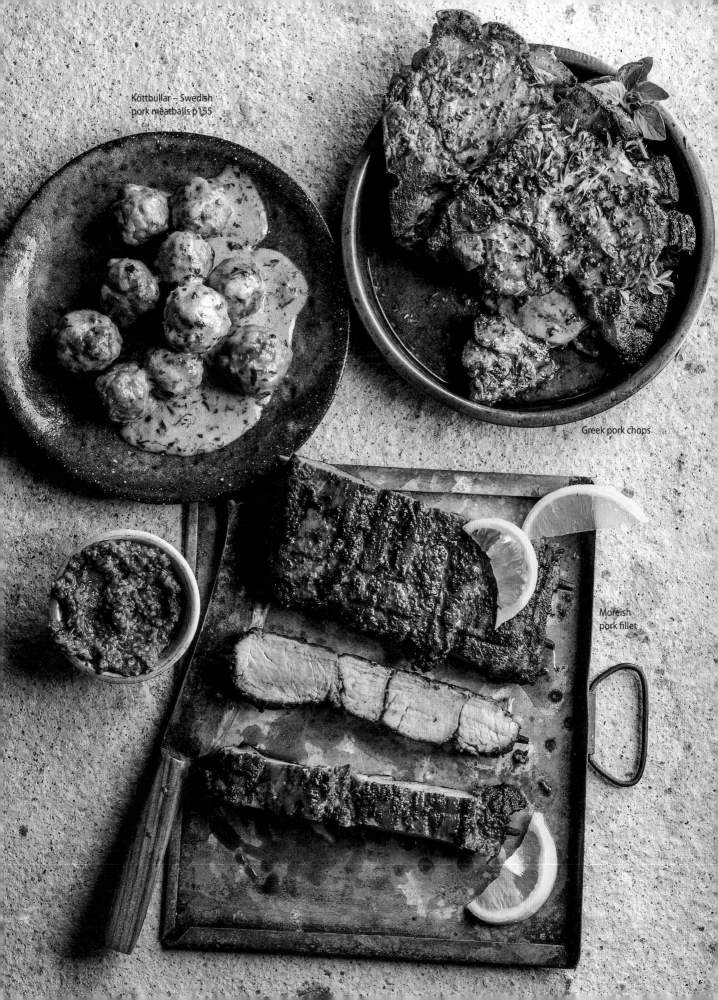

Köttbullar – Swedish
pork meatballs p155

Greek pork chops

Moreish
pork fillet

FENNEL SAUSAGE WITH PEPPERS AND BASIL

Serves 4

4 tbsp olive oil

6 sausages (any kind), whole

1 red onion, thinly sliced

2 red peppers, thinly sliced

2 tsp fennel seeds, lightly crushed

4 cloves garlic, minced

3 tbsp tomato paste

8 plum tomatoes, skin removed, grated

125ml chicken stock or broth
(see page 232)

1 small handful fresh basil leaves,
shredded

Salt and pepper

1 Get half the olive oil up to a medium heat in a large frying pan and add the sausages to cook until they are golden-brown on both sides. They don't need to be cooked through at this stage.

2 Once the sausages are brown, set them aside and add the remaining oil and the onion, peppers and fennel seeds and sauté them until the onions are golden-brown.

3 Now add the garlic and stir until fragrant.

4 Add the tomato paste and the grated tomato and stir for about 5 minutes, then add the stock and bring to the boil.

5 Reduce the sauce by half.

6 While the sauce is reducing, cut the sausages into four chunks per sausage, then add them back to sauce (once it has reduced) and simmer them gently until they are cooked through.

7 Season the sauce with salt and pepper and stir through the basil, then serve immediately.

GOES WELL WITH: Cauliflower Colcannon, Carciofi alla Romana, Buttered Broccoli.

BANGING MUSTARD BANGERS

Serves 4

I can't tell you how many times I've had friends and family text me with a question about Banting (LCHF), only to have their autocorrect interfere. 'Jonno, I'm really struggling. I'm Banging really hard and I can't seem to lose weight.' But these bangers really are banging!

2 tbsp butter

3 large leeks, washed and cut
into chunks

2 tbsp hot English mustard

1 sprig thyme

250ml white wine

250ml cream

6 pork bangers (ask your butcher
for 'no cereal')

Salt and pepper

1 Preheat your oven to 220°C and pop the grill setting on.

2 Heat the butter in a medium-sized ovenproof pan and add the leeks.

3 When the leeks are caramelised, add the mustard, thyme and wine and reduce it by half while stirring.

4 Once the wine is reduced, add the cream and bring to the boil. Reduce the sauce by a third, then remove from the heat.

5 Arrange the bangers, evenly spaced, in a tray and pop them in the oven until they are dark-brown on top. Then flip them over and grill them until they are brown on the other side – probably 5 minutes a side.

6 Once they are brown on both sides, add them (juices and all) to the pan and bring the pan back up to a gentle simmer for the sausages to cook through in the sauce – about 1 or 2 minutes.

7 Season with salt and pepper and serve immediately.

GOES WELL WITH: Cauliflower Colcannon, Buttered Courgettes, Roasted Broccoli.

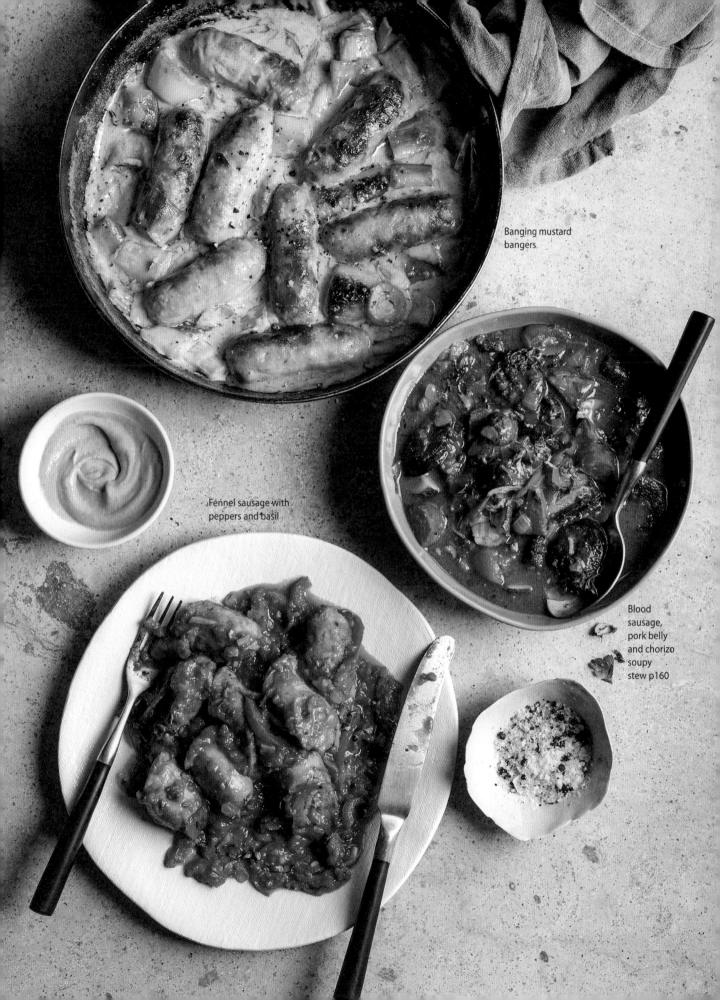

Banging mustard bangers

Fennel sausage with peppers and basil

Blood sausage, pork belly and chorizo soupy stew p160

BLOOD SAUSAGE, PORK BELLY AND CHORIZO SOUPY STEW

See page 159

Serves 4

200g cherry tomatoes, cut in half

200g courgettes, cut into pieces the
    same size as the tomato halves

4 sprigs thyme

2 garlic cloves, roughly chopped

4 tbsp olive oil

1 large onion, roughly chopped

240g cured chorizo, peeled and
    cut into chunks

1 litre pork stock or bone broth
    (see page 232)

1 bay leaf

1 pinch saffron

1 tsp sweet smoked paprika

250g cooked, sliced (leftover) pork
    belly or shoulder

350g thick-sliced morcilla or
    black pudding, cut into chunks

Juice of ½ lemon

1 small handful flat-leaf parsley,
    roughly chopped

1 small handful oregano,
    roughly chopped

Salt and pepper

1 Preheat your oven to 180°C.

2 Toss the cherry tomatoes, courgettes, thyme, garlic, olive oil and a liberal sprinkling of salt and pepper in a large bowl, then tip them out into a roasting pan so that they lie in one layer.

3 Pop the pan in the oven and roast for about 20 minutes. The tomatoes should be caramelised slightly and the courgettes soft.

4 While the tomatoes and courgettes are roasting, get a medium-sized pot on the heat, add a little oil and add the onion to caramelise until golden.

5 Add the chorizo and stir for another 5 minutes or so.

6 Add the stock, bay leaf, saffron and smoked paprika and bring it all up to a gentle simmer, then let it tick away for about 10 minutes. (If the vegetables aren't ready when you reach this point, turn off the heat on the stock.)

7 When the vegetables are done, add them to the stew along with the cooked pork belly and the chunks of blood sausage and bring to the boil again.

8 Season with salt, pepper and lemon juice, and stir in the herbs before serving.

GOES WELL WITH: Deconstructed Ratatouille, Buttered Spinach.

PERUVIAN-STYLE CHICKEN LIVERS WITH CHIPOTLE MAYONNAISE

See page 163

Serves 4

125ml mayonnaise (see page 274)

1 tbsp ground chipotle chilli,
   or your favourite smoky chilli sauce

4 tbsp olive oil

1 tbsp ground cumin

1 tbsp ground coriander

¼ tsp black pepper

4 tbsp lime juice

1 garlic clove, minced

½ tsp chilli flakes

½ tsp salt

1 tbsp tomato paste

500g chicken livers, membranes
   removed and cut into thirds

4 bamboo skewers, soaked in water

1 Make the dipping sauce by whisking together the mayonnaise and chipotle. Store the sauce in the fridge until required.

2 Warm the oil in a small pan and add the cumin, coriander and pepper, letting it sizzle for about 5 minutes.

3 Pour the spiced oil with the lime juice, garlic, chilli flakes, salt and tomato paste into a small jug and blitz with a stick blender until smooth. Pour the mix over the chicken livers to marinate.

4 After an hour, thread the livers on the skewers. Light a barbecue with enough coals to make a stinking-hot fire or get a griddle pan super-hot.

5 When the coals or griddle pan are ready, place the skewers on the heat. They should spit and hiss while they char.

6 Cook them for about 3 minutes on each side, basting them with whatever marinade is left when you turn them.

7 If you're not a pink liver fan, give them an extra 3 minutes on each side.

8 Remove them from the heat and serve immediately with the smoky mayo for dipping.

GOES WELL WITH: Winter Salad of Radicchio with Parsley and Sweet Sautéed Onion.

STEAK AND KIDNEY NO-PIE PIE

Serves 4

2 tbsp butter

1 onion, roughly chopped

2 celery stalks, roughly chopped

2 carrots, roughly chopped

500g beef brisket, cut into 3cm chunks

250ml red wine

1 bay leaf

2 tbsp hot English mustard

2 tbsp tomato paste

300g beef or lamb kidney, sheaths
  removed, sinews cut out, and cut
  into 2cm chunks

1 litre beef stock

4 large black mushrooms, cut into ⅛

1 handful flat-leaf parsley,
  roughly chopped

Salt and pepper

1   Preheat your oven to 180°C.

2   Heat the butter in a medium casserole or ovenproof pot and add the onions, celery and carrots to sauté until they are soft.

3   Add the beef and sauté until it is cooked through. It may release juices but this is fine, just make sure the juices have evaporated before the next step.

4   Add the red wine, bay leaf, mustard, tomato paste and kidneys and stir them occasionally, while you wait for the wine to reduce by half.

5   Add the stock and bring to the boil, then pop the lid on and put the whole thing in the oven for 1 hour.

6   After 1 hour, take out the pot, mix through the mushrooms, cover it and put it back in the oven for 1 more hour.

7   After the second hour, take it out and check the thickness of the sauce. If it needs to be thickened, pop it on the stove and reduce on a gentle heat.

8   When you're ready to serve, fire up the heat, season it with salt and pepper to taste and mix through the parsley.

GOES WELL WITH: Buttered Broccoli, Creamy Brussels Sprouts, Braised Fennel.

CALVES' LIVER WITH ONIONS

Serves 4

1 tbsp olive oil

250g streaky bacon, roughly chopped

1 onion, thickly sliced

5 fresh sage leaves, finely shredded

1 tbsp tomato paste

125ml red wine

300ml beef stock or broth
  (see page 232)

500g calves' liver, peeled and cut into
  1.5cm slices

2 tbsp olive oil

2 fingers butter

Salt and pepper

1   Heat the oil in a large pan over a medium heat and add the bacon, onion and sage and sauté until they are dark and caramelised.

2   Add the tomato paste and stir until a sediment collects on the base of the pan.

3   Pour in the wine. As it boils, use a wooden spoon to scrape the bits off the base of the pan.

4   Once the wine has reduced by two-thirds, add the stock and reduce the sauce by half. At this point, season with salt and pepper to taste.

5   Pour the sauce into a bowl, wipe the pan clean and add the 2 tablespoons of olive oil. Turn the heat up to very high.

6   Season the slices of liver with salt and pepper, then put them in the smoking-hot pan.

7   After 2 minutes, turn each piece (only once), leave for another two minutes, then pour in the sauce.

8   The sauce should boil immediately from the heat of the pan. Let it boil for an extra minute or 2, then remove from the heat and stir in the butter. It should be shiny.

9   Season to taste and serve immediately.

GOES WELL WITH: Buttered Brussels Sprouts, Spaghetti Squash Fritters,
Steamed Gem Squash.

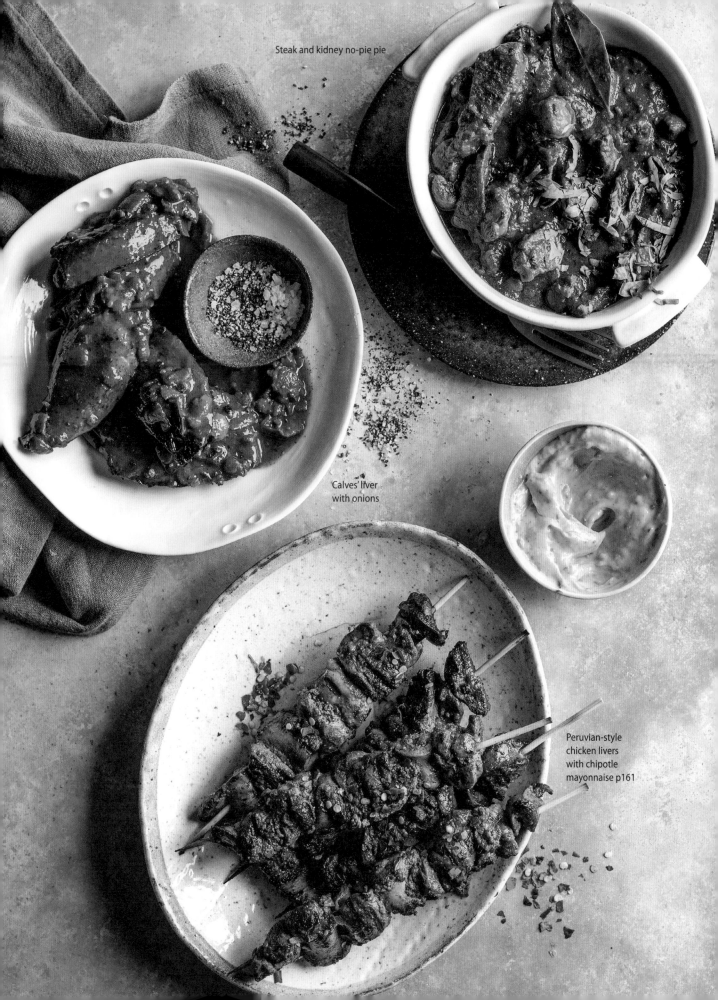

Steak and kidney no-pie pie

Calves' liver with onions

Peruvian-style chicken livers with chipotle mayonnaise p161

SMOKED BONE MARROW WITH GREMOLATA

Serves 4

If you don't have a coal fire, this recipe works just as well in an oven at 180°C.
If you go this route, skip all steps that call for oak shavings. So, basically, season the
marrowbones and roast them for 20 minutes.

2 tbsp lemon zest, preferably
    microplaned
2 garlic cloves, finely chopped
2 large handfuls flat-leaf parsley,
    roughly chopped
8 beef bones, centre-cut and vertically
    halved (ask your butcher)
1 large handful of oak shavings
250ml water
Multiple glugs of olive oil
Juice of 1 lemon
Salt and black pepper

1 Prepare the barbecue for a medium heat, with a fire on one side only as shown in the barbecue lesson on page 35.
2 Make the gremolata by mixing the lemon zest, chopped garlic and parsley and set it aside.
3 Season the marrowbones and place the bones, marrow facing up, on the opposite side of the grill from the coals in a small dish and pop the lid on for 10 minutes.
4 While the bones are roasting, mix the water with the wood chips and keep them at hand.
5 After 10 minutes, open the Weber and spread the oak shavings evenly over the coals, then quickly replace the lid.
6 Leave it for another 15 minutes to smoke away, then take off the lid, remove the bones and serve immediately with glugs of olive oil, a squeeze of lemon and gremolata sprinkled over the marrowbones.

GOES WELL WITH: Shaved Radish Salad, Turnip Skordalia, Celery Pickle.

GYU TAN DON – CHINESE OX TONGUE

Serves 4

500g raw ox tongue, peeled and
    thinly sliced
4 tbsp soy sauce
2 tbsp mirin
2 tbsp sesame oil
2 tbsp avocado oil
6 spring onions, finely chopped
2 red chillies, chopped
White pepper

1 Toss the tongue, soy sauce, mirin and sesame oil together in mixing bowl and leave it to sit in the fridge for an hour.
2 Heat the avocado oil in a large pan and drop in the tongue.
3 Spread the tongue out and let it fry for 5 minutes on each side. It will initially release its juices, but over the 10 minutes of cooking time they will reduce, and you will end up with the dry and sticky tongue.
4 Add the spring onions, the chillies and pepper and sauté, stirring constantly for another 2 or 3 minutes. Serve immediately.

GOES WELL WITH: Broccolini in Oyster Sauce, Stir-fried Spring Onions and Pak Choi.

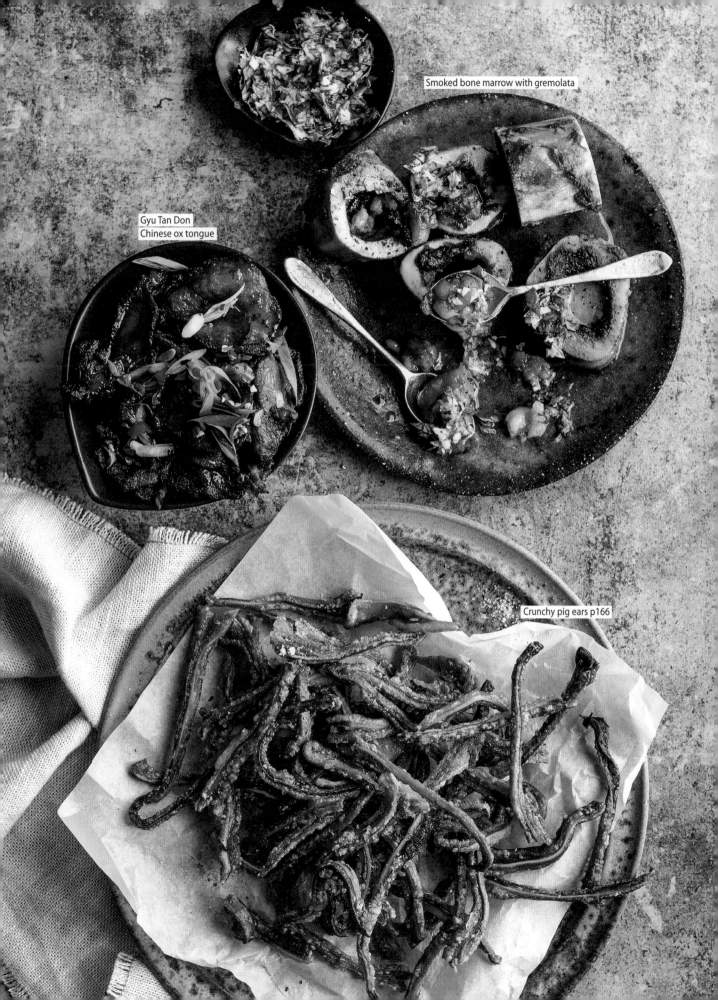

Smoked bone marrow with gremolata

Gyu Tan Don
Chinese ox tongue

Crunchy pig ears p166

CRUNCHY PIG EARS

See page 165

Serves 4

6 pig ears, washed, hair burnt off with
   blow torch (ask your butcher)
2 garlic cloves, peeled
1 tsp dried thyme
1 tsp black peppercorns
250ml avocado oil
Salt

1   Simmer the ears, garlic, thyme and peppercorns in a pot of water for 3 hours.
2   Take the ears out, discarding the poaching liquor, pat them dry and leave them in the fridge on a drying rack overnight.
3   Preheat your oven to 200°C.
4   Now, slice the ears into thin strips and toss them in a bowl with the oil and a liberal sprinkling of fine salt.
5   Lay them out in single layers on roasting trays and pop them into the oven for about 20 minutes. You'll have to watch them. Only take them out once every piece has crackled and spat.
6   Drain them on paper towel and serve them as a snack with drinks, or a snack whenever.

GOES WELL WITH: Classic Slaw, Fennel and Sour Cream Salad, Mayonnaise.

PORK CHEEKS IN CIDER

See page 169

Serves 4

600g pork cheeks, fat on and cut in half

2 tbsp olive oil

2 tbsp butter

1 onion, chopped

1 carrot, chopped

1 leek, chopped

1 celery stalk, chopped

250g streaky bacon, sliced

2 garlic cloves, finely chopped

½ handful thyme sprigs, leaves
   removed and chopped

2 bay leaves

3 tbsp tomato paste

500ml very dry cider

500ml beef stock or broth (page 232)

1 handful flat-leaf parsley, chopped

Salt and pepper

1 Heat your oven to 160°C.

2 Season the pork cheeks with salt and pepper and brown them on a medium heat in the olive oil in a medium-sized ovenproof pot or casserole.

3 Remove the cheeks and set them aside and melt the butter in the same pot.

4 Now, add the onion, carrot, leek, celery, bacon, garlic, thyme and bay leaves and sauté them for about 10 minutes, or until they are caramelised.

5 Now stir in the tomato paste, and leave it to cook a bit before adding the cider and the beef broth.

6 Return the cheeks to the pot, bring to the boil, cover it all with foil or a lid, and place it in the oven for 2 hours.

7 After 2 hours, remove it from the oven, take the lid off, stir through the parsley, season to taste with salt and pepper and serve immediately.

PAN-FRIED SWEETBREADS PICCATA

See page 169

Makes 2 mains, 4 starters

400g veal sweetbreads

Milk

Juice of 2 lemons

4 tbsp butter

4 tbsp olive oil

2 tbsp capers, drained

½ handful celery leaves

½ handful flat-leaf parsley

Salt and black pepper

1 Place the sweetbreads in a small container, cover with milk and leave them overnight in the fridge.

2 Discard the milk, rinse the sweetbreads and cut out any veins or dark bits.

3 Pop them into a small pot, cover them with water, add a tablespoon of salt and ¼ of the lemon juice, and bring to the boil for 5 minutes.

4 After 5 minutes take them out and refresh them in ice water. Once they're cool, pat them dry with paper towels and season with salt and pepper.

5 Now melt the butter in a large pan over a medium heat, and once it begins to bubble, add the sweetbreads.

6 In the meantime, combine the remaining ingredients in a bowl and season with salt and pepper.

7 Cook the sweetbreads for 5 minutes on each side, then pour in the sauce and let it come to a boil.

8 Serve the sweetbreads immediately on a platter, covering them in the saucy pan juices.

GOES WELL WITH: Sautéed Mange Tout with Mint, Lemon and Ricotta, Buttered Kale, Roasted Cherry Tomato Caprese.

TRIPE

I remember my nanny boiling tripe in our kitchen when I was a child and moaning about the smell. It wasn't until I learned to make it properly at college that I thought it was something I might choose to eat one day. Then I worked a harvest in Champagne, near Troyes, France. Troyes is famous for its *andouillette*, a sausage made of pork, tripe and/or chitterlings. It is an acquired taste, but the French absolutely love it. At first I needed lots of strong mustard to get it down, but eventually, I could eat it neat, and enjoy it that way. The climax of my tripe-eating career? That was definitely in Argentina at a wedding, where they treated us to *chinchulines* or, simply, BBQ 'baby tripes' with a twist of lemon juice, salt and pepper. And it was great.

While the benefits of tripe are becoming better known, it is still an acquired taste. And to acquire a taste for something, you have to start small. This curry is a very soft landing into tripe. The spices are powerful, the coconut milk adds depth and richness, while the tamarind offers a nice balance of acidity. The tripe flavour itself ends up being slightly masked and quite subtle. So if you're new to tripe, this is the right recipe to choose for your first time.

SRI LANKAN TRIPE CURRY

Serves 4

120g butter
2 tbsp ground coriander
2 tbsp ground cumin
2 tsp ground turmeric
3 tsp ground ginger
2 tsp ground cardamom
¼ tsp ground cloves
1 cinnamon stick
20 dried curry leaves
2 lemongrass stems, finely chopped
1 onion, roughly chopped
4 garlic cloves, roughly chopped
2 thumbs of ginger, grated
600g honeycomb tripe, washed and cut
  into 5cm squares
1 litre chicken stock
1 tsp chilli powder
2 tbsp lime juice
1 tsp salt
1 x 400ml can coconut milk
1 tbsp smooth tamarind paste
1 red chilli, finely chopped
1 big handful fresh coriander,
  roughly chopped

1 Melt the butter in a medium pot and add the spices, curry leaves, lemongrass, onion, garlic and ginger and sauté for about 10 minutes.
2 Now add the tripe, give it a stir around, then add the stock, chilli powder, lime juice and salt and bring to the boil.
3 Place the lid on and simmer very gently on a low heat for 3 hours. Check it every 30 minutes to give it a stir, and top it up with water if necessary. Make sure it isn't catching.
4 After 3 hours, add the coconut milk, tamarind and chilli and stir, then let it simmer until it has reduced to a thick curry consistency.
5 Just before serving, check the seasoning and adjust with salt, pepper and lime juice and add freshly chopped coriander.

GOES WELL WITH: Fried Curry Cabbage, Peri-Peri Chard.

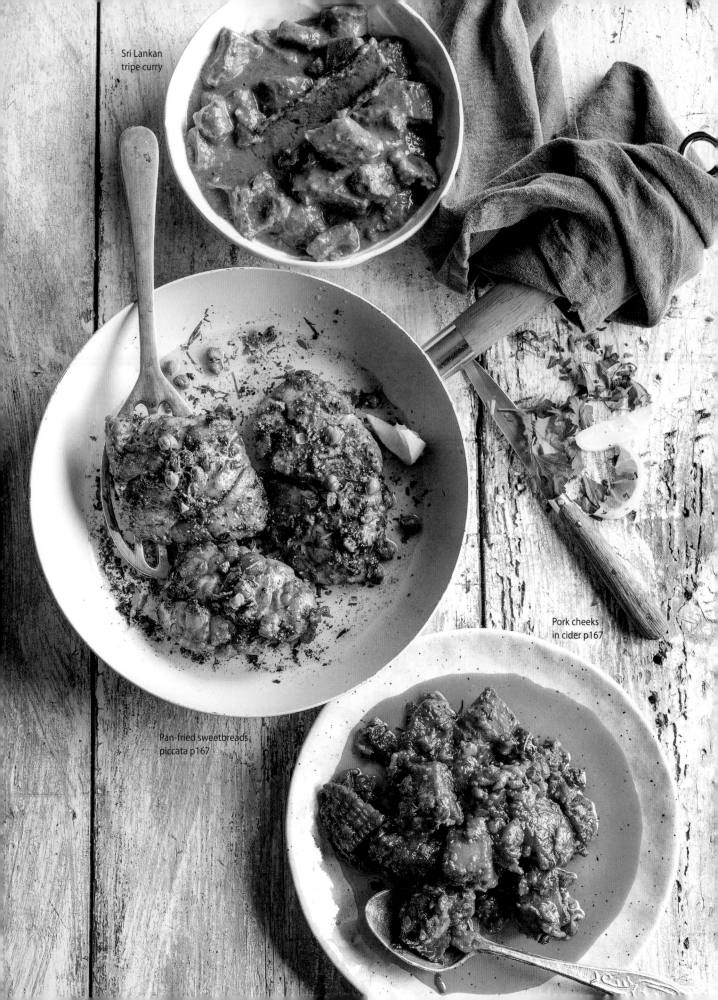

Sri Lankan
tripe curry

Pork cheeks
in cider p167

Pan-fried sweetbreads
piccata p167

CHICKEN PARMIGIANA

The national dish of Australia! (Well, it might as well be.)

Serves 4

1 x 400g tin whole peeled or
   chopped tomatoes

125ml + 4 tbsp olive oil

1 onion, roughly chopped

2 celery stalks, roughly chopped

3 garlic cloves, peeled

1 bay leaf

1 handful fresh basil leaves

4 chicken breasts, bone off, skin on

180g Parmigiano Reggiano, grated

Salt and black pepper

1 Preheat your oven to 140°C.

2 Use your hands to squash and mix the tinned tomatoes and 125ml olive oil with the onion, celery, garlic and bay leaf. Season with salt and pepper.

3 Pop the mix into a tray, cover it with foil and place it in the oven for 90 minutes.

4 Remove the foil, turn the grill to full blast, and return the sauce to the oven until bits of the sauce start to char. Max 10 minutes.

5 Tip the contents into a jug or mixing bowl, add the basil, season with salt and pepper and blitz it with a stick blender until smooth.

6 Now heat the oven up to 180°C and get the chicken ready.

7 Heat the remaining olive oil to a medium-high heat in a large pan.

8 Season the chicken breasts with salt and pepper and fry for 4 minutes on each side, then set aside to cool. It's fine if they are not cooked through.

9 Spread half of the sauce over the bottom of a small baking tray.

10 Place the chicken on top of the sauce in a single layer. Cover with the remaining sauce and top with the cheese.

11 Pop the tray in the oven and bake for 10 minutes or until the cheese is dark-brown, and serve immediately.

GOES WELL WITH: Roasted Artichokes with Lemon and Dill Vinaigrette, Courgetti with Mint, Basil and Pine Nuts, Caprese Salad.
For the full recipe for The Easiest Tomato Sauce, see page 303.

ROMESCO CHICKEN TRAY BAKE

Serves 4

4 drumsticks and 4 thighs, bone in,
   skin on

2 red peppers, cored, seeded and cut
   into 8 chunks

8 big garlic cloves, unpeeled

3 tbsp tomato paste

2 tbsp sherry vinegar

1½ tsp smoked paprika

½ tsp cayenne pepper

125ml olive oil

1 large lemon, cut into quarters

1 small handful flat-leaf parsley,
   roughly chopped

40g flaked almonds, toasted

Salt and black pepper

1 Preheat your oven to 180°C and lightly grease a baking tray.

2 Add the drumsticks, peppers, garlic cloves, tomato paste, sherry vinegar, smoked paprika, cayenne pepper, olive oil, lemon quarters and a good whack of seasoning to a large mixing bowl, and use your hands to mix everything until well coated.

3 Tip the chicken pieces and the peppers onto the baking tray and pop them in the oven for 40 minutes.

4 Remove the tray from the oven and use your tongs to pick out the garlic cloves and lemon wedges before tipping everything else into a large mixing bowl.

5 Add the parsley, then squeeze the flesh from the garlic cloves and the 'meat' of the lemon wedges over the chicken and mix well.

6 Tip it out onto a serving platter and scatter with toasted almonds.

GOES WELL WITH: Carciofi alla Romana, Buttered Broccoli, Sautéed Chard and Almonds.

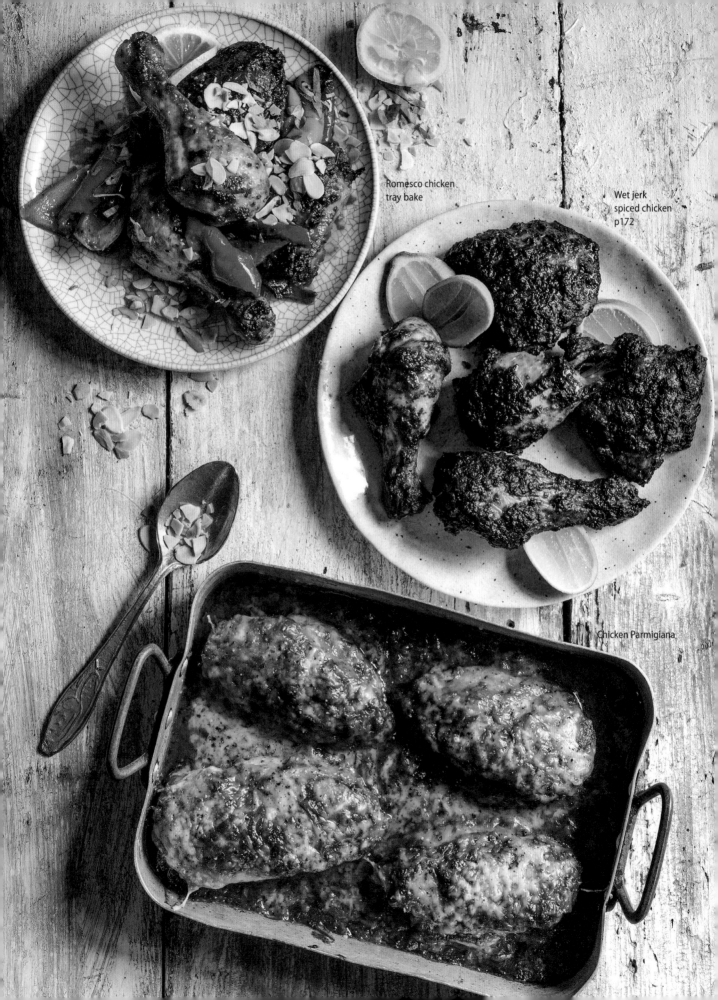

Romesco chicken
tray bake

Wet jerk
spiced chicken
p172

Chicken Parmigiana

WET JERK SPICED CHICKEN

See page 171

Serves 6

8 spring onions, chopped

1 red chilli, destemmed and finely chopped

125ml avocado oil

Juice of 3 limes

3 garlic cloves, finely chopped

10 sprigs thyme, leaves picked

1 small handful basil leaves

1 small handful fresh coriander, roughly chopped

2 tbsp smoked paprika

2 tsp ground ginger

½ tsp cayenne pepper

½ tsp allspice

½ tsp ground cinnamon

½ tsp ground cloves

½ tsp ground nutmeg

½ tsp ground cumin

1 tsp black pepper

1 tsp salt

6 drumsticks and 6 chicken thighs, bone in

2 limes cut into wedges

1 Whizz everything except for the chicken and the lime wedges up in a blender.

2 Preheat your oven to 180°C.

3 Mix the jerk sauce with the chicken pieces in a bowl, then spread them evenly over a medium-sized baking tray and place them in the oven for 35 minutes.

4 Place them on a serving platter and serve with fresh lime wedges.

GOES WELL WITH: Spicy Roasted Cabbage Wedges, Whole Roasted jerk Cauliflower, Kale and Cabbage Salad.

For the full recipe of Wet Jerk marinade, see page 295.

TARRAGON ROASTED CHICKEN

See page 175

Serves 4

100g butter

1 large handful fresh tarragon, picked
and roughly chopped

2 garlic cloves, minced

1 whole chicken

375ml white wine

Salt and pepper

1 Preheat your oven to 220°C.

2 Blend the butter, two-thirds of the tarragon and garlic together in a food processor or in a bowl with your hands.

3 Smear the butter all over the chicken, pushing it under the skin in places where it is loose, then give it a liberal sprinkling of salt and pepper.

4 Place the chicken in a small roasting tray, pour in the wine and pop the chicken into the oven for 15 minutes.

5 Lower the heat to 180°C then roast for another 45 minutes.

6 When the chicken comes out, add the remaining tarragon to the pan juices, shake them around, then leave the whole tray for 10 minutes for the juices to infuse and for the chicken to rest.

7 Portion the chicken and serve when ready with the pan juices as gravy.

GOES WELL WITH: Provençal Mushrooms, Deconstructed Ratatouille.

DAK GALBI KOREAN CHICKEN STIR FRY

Serves 4

3 tbsp gochujang (Korean chilli paste)

1 tsp ottogi (Korean curry powder)

1 tbsp gochugaru (Korean chilli flakes)

2 tbsp soy sauce

2 tbsp rice wine

1 garlic clove, minced

1 tsp minced ginger

1 onion, grated

500g deboned chicken thighs, cut into bite-sized pieces

3 tbsp coconut oil

1 large carrot, peeled and very thickly sliced on the diagonal

¼ head green cabbage, shredded

10 Korean perilla leaves, thinly sliced (or 1 handful basil, torn)

1   In a large bowl mix together the chilli paste, curry powder, chilli flakes, soy sauce, rice wine, garlic, ginger, onion and chicken pieces, then leave for 4 hours to marinate.

2   Heat the coconut oil to very hot in a large pan.

3   Add the carrot, cabbage and the chicken to the pan and cook, stirring continuously until the chicken is cooked through (probably about 9 minutes), then mix through the shredded perilla leaves or basil, and cook for another minute.

GOES WELL WITH: Spicy Cucumber Salad, Korean Spring Onion Salad.

CASABLANCA CHICKEN CASSEROLE

Serves 4

3 garlic cloves, chopped

1½ tsp smoked paprika

1½ tsp ground turmeric

1 tsp cumin seeds

4 tbsp olive oil

8 chicken thighs, bone in, skin on

2 onions, chopped

500ml chicken stock

1 lemon, thinly sliced

100g pitted green olives

1 pinch saffron

1 handful fresh coriander, chopped

Salt and black pepper

1   Blend the garlic, paprika, turmeric, cumin seeds, some salt and half the olive oil in a food processor into a smooth paste.

2   Massage the paste into the chicken pieces and leave them to marinate for 4 hours.

3   Heat the remaining olive oil in a large pan and add the onions and chicken thighs to cook on each side until golden-brown.

4   Then, add the stock (and enough water to reach halfway up the chicken if needed), the lemon slices, olives and saffron and bring it to a simmer.

5   Leave it to simmer uncovered for 30 minutes, then stir through the coriander, season with salt and pepper, and serve.

GOES WELL WITH: Charred Asparagus with Lemon, Beans with Caper Dressing, Roasted Kale.

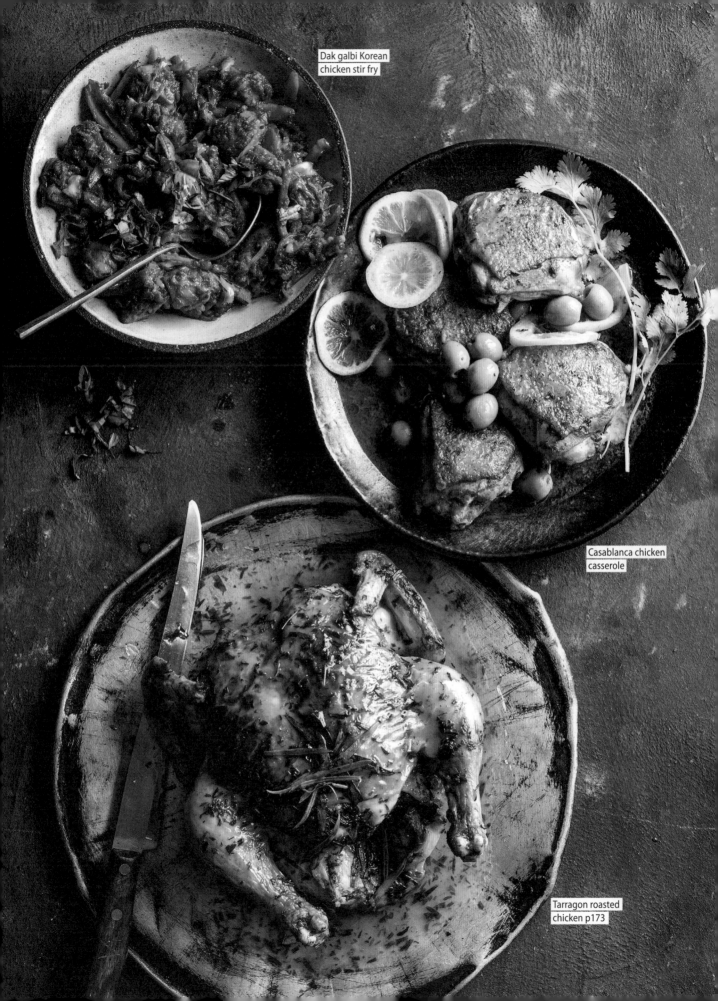

Dak galbi Korean
chicken stir fry

Casablanca chicken
casserole

Tarragon roasted
chicken p173

BUTTERFLYING A CHICKEN

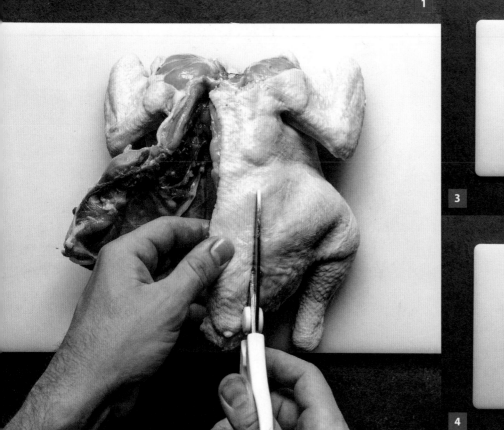
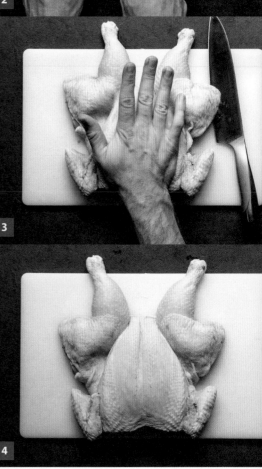

1 Place the chicken breast-down on a board and cut down either side of its spine with a pair of heavy-duty kitchen scissors. Remove spine completely.
2 Open up the rib cage and place the butt of your knife down the centre of the breast bone. Use the palm of your hand to hammer the blade into the bone until about halfway.
3 Flip the bird breast-side up and use the palm of your hand again to press down hard to break the breast apart.
4 Now follow the recipe.

TAKEAWAY CHICKEN

See page 179

Serves 4

One of my first jobs was as a cashier in a Portuguese takeaway near my school in Cape Town. Until that point I had always wondered why it took us so long to cook a chicken on the barbecue at home, while this place and many others could serve you a fully cooked bird in 10 minutes. On my first day, I saw them steaming about a hundred chickens in a massive steamer, and it all made sense: they pre-steamed their chickens so they were perfectly juicy and falling-off-the-bone. Then, all the chickens needed before they were ready to eat was a little run over the grill to heat them through, and a generous basting. If you're nervous that a massive chicken won't be thoroughly cooked on the barbecue, use this recipe.

1 large butterflied chicken (see opposite page)

2 garlic cloves, peeled

Zest and juice of 2 lemons

1 tsp dried chilli flakes

1 small handful fresh oregano, leaves picked and chopped

1 small handful flat-leaf parsley, roughly chopped

4 tbsp olive oil

3 tbsp sweet paprika

Salt and black pepper

1 extra lemon, to serve

1 Preheat your oven to 180°C.

2 Butterfly your chicken following the steps on the opposite page.

3 Pop it on a rack in a deep tray and fill the tray with water until it reaches just below the chicken. Then wrap the tray in foil and pop it in the oven for 1 hour.

4 Prepare a barbecue (Weber) to a medium-high heat.

5 Blitz the remaining ingredients, except for the serving lemon, in a small jug with a stick blender and keep it on hand while you grill the chicken.

6 When the coals are ready, gently place the chicken on the grid and leave it to brown. You can leave it for about 4 minutes on each side.

7 Once it is nicely charred on both sides, give it a basting of the marinade and flip it over. Baste the other side, then flip it again after a couple minutes. After about 3 bastings on each side, the bird should be charred and basted enough to devour.

8 Transfer the chicken onto a serving platter, splash with the remaining marinade and the juice from the extra lemon and serve immediately.

GOES WELL WITH: Classic Coleslaw, Peri-Peri Chard, Tzatziki.

CHOCOLATE MOLE CHICKEN

Serves 4

4 tbsp olive oil

½ tsp black peppercorns

½ tsp aniseed

½ tsp cumin seeds

3 cloves

½ tsp ground cinnamon

2 onions, thinly sliced

5 garlic cloves, roughly chopped

35g almonds

35g pecan nuts

35g hazelnuts

1 tbsp sesame seeds

1 litre chicken stock or broth
(see page 232)

1 tsp cayenne pepper

1 tsp sweet paprika

3 tbsp cocoa powder

Splash of olive oil

8 chicken pieces (a good mix)

Salt and black pepper

Fresh oregano, to serve

1 Heat the oil in a large pan over a medium heat and add the peppercorns, aniseed, cumin, cloves and cinnamon to the pan and cook for a minute until fragrant.

2 Then add the onion and garlic to the pan and sauté until golden-brown.

3 Now add the almonds, pecans, hazelnuts and sesame seeds and cook until the sesame seeds are toasted.

4 Add the chicken stock, cayenne pepper, paprika and cocoa powder and let it simmer until the liquid has reduced by half.

5 Tip the whole thing into a food processor and whizz it until it forms a smooth sauce.

6 Preheat your oven to 180°C.

7 Heat some olive oil in a casserole and brown the chicken pieces, turning them every few minutes.

8 Once they are brown on all sides, pour over the mole sauce and pop them in the oven for 45 minutes.

9 Season to taste, and serve immediately with a scattering of fresh oregano.

GOES WELL WITH: Guacamole, Classic Slaw, Berbere Cauliflower with Tarator.

ONE-PAN CHICKEN AND MUSHROOM STEW

Serves 4

4 chicken breasts, bone in, skin on

2 tbsp butter

2 tbsp olive oil

1 shallot, finely sliced

1 tsp fresh thyme leaves, chopped

1 tbsp minced garlic

240g button mushrooms, quartered

250ml white wine

250ml chicken stock or broth
(see page 232)

½ tsp dried chilli flakes

125ml cream

1 handful flat-leaf parsley, roughly
chopped

Salt and pepper

1 Preheat your oven to 180°C and season the chicken with salt and pepper.

2 Heat the butter and olive oil in a large pan and add the chicken breasts, turning them every couple of minutes, until golden-brown on each side. Set aside.

3 Add the shallot and thyme and sauté until the shallots are softened.

4 Add the garlic and stir it around for a minute, then add the mushrooms and cook them for 5 minutes, until they are soft.

5 Pour in the wine and reduce it by half, then add the stock and the chilli flakes and reduce the sauce by half again.

6 Now add the cream, bring it to the boil. Add the chicken pieces back in and pop the pan in the oven for 15 minutes.

7 Remove from the oven, season to taste with salt and pepper and mix through the chopped parsley before serving.

GOES WELL WITH: Buttered Courgettes, Confit Leeks.

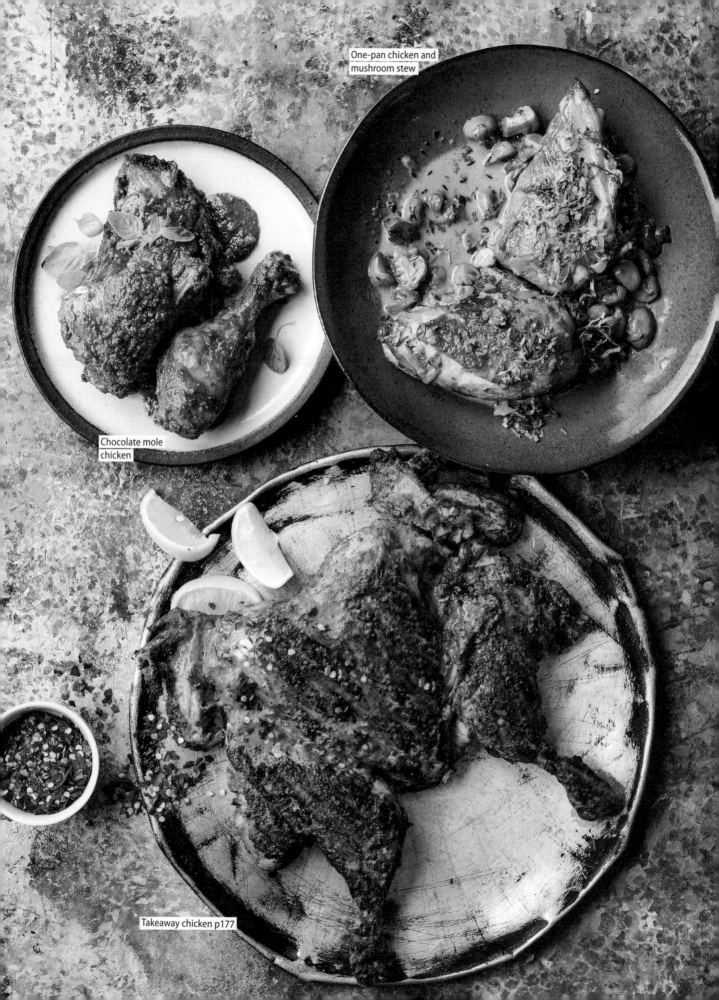

One-pan chicken and mushroom stew

Chocolate mole chicken

Takeaway chicken p177

ANGRY HARISSA CHICKEN WINGS

Serves 4

4 tbsp coconut oil

3 garlic cloves, roughly chopped

1 tbsp fresh red chilli, deseeded and chopped

1 tsp ground caraway seeds

2 tsp ground cumin

1 tsp ground coriander

1 tsp salt

3 tbsp tomato paste

1 tbsp sweet paprika

1 handful fresh coriander, finely chopped

800g chicken wings

1 Preheat your oven to 200°C.

2 Melt the coconut oil in a small saucepan or frying pan. Once the oil is warm but not too hot, add the garlic, chilli, caraway, cumin, ground coriander and salt.

3 Gently fry the ingredients in the oil until they become fragrant (about 3 or 4 minutes).

4 Add the tomato paste and sauté gently for a few more minutes.

5 Remove from the heat and scrape the contents of the pan into a narrow container (because you'll be blending a small volume; the jug that comes standard with a stick blender is a great option).

6 Now add to this mixture the sweet paprika and the fresh coriander and blend with a stick blender.

7 Mix the harissa sauce and the chicken wings well with your hands in a mixing bowl.

8 Lay the wings out on a cooling rack, on top of a roasting tray, and place them in the oven for 30 minutes.

9 Once they're cooked, arrange them on a serving platter.

GOES WELL WITH: Classic Slaw, Tzatziki, any yoghurt dip.

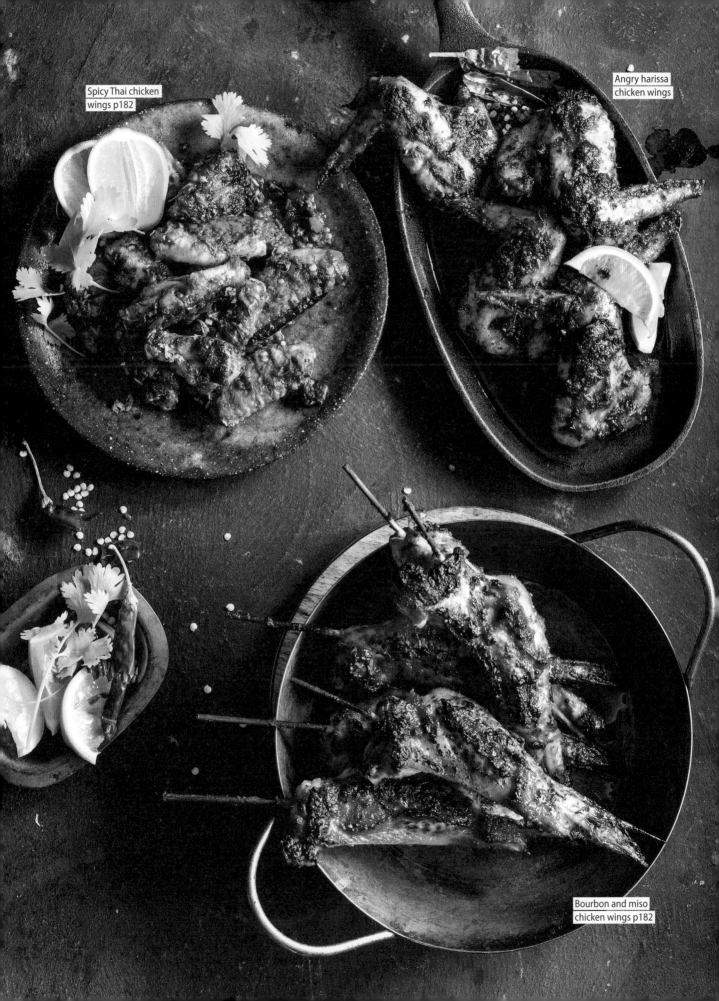

Spicy Thai chicken wings p182

Angry harissa chicken wings

Bourbon and miso chicken wings p182

BOURBON AND MISO CHICKEN WINGS

See page 181

Serves 4

100g miso paste

3 tbsp bourbon or Tennessee whiskey

1 tbsp chilli paste

2 tbsp apple cider vinegar

2 tbsp wholegrain mustard

1 tbsp minced ginger

1 tbsp minced garlic

800g chicken wings

2 limes, quartered, to serve

1 In a small jug, blitz everything except the chicken and limes with a stick blender.

2 Place the chicken wings in a medium mixing bowl and cover them with the marinade. Leave for an hour.

3 Prepare a barbecue to a gentle heat.

4 Grill the wings for 20 minutes, turning occasionally and basting with the remaining marinade.

5 Serve with fresh limes.

GOES WELL WITH: Nasu Dengaku – Grilled Miso Aubergine, Classic Slaw, Lime, Chilli and Sesame Stir-fried Mange Tout.

SPICY THAI CHICKEN WINGS

See page 181

Serves 4 as a starter

12 chicken wings, cut at the joint, tips discarded

1 tbsp fish sauce

Juice of 1 lemon

2 garlic cloves, crushed

1 tbsp avocado oil

6 tbsp rice vinegar

2 tbsp soy sauce

1 small red chilli

1 handful coriander, roughly chopped

1 Get a griddle pan smoking-hot.

2 Without seasoning or oil, char the wings on the griddle pan on both sides so they get grill lines and some of the charred flavour.

3 While you're charring the wings, blitz the remaining ingredients (apart from the coriander) in a small jug with a stick blender.

4 When the wings are done, transfer them to a small roasting dish, toss them in the sauce and pop them into the oven for 15 minutes.

5 As they come out of the oven, scatter the coriander in the dish and stir before tipping them, juices and all, onto a platter to serve.

GOES WELL WITH: Nuoc, Thai prawn cakes with Thai mayo.

MACADAMIA SATAY

See page 185

Serves 4

1 tsp turmeric

1 tsp cumin

1 tsp white pepper

1 tsp minced ginger

1 small onion, chopped

2 cloves garlic, peeled

½ tsp salt

600g deboned chicken thighs, cut into
   bite-sized pieces

80ml coconut oil

1 red onion, cut into chunks

4 big garlic cloves, peeled

2 tbsp Thai chilli paste

2 lemongrass stalks, finely chopped

½ tsp shrimp paste

500ml coconut milk

1 tbsp tamarind paste

120g macadamia nut butter

1. Blend the turmeric, cumin, pepper, ginger, onion, garlic and salt in a small jug with a stick blender and rub it into the chicken pieces.
2. Thread the chicken pieces onto bamboo skewers, then cover and refrigerate for 3 hours.
3. After the meat has marinated, prepare a barbecue to a medium-high heat, or a griddle pan to smoking-hot.
4. Blend the coconut oil, red onion, garlic, chilli paste, lemongrass and shrimp paste in small jug with a stick blender until it is very smooth.
5. Add the paste to a medium-sized frying pan and sauté on a medium heat until the oil has seeped out and the paste is well caramelised.
6. Add the coconut milk to the pan along with the tamarind paste and the macadamia butter and bring to the boil, then simmer for about 15 minutes on a gentle heat to thicken. Set aside until ready to serve.
7. When the coals are ready, place the skewers on the barbecue and grill for 10 minutes, turning regularly.
8. Remove the skewers from the grill and serve with the satay sauce.

GOES WELL WITH: Lime, Chilli and Sesame Stir-fried Mange Tout, Stir-fried Cucumber with Sesame Seeds, Stir-fried Spring Onions and Pak Choi.

SHANGHAINESE POACHED CHICKEN

Serves 4

500ml chicken broth or stock

500ml Shaoxing rice wine

2 thumbs of ginger, peeled and halved

6 spring onions (4 quartered, 2 finely chopped)

4 chicken breasts, skin attached

Salt and white pepper

1 Add the broth, rice wine, ginger, quartered spring onions, and salt and pepper to a small pot and bring it to the boil.

2 Add the chicken breasts and cook for 10 minutes, then transfer to cold water.

3 Keep the heat of the broth up, and reduce it by two-thirds.

4 Slice the chicken breasts into 1cm slices, divide them between serving bowls, and cover them with the broth and chopped spring onions.

GOES WELL WITH: Steamed Asparagus with Miso and Ginger Dressing, Stir-fried Spring Onions and Pak Choi.

MOTHER-IN-LAW'S CORONATION CHICKEN

Makes 1kg

This is literally my mother-in-law's Coronation Chicken. I was trying to think of something funny to write about it, but it is so good there is actually nothing funny to say. This is best used in salads or for a cold buffet.

1 whole chicken

1 tsp curry powder

1 tsp ground coriander

½ tsp turmeric

125ml mayonnaise (see page 274)

125ml double thick yoghurt

1 handful fresh coriander, roughly chopped

4 tbsp toasted almonds

1 Put the chicken in a small or medium pot and cover it with water.

2 Simmer it gently for 40 minutes, or until it is completely cooked through, then leave it to cool in the water until it reaches room temperature.

3 While the chicken is poaching, combine the curry powder, ground coriander, turmeric, mayonnaise and yoghurt in a bowl and leave to infuse in the fridge.

4 When the chicken is cooled, set the broth aside for another meal, and use your hands to pull the meat off the chicken. Then use your fingers to shred it into bite-sized chunks.

5 Mix the sauce through the chicken with the fresh coriander and dish it onto a platter.

6 Scatter with toasted almonds and some extra coriander leaves and serve.

GOES WELL WITH: Edamame Bean and Radish Salad.

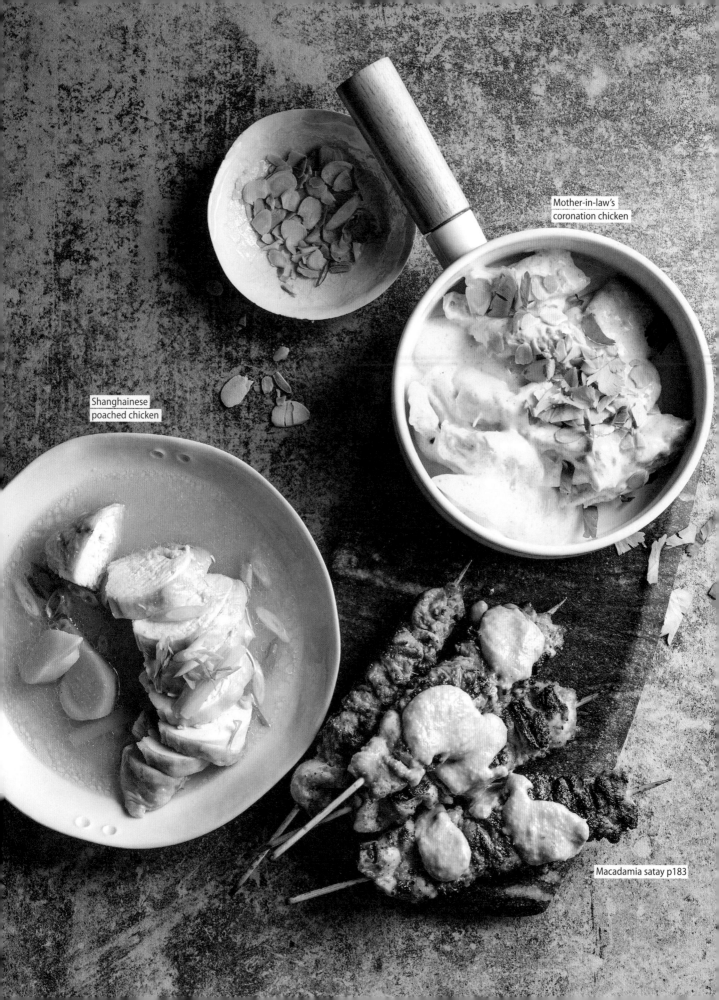

Mother-in-law's coronation chicken

Shanghainese poached chicken

Macadamia satay p183

DUCK BREASTS WITH COS LETTUCE WRAPS

Serves 4

4 duck breasts

3 tbsp rice wine

1 tsp Chinese five spice

6 tbsp soy sauce

1 garlic clove, minced

2 tbsp grated ginger

1 tbsp Chinese chilli sauce

1 tbsp sesame oil

3 tbsp oyster sauce

2 heads cos lettuce, leaves separated

50g spring onions, cut into thin strips

1 cucumber, thinly sliced

1 Preheat your oven to 200°C, while you score the skin of the duck breasts in a 1cm diamond pattern.

2 Mix the duck breasts, rice wine, five spice and 3 tablespoons of soy sauce in a large bowl and leave to marinate for an hour in the fridge.

3 Remove from fridge, pat the breasts dry with a kitchen towel, then place skin-side down in a cold pan.

4 Light the hob or turn it onto 'hot' and let the pan heat until the fat starts to render from the skin. Keep it cooking until the breasts are spitting and crackling in the pan and the skin is very crispy and a dark golden-brown.

5 Now flip them over and pop the whole pan in the oven for 5 minutes.

6 Quickly make the dipping sauce by mixing the garlic, ginger, Chinese chilli, sesame oil, oyster sauce and soy sauce together.

7 Remove the pan from the oven. Quickly remove the breasts from the pan and place them on a cool plate or board to rest for 10 minutes. Keep the fat for roasting another dish.

8 Slice the duck breasts into thin slices and arrange them on platter, along with bowls with lettuce leaves, spring onion and cucumber.

9 Give each guest their own bowl of dipping sauce and show them how to build the wraps: start with a lettuce leaf then add some cucumber, spring onion and a good slice or two of duck, then top it with the dressing.

CONFIT DUCK

Serves 4

4 duck legs, rinsed and patted dry

1 tsp coarse salt

1 tsp fine salt

1 tsp whole black pepper, lightly cracked

1 tbsp coriander seeds, lightly crushed

1 bay leaf, shredded

Extra duck fat

1 Massage all of the ingredients into the duck legs and leave them overnight in a tray in the fridge.

2 Preheat your oven to 120°C.

3 Rinse the rub off the legs, pack them very tightly into a small pot or tray. Cover them with the extra duck fat, pop the lid on, or cover the tray with foil and place them in the oven for 5 hours.

4 Remove the duck from the oven and remove the legs from the fat in the pan.

5 To serve, pan-fry the duck legs on a medium heat to drain off the extra fat. Serve as is or flake the duck into salads, or press into a terrine and cover with fat to make rillettes.

GOES WELL WITH: Braised Fennel, Provençal Mushrooms, Shaved Radish Salad.

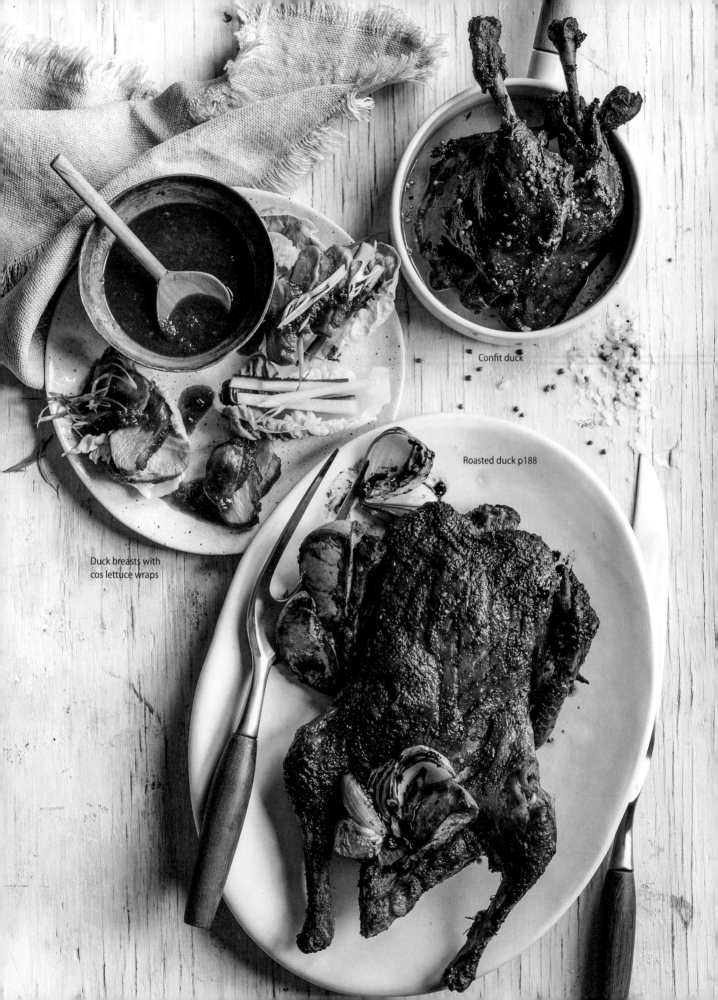

Confit duck

Roasted duck p188

Duck breasts with
cos lettuce wraps

ROASTED DUCK

See page 187

Serves 4

There are thousands of duck recipes out there with loads of flavour combinations. For the most part, the flavour profiles are divided between Western, which usually includes orange peel and cinnamon, and Asian, which usually includes soy sauce, ginger, star anise, cinnamon and, funnily enough, orange peel. Regardless of the flavour, the method of roasting a duck is similar everywhere. This is how it's done.

1 whole 3kg duck, fully defrosted,
   giblets removed
2 tbsp coarse salt
Seasoning of your choice (Asian, BBQ,
   French, Italian or general duck rub)
Stuffing of your choice (usually includes
   onion, apple, cinnamon or orange, or
   all of the above)
350ml water

1 Preheat your oven to 180°C.
2 Place the duck breast-side up on a cutting board and use a Stanley knife to score the skin in a 1cm grid. You want to cut about halfway into the skin, and the grid should cover the entire top half of the bird.
3 Then, use a skewer or sharp knife to poke holes in the skin in areas that you couldn't reach with the neat grid. This could be all of the legs, in the fatty parts of joints and around the wings.
4 Now massage the entire bird with the salt and seasoning and fill the cavity with the ingredients for the stuffing.
5 I don't truss ducks because they render more fat if they are 'free'.
6 Pour the water into a small, deep roasting dish, place the duck, breast-side up, in the dish, and pop in the oven.
7 Turn the duck after an hour to breast-side down.
8 After another hour, turn the heat up to 200°C, then flip the duck to breast-side up again.
9 Throughout the entire 3 hours, be sure to baste the duck with the juices from the tray. Every 20 minutes should be fine.
10 After 3 hours, remove the tray from the oven and leave the duck to rest.
11 Now it's time to make the gravy, if you're having one. Carve and serve.

GOES WELL WITH: Broccolini in Oyster Sauce, Fried Garlic Green Beans, Stir-fried Mushrooms with Bamboo Shoots.

FISH & SEAFOOD

Different fish are 'sustainable' in different countries. We have readers all over the world, notably the UK, US, Canada, Australia, New Zealand, the UAE and of course South Africa. If salmon, for instance, is not sustainable in your country, substitute it with another oily fish.

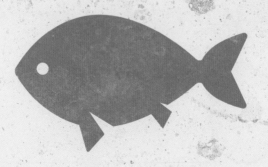

COD AU GRATIN

See page 193

Serves 4

2 tbsp butter

4 fresh cod or hake fillets, scaled and
   cleaned (about 4x180g)

1 tbsp Dijon mustard

500ml cream

1 large pinch ground nutmeg

90g grated Parmigiano Reggiano

120g grated Cheddar

1 small handful fresh dill,
   finely chopped

Salt and white pepper

2 egg yolks

1   Preheat your oven to 180°C.
2   Melt the butter in a saucepan over medium heat and wait for it to bubble.
3   Add the fish fillets and fry them for 3 minutes on each side. Remove the pan from the heat, then pack the fillets tightly in a small, deep baking tray.
4   Return the pan to the heat, add the mustard and fry gently for a minute or two in the remaining butter, then pour in the cream and nutmeg and bring to the boil.
5   Once the mixture has reduced by half, remove from the heat and stir in half the cheese and the dill. Keep mixing until the cheese is totally melted.
6   Once this has cooled a bit, season to taste with salt and pepper, then mix in the egg yolks.
7   Pour the sauce evenly over the fish, top with the remaining cheese, and pop it all in the oven for 20 minutes until the cheese is bubbling and dark-brown.

CULLEN SKINK (SCOTTISH HADDOCK SOUP)

See page 193

Serves 4 as a starter

*When I was looking for interesting things to do with haddock and I came across
this dish, I had to put it in. I don't think I have ever heard a cooler name for a soup
in my life. My hair goes a little bit ginger every time I say it out loud.*

500g smoked haddock fillets

1 litre fish stock or broth (see page 232)

300g turnips, peeled and diced

2 tbsp butter

1 large onion, finely chopped

1 bay leaf

250ml cream

1 handful flat-leaf parsley, chopped

Salt and black pepper

1   Place the haddock fillets skin-side down in a medium-sized pot or pan and cover with stock.
2   Simmer for 4 minutes on each side, then remove the fillets, take the skin off, pick the bones out and flake the meat.
3   Keep the cooking liquid in the pan and add the turnips. Cook, covered, for 15 minutes, until mushy.
4   Scoop the turnips out with a slotted spoon and blitz them in a small jug with the butter until smooth and silky.
5   Now add the onion and bay leaf to the stock and let them simmer until the onions are translucent.
6   Add the cream and the mashed turnips and simmer gently until it reaches a thick soupy, chowdery consistency.
7   Finally, mix through the haddock, the parsley and add a good dose of salt and pepper for seasoning, then serve hot.

PAN-FRIED HADDOCK WITH OLIVES AND TOMATOES

See page 192

Serves 4

4 fresh haddock fillets (about 180g each)

125ml olive oil

1 onion, finely chopped

2 garlic cloves, minced

80ml dry white wine

80g cherry tomatoes, halved

3 tbsp pitted black olives

1 tbsp capers, roughly chopped

4 tbsp chicken broth (see page 232)

1 tbsp chopped flat-leaf parsley

½ handful basil, chopped

Salt and black pepper

1 Season the fillets liberally with salt and pepper.

2 Heat half the olive oil in a large pan and add the fillets to cook for 4 minutes on each side, then set aside.

3 Add the remaining olive oil to the same pan and add the onion to sauté until it begins to caramelise, then add the garlic and keep stirring until it becomes fragrant.

4 Add the wine and use a wooden spoon to scrape the bits free from the bottom of the pan.

5 Once the wine has reduced by half, add the tomatoes, olives and capers, and simmer until the wine has cooked away.

6 Now stir in the chicken broth and let it reduce by half before checking the seasoning and mixing through the parsley and basil.

7 Finally, add the fish back into the pan and keep spooning over the sauce until the fish is warmed through.

GOES WELL WITH: Roasted Artichokes with Lemon and Dill Vinaigrette, Buttered Kale, Caprese Salad.

SOLE MEUNIÈRE

See page 192

Serves 4

Sole, in my opinion, is one of the most underrated fish out there. It's so easy to cook. It's almost as though the less you do to it, the better.

4 large sole fillets, boned and skinned

5 tbsp butter

1 lemon, thinly sliced

2 tbsp capers, drained and roughly chopped

1 handful flat-leaf parsley, roughly chopped

Salt and black pepper

1 Season the sole with salt and pepper on both sides.

2 Heat 2 tablespoons of butter to a medium-high heat in a large pan and add the fillets (preferably in a pan big enough to take all 4 at once).

3 Fry them for 4 minutes on each side, then remove them from the pan, and place on plates or a platter.

4 Keep the heat on and add the remaining butter to the pan, along with the lemon slices and capers.

5 Cook the lemon pieces until they are translucent, then add the parsley to the butter sauce and spoon the it all over the fish just before serving.

GOES WELL WITH: Roasted Brussels Sprouts, Caramelised Garlic Fennel.

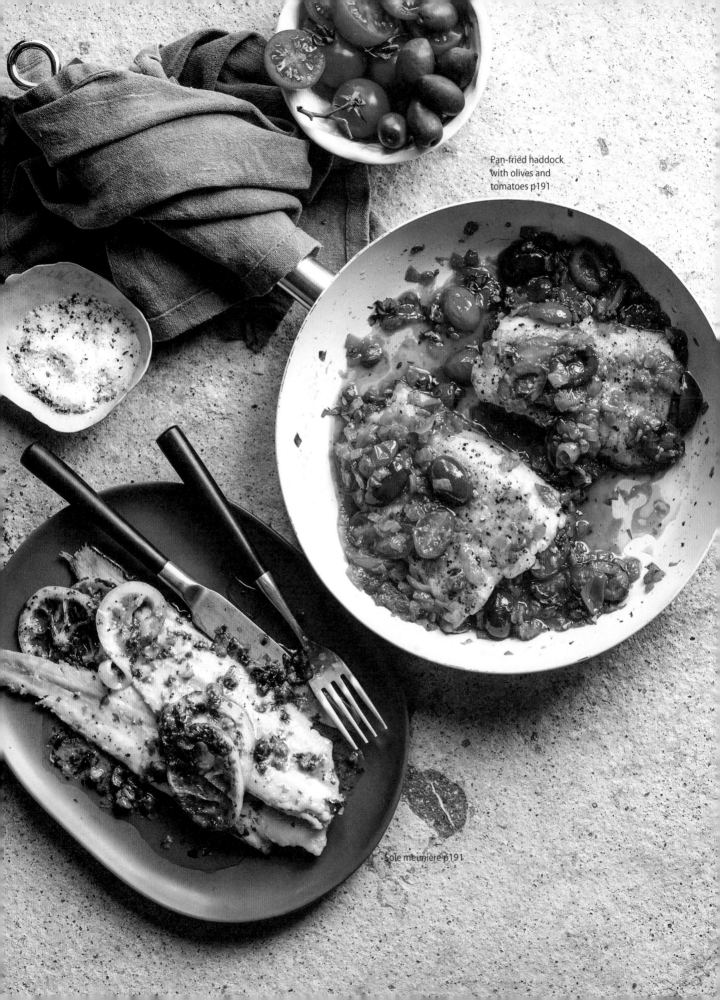

Pan-fried haddock
with olives and
tomatoes p191

Sole meunière p191

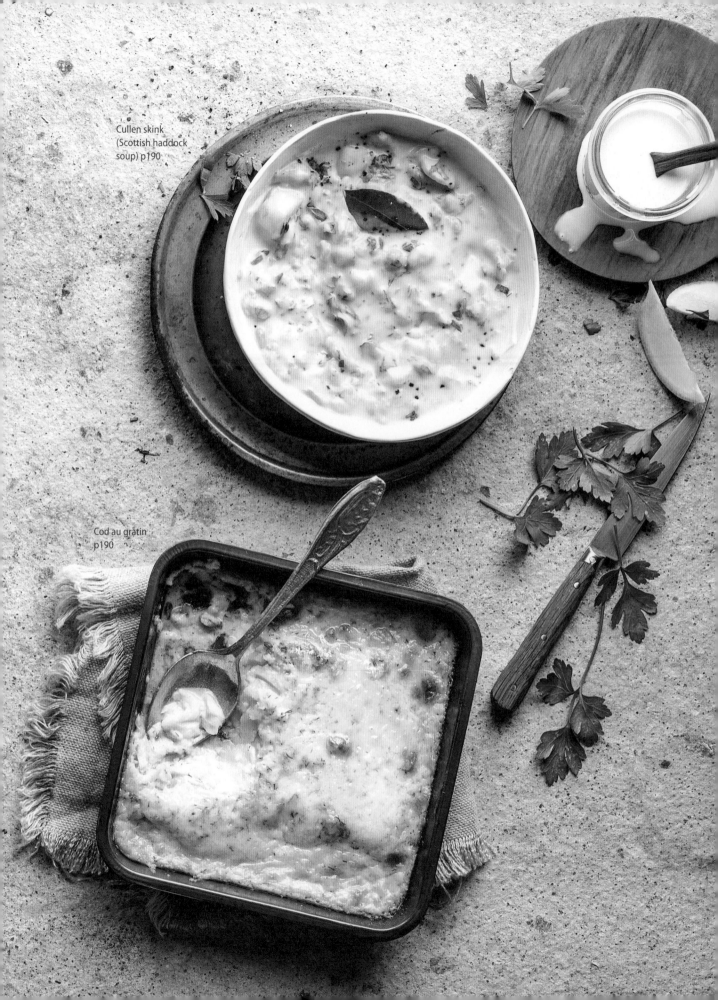

Cullen skink
(Scottish haddock
soup) p190

Cod au gratin
p190

CRACKED BLACK PEPPER CRAB WITH LEMONGRASS AND BASIL

Serves 4

3 stalks fresh lemongrass, ends
   trimmed, cut into chunks
2 thumbs ginger, peeled
3 garlic cloves, peeled
5 tbsp soy sauce
1 tbsp black pepper, cracked
4 steamed Dungeness (or similar) crabs,
   cleaned, bodies quartered and
   legs cracked
3 tbsp avocado oil
1 small handful fresh coriander, roughly
   chopped
1 small handful Thai basil leaves,
   roughly chopped

1 Whizz the lemongrass, ginger and garlic together in a food processor until smooth. You may want to add a little water to help it blend better.
2 Pour the soy sauce and the black pepper into a bowl, add in the paste from the blender and mix.
3 Mix in the crab pieces and leave them in the fridge for 1 hour.
4 Get a large, heavy-based pot very hot and add the oil.
5 Use a slotted spoon to lift the crab pieces out of the bowl, letting the marinade drain, and drop them into the pot.
6 Stir them around to heat them through for 3 to 4 minutes, then pour in the marinade and let it steam and bubble for 1 to 2 minutes.
7 Finally, add the coriander and basil, remove from the heat and mix well before serving.

GOES WELL WITH: Fried Garlic Green Beans, Spinach in Sesame Dressing.

LOBSTER THERMIDOR-ISH

Serves 2

Lobster thermidor usually contains wheat flour and bakes the same way as Welsh rarebit would. There is no flour in my recipe; although the flavours are the same, the final texture is somewhat different.

3 tbsp butter
½ red onion, finely chopped
1 shot cognac
1 tbsp Dijon mustard
300ml fish stock (see page 232)
1 tbsp ground almonds or almond flour
125ml cream
1 handful fresh tarragon, roughly
   chopped
40g Gruyère, grated
1 pinch nutmeg
2 lobsters or crayfish, cut in half
   lengthways, intestines removed
2 egg yolks
Salt and black pepper

1 Preheat your oven to 220°C.
2 Get the butter bubbling in a small pot and sauté the onion until it has softened.
3 Add the cognac (you can light it, if you want to be fancy) and boil until it has completely evaporated.
4 Add the mustard, fish stock and almonds or almond flour, and let the sauce reduce to a quarter of its original volume.
5 Add the cream and reduce the sauce further.
6 Add the tarragon, remove the pot from the heat and stir in the Gruyère and nutmeg.
7 Keep stirring until the cheese has completely melted, then adjust the seasoning to taste. Remove from the heat and leave it to cool for about 10 minutes.
8 Place the crayfish or lobsters in a baking dish.
9 Mix the egg yolks into the sauce mixture. Blend thoroughly and spoon the sauce over the meat of the crayfish, then pop the dish in the oven for 12 minutes. Remove and serve immediately.

GOES WELL WITH: Braised Fennel, Caramelised Endive and Leeks.

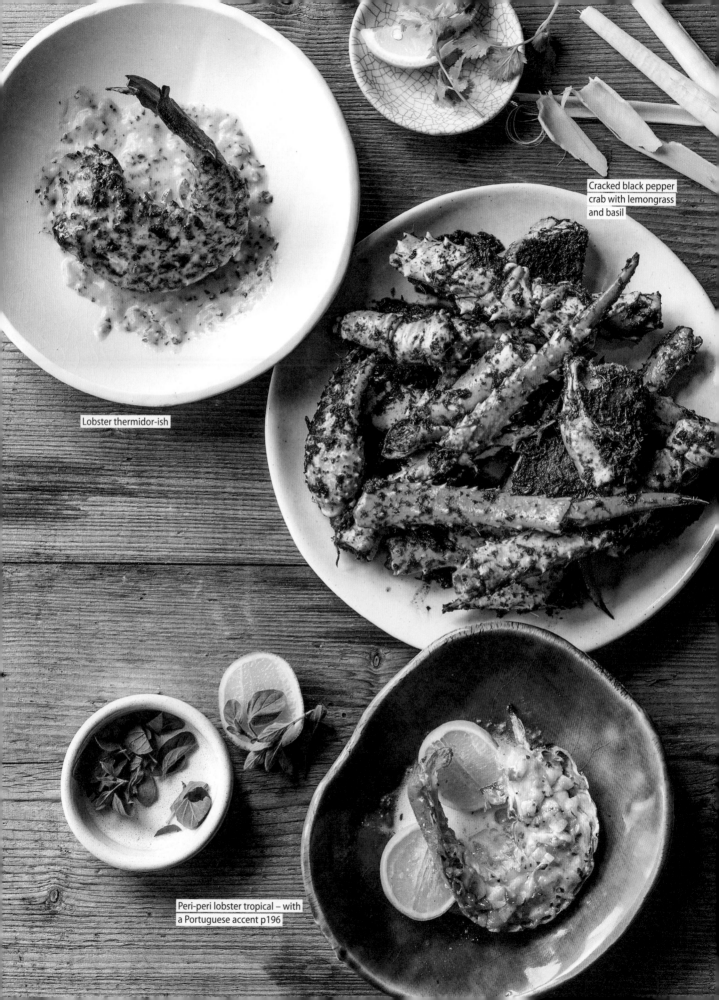

Cracked black pepper crab with lemongrass and basil

Lobster thermidor-ish

Peri-peri lobster tropical – with a Portuguese accent p196

PERI-PERI LOBSTER TROPICAL – WITH A PORTUGUESE ACCENT

See page 195

Serves 2

In 2010 I went on a boys' mission with my dad to Mozambique. We met a local baker, Carlos, who sold us ciabatta that he made by hand from cassava flour. His oven was made out of a decommissioned fridge and he fuelled it with coconut husks that he collected from the surrounding groves. Intrigued by his resourcefulness, we asked him what he could do with a lobster (they are dirt-cheap in Mozambique). This is what he made; except he used his fridge-oven-barbecue to cook it.

2 tbsp coconut oil

2 garlic cloves, roughly chopped

1 red chilli, roughly chopped

1 big pinch ground cardamom

125ml coconut cream

1 lime, cut in half

¼ tsp sweet paprika

¼ tsp dried oregano

1 big pinch salt

2 raw lobsters, cut down the middle, intestines removed

1 Build your barbecue up to a ferocious heat.

2 Heat the coconut oil up to a medium heat in a medium-sized pan.

3 Add the garlic, chilli and cardamom and fry gently for 3 minutes.

4 Add the coconut cream, juice of one half of the lime, paprika, oregano and salt, and reduce the sauce slightly – just enough to thicken a bit and have all the flavours nicely infused.

5 Now season the lobster meat, give it a light basting with the sauce and slap it meat-side down on the grill on the hottest part of the fire. Leave them to char for 3 minutes.

6 Flip them over, then distribute the remaining marinade between the four halves.

7 Now watch the meat carefully. Once you see the juices between the meat and the shell begin to bubble, they are ready to take off the grill.

8 Leave them to rest for a few minutes, then give them a twist of that other lime half and eat immediately.

GOES WELL WITH: Charred Asparagus with Lemon, Peri-Peri Chard, Buttered Garlic Spinach.

TUNA POKE BOWLS

See page 199

Serves 4

You're probably thinking, 'What about the pineapple?' What you get in carbs in this small amount of pineapple, you get a million times more in digestive enzymes. But that's not a licence to be naughty. With the pineapple included, this is a once-a-week or month kind of dish. Unless of course you don't give a toss about carbs. Then you can eat it whenever you like.

800g fresh, raw tuna, cut into
  2.5cm cubes

150ml sesame oil

4 tbsp soy sauce

3 tbsp lime juice

2 tbsp rice vinegar

2 tbsp any good Asian chilli garlic sauce

1 thumb ginger, grated

250g fresh pineapple cut into
  2cm cubes

680g finely shredded purple cabbage

1 English cucumber, cut in quarters
  lengthways, then cut into 2cm chunks

150g steamed edamame beans

4 spring onions, chopped

2 avocados, peeled and cubed

2 red chillies, finely chopped

2 tbsp toasted black or white
  sesame seeds

1 In a large mixing bowl, stir the tuna, sesame oil, soy sauce, lime juice, rice vinegar, chilli garlic sauce and ginger together, and leave it for half a day – or an hour, at least.

2 Mix the remaining ingredients, except the sesame seeds, together in another large mixing bowl and divide them between four serving dishes.

3 Finally, top the bowls with the marinated tuna and sprinkle each bowl with some sesame seeds.

GAME FISH TIRADITO

Serves 4

Similar to ceviche, tiradito reflects the Japanese influence on Peruvian cuisine, the main differences being that the sauce goes on at the end (ceviche is marinated) and tiradito is sliced sashimi-style (ceviche is cubed).

Juice of 5 limes

1 red chilli, finely chopped

1 tsp amarillo paste (or any medium-strength chilli paste)

1 garlic clove, chopped

4 tbsp olive oil

1 small handful fresh coriander, roughly chopped

500g barramundi, yellowtail or yellowfin tuna fillet, boned and skinned

1 tbsp toasted white sesame seeds

1 tbsp toasted black sesame seeds

Salt and pepper

1 To make the marinade, blitz the lime juice, chilli, amarillo paste, garlic and oil in a small jug with a stick blender.

2 Mix through the coriander and season to taste with salt and pepper.

3 Slice the fish into sashimi-style slices and lay the slices neatly on a serving dish.

4 Pour the marinade over the fish, and sprinkle with sesame seeds and any leftover coriander.

BLACKENED SWORDFISH WITH GUACAMOLE

Serves 4

1 tbsp fine salt

1 tbsp cayenne pepper

1 tbsp black pepper

1 tbsp smoked paprika

1 tbsp garlic powder

2 tsp onion powder

2 tsp dried oregano

2 tsp dried thyme

4 x 200g swordfish steaks, patted dry

3 tbsp coconut oil

2 limes, cut into wedges

1 batch of guacamole (see page 278)

1 Mix the spices and herbs together in a small mixing bowl, then pour them on a flat tray or plate.

2 Dunk the fish steaks in the spice and herb mixture, one decent dab per side, then set aside.

3 Get the coconut oil ridiculously hot in a large frying pan.

4 As it is about to smoke, add the steaks and sear for 2 minutes on each side. The cayenne pepper and paprika should blacken from the heat (open a window, this could get smoky).

5 Remove the steaks from the heat and serve them immediately with some lime wedges and guacamole.

GOES WELL WITH: Spicy Roasted Cabbage Wedges, Classic Slaw, Spicy Roasted Okra.

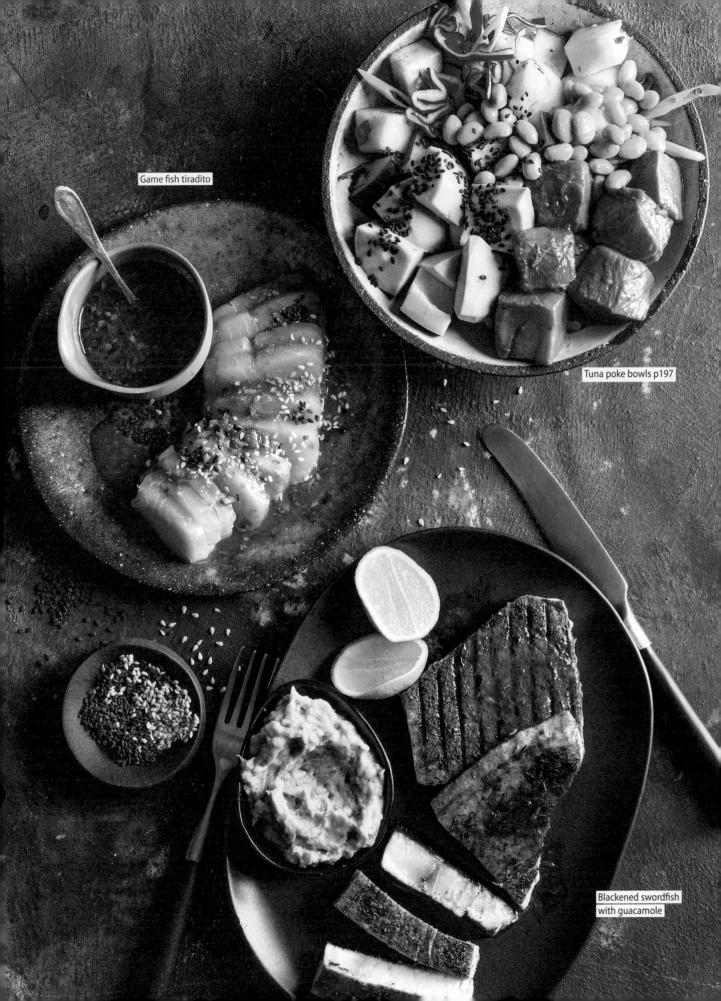

Game fish tiradito

Tuna poke bowls p197

Blackened swordfish
with guacamole

COURGETTI VONGOLE – CLAM COURGETTI

See page 203

Serves 2

It's tough to cook courgetti for more than two people. Either serve this for two only, or do it in two batches. Although not traditional, you could mix 2 tablespoons of crème fraîche or double cream through it at the end to make a richer, creamier version.

3 tbsp olive oil

400g courgetti (see page 66)

½ onion, finely chopped

½ red chilli, seeded and finely chopped

2 garlic cloves, finely chopped

125ml dry white wine

500g small clams, cleaned and rinsed

1 small handful flat-leaf parsley,
   roughly chopped

Salt and black pepper

½ lemon, cut into wedges

1 Heat half of the olive oil to almost smoking-hot in a large frying pan that has a lid.

2 Add all the courgetti at once and stir-fry it until it is lightly cooked, then tip it out into a bowl. See note on page 67 about searing courgette noodles.

3 Now add the rest of the olive oil to the pan and lower the heat.

4 Add the onions, chilli and garlic and sauté for about 3 minutes until softened. For once, we're going to avoid caramelisation here.

5 Pour in the wine and reduce it by half, then add the clams and pop the lid on for 3 minutes, until the shells have opened.

6 Discard any broken clams and clams that didn't open.

7 Finally, add the courgetti and the parsley and toss to combine.

8 Check the seasoning and adjust with salt and pepper.

9 Dish it up and finish it off with a crack of black pepper, a good splash of olive oil and a twist of lemon.

GREAT AS A MEAL ON ITS OWN.

MUSSEL CHOWDER

See page 203

Serves 4

In Cape Town the only clams we get are the frozen kind. Black mussels, however, can literally be picked off the rocks just a few kilometres from my house. If you're in a clam region, you can swap mussels for clams in the same quantity and at the same point in the recipe.

3 tbsp butter

250g streaky bacon, diced

2 large onions, roughly chopped

4 celery stalks, finely chopped

3 garlic cloves, roughly chopped

4 medium turnips, cut into 1.5 cm cubes

750ml fish stock or broth (see page 232)

250ml thick cream

½ lemon

1 red chilli, cut in half lengthways

1.2kg black mussels, washed and debearded

1 handful fresh dill, finely chopped

1 handful flat-leaf parsley, chopped

Salt and black pepper

1 Heat a large pot to a medium heat. Add the butter, bacon, onions, celery, garlic and turnips, and sauté until they are soft and well caramelised. This could take 20 minutes.

2 Add the stock and let it simmer gently with the lid on until the turnips are mushy.

3 Use a potato masher to roughly crush the turnips.

4 Now add the cream, half lemon and chilli and gently simmer until the cream begins to thicken.

5 Add the mussels and pop the lid on for about 4 minutes for the mussels to cook. They should all be open when the lid comes off. If none of them are open, pop the lid back on for a few more minutes.

6 When it seems as though no more are going to open, discard the unopened ones, then mix through the dill and parsley, and check the seasoning before serving.

GREAT AS A MEAL ON ITS OWN.

GUMBO

See page 203

Serves 4

3 tbsp olive oil

1 onion, finely chopped

½ green pepper, roughly chopped

½ red pepper, roughly chopped

2 big stalks celery, roughly chopped

3 garlic cloves, chopped

750ml chicken stock or broth (see page 232)

2 tbsp Cajun spice mix (see page 308)

1 x 400g tin chopped tomatoes

200g okra, sliced

300g tiger prawns, heads removed, peeled and deveined

200g baby shrimps, heads removed, peeled and deveined

1 handful flat-leaf parsley, chopped

2 spring onions, thinly sliced

1 Heat the oil in a large saucepan over a medium heat. Add the onion, peppers and celery and sauté until softened.

2 Add the garlic and keep stirring until it becomes fragrant.

3 Now add the stock, Cajun spice mix and tomatoes and bring to the boil, then reduce the heat to a gentle simmer and let it tick away for 1 hour.

4 Add the okra and simmer for another 15 minutes.

5 A few minutes before serving, add the prawns and shrimps and let the mix simmer for 5 minutes.

6 Finally, stir in the parsley and spring onions and serve immediately.

GREAT AS A MEAL ON ITS OWN.

DIRTY MUSSELS

Serves 4

We have a family holiday house in Betty's Bay just outside Cape Town. Whenever we get together and there's a spring tide, we head out to pick mussels to cook. These days, instead of the creamy mussel pots of old, we just slap the mussels straight on the grill, kelp and all, and when they pop open, we baste them in heavenly herby butter and put them back on the fire to finish off. A few minutes later we eat them right off the grill with our hands, and slurp the buttery juices straight from the shells.

500g melted butter

50g fresh basil

50g fresh parsley

50g fresh coriander

4 tbsp Asian chilli paste

3 thumbs ginger, roughly chopped

6 garlic cloves, peeled

125ml lemon juice

2kg black mussels, beards in,
  kelp on (if any)

Lots and lots of salt and black pepper

1   Light your Weber (or pizza oven) and bring up to a very high heat.

2   Use a stick blender to blend everything except for the mussels in a medium-sized jug.

3   Place the mussels on the griddle and wait for them to start spitting. As they are about to start opening properly, use your tongs to transfer them to a tray. Repeat this with all of them.

4   Now use your fingers or a butter knife to pry each mussel all the way open, breaking off and discarding each empty half-shell.

5   Arrange the meaty half-shells flesh-side up in small roasting trays, and fill each shell with a teaspoon of the butter sauce.

6   Now one tray at a time (depending on how many will fit in the Weber at once), pop the mussels back on the heat and put the lid on for about 3 minutes.

7   Remove the lid and serve the mussels immediately. They should be sizzling in the herb butter.

8   This recipe also works brilliantly in a pizza oven if you're lucky enough to have one. Obviously, you would do the first step on a baking tray in the oven, rather than cooking them straight on the bricks in the oven

GOES WELL WITH: Steamed Asparagus with Miso and Ginger Dressing, Fried Garlic Green Beans, Lime, Chilli and Sesame Stir-fried Mange Tout.

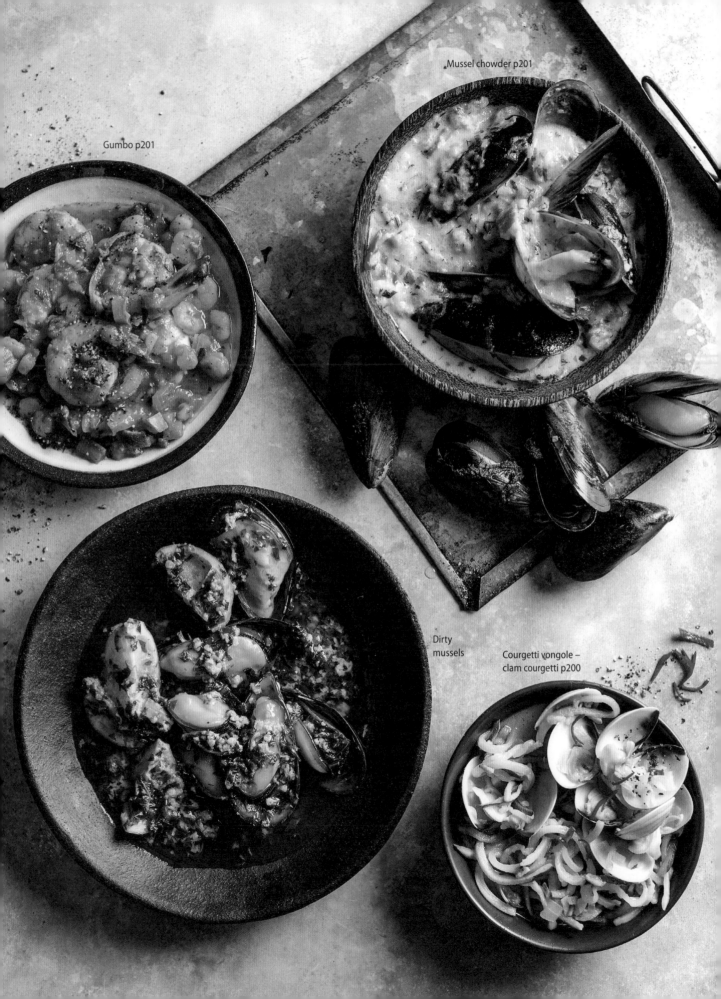

Gumbo p201

Mussel chowder p201

Dirty
mussels

Courgetti vongole –
clam courgetti p200

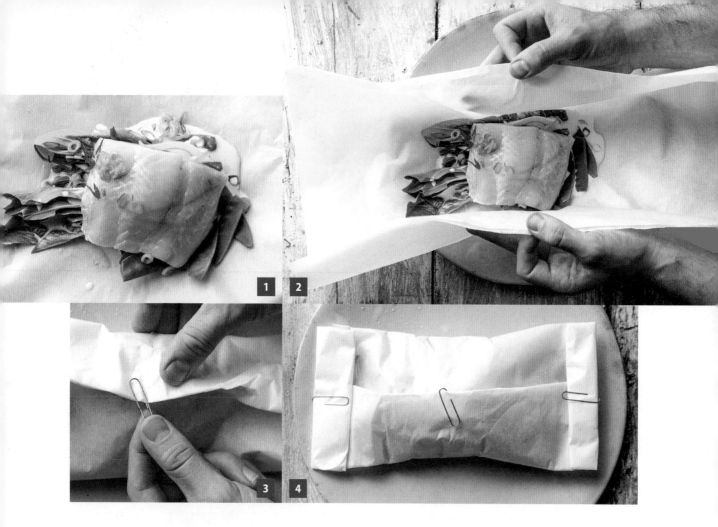

MAKING A PARCEL

1 Place the filling in the centre of the paper and top with the sauce.
2 Fold two sides of the paper together, then roll them all the way down until the paper is tightly wrapped around the filling, and fasten with a paper clip.
3 Roll the ends all the way up to the filling and fasten them with a paper clip.
4 Pop the parcel on a tray and bake in the oven for 12 minutes.
5 If you want to cook your parcel on the barbecue, wrap the parcel in foil as well, so the paper doesn't burn. Place the parcel directly on the heat for 8 to 10 minutes.

'GOOD FOOD IS THE FOUNDATION OF GENUINE HAPPINESS.'

– AUGUSTE ESCOFFIER

STEAMY MUSSEL PARCEL

Serves 1

600g fresh mussels

12 medium cherry tomatoes, diced

1 bulb fennel, thinly sliced

2 garlic cloves, roughly chopped

1 medium leek, sliced

4 tbsp butter

60ml white wine

1 handful of flat-leaf parsley, chopped

2 lemons, cut into wedges

1 Preheat your oven to 200°C.

2 Mix together all the ingredients, except the parsley and lemon wedges, then place the mix in a parcel as per the parcel lesson on page 204.

3 Bake the parcel on a tray in the oven for 12 minutes.

4 If you prefer to cook your mussels on the barbecue, wrap the parcel in foil as well, so the paper doesn't burn. Place the parcel directly on the heat for 8 to 10 minutes.

5 Serve with chopped fresh parsley and a lemon wedge.

CHILLI AND LEMON PRAWN PARCEL

Serves 2

600g prawns (21 to 25 prawns, shells on, veins removed)

4 tbsp butter

50ml lemon juice

Zest of 1 lemon

2 tbsp parsley, chopped

3 garlic cloves, sliced

1 whole red chilli, sliced

60ml white wine – a wooded Chardonnay for the discerning palate

1 Preheat your oven to 200°C.

2 Mix all the ingredients together, then pack them into a parcel as per the parcel lesson on page 204.

3 Bake in the oven for 12 minutes.

4 If you want to cook your prawn parcel on the barbecue, wrap the parcel in foil as well, so the paper doesn't burn.

5 Serve with extra freshly chopped garlic and a wedge of lemon.

BAKED ASIAN FISH PARCEL

Serves 4

1 tbsp fish sauce

1 tsp red curry paste

100ml coconut cream

Juice of half a lime

1 handful fresh coriander, chopped

3 stalks tenderstem broccoli

50g mange tout

1 large spring onion

1 head pak choi, cut in half lengthways

200g white fish fillets, preferably cod, hake or a mild fish

1 Preheat your oven to 200°C.

2 Pop the fish sauce, curry paste, coconut cream, lime juice and coriander in a bowl and whisk it until the curry paste is dissolved.

3 Place the broccoli, mange tout, spring onion and pak choi in the centre of the paper and top with the fish. Pour the sauce over everything and roll the parcel up into a package as per the parcel lesson on page 204.

4 Bake the parcel on a tray in the oven for 12 minutes or, if using a barbecue, wrap the parcel in foil and pop it straight onto the coals.

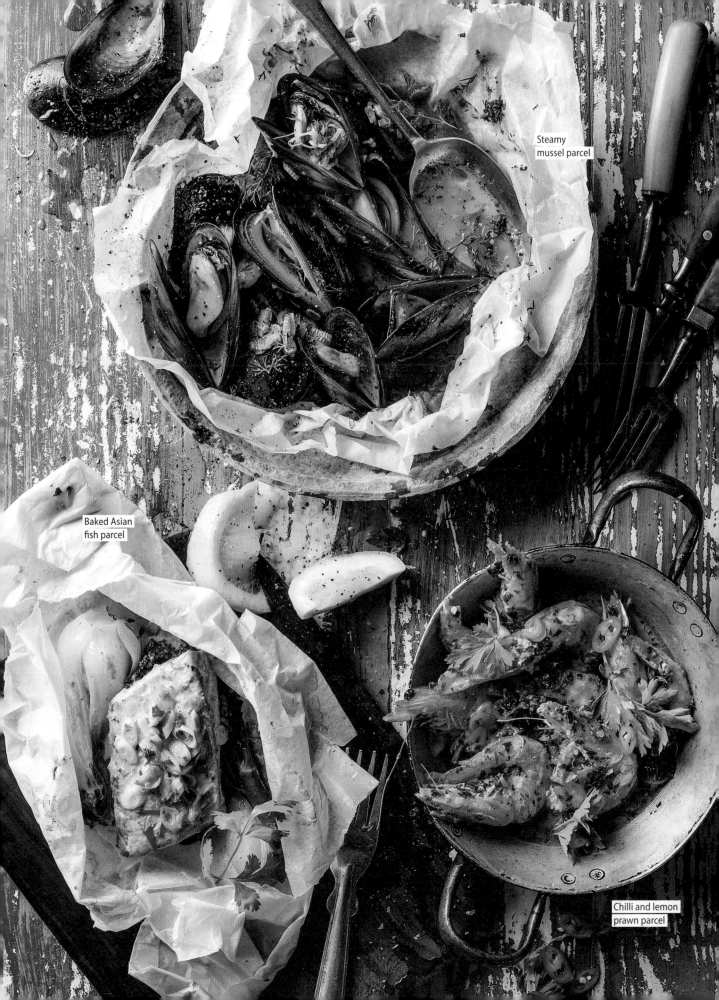

Steamy
mussel parcel

Baked Asian
fish parcel

Chilli and lemon
prawn parcel

CLEANING SQUID

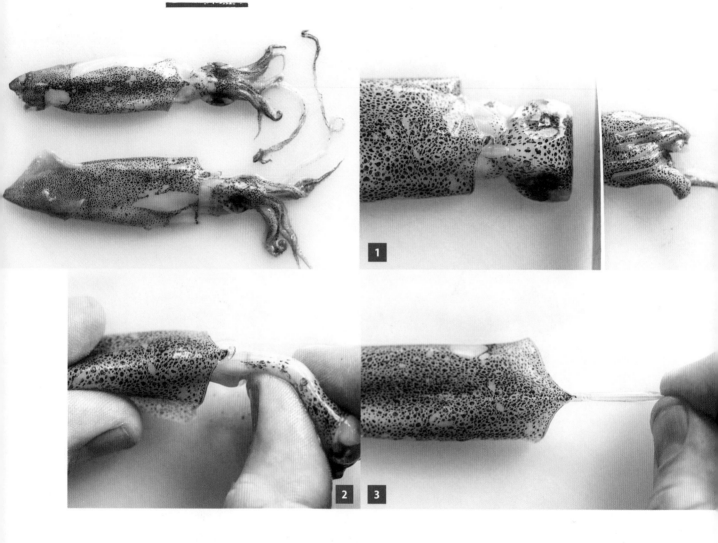

I find that the squid I can get from my fishmonger (or supermarket) already cleaned often ends up tough, while the stuff I get fresh, and clean myself is usually tender and more delicious. I think it's worth the effort. So this lesson is for those of you who agree and would prefer to get your squid uncleaned.

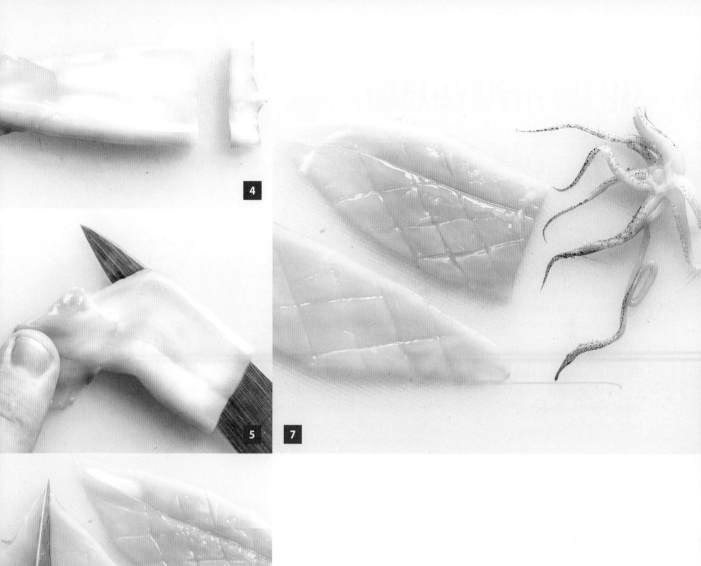

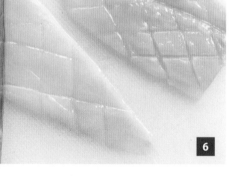

1 Cut off the tentacles above the beak.

2 Grab the head and pull it out of the tube.

3 Find the plasticky spine in the tube and pull that out with your finger.

4 Wash the colour off with a cloth and some fresh running water, and cut off the rough bit at the end. You don't *have* to cut it off, but it does look neater.

5 Insert your knife into the tube, slide it up to split it open, then cut it in two lengthways.

6 Gently score the tubes by running your blade over the surface, being careful not to cut all the way through.

7 Now follow the steps in the recipe.

SALT AND PEPPER CALAMARI

See page 213

Serves 2

I've made this recipe to serve two, because more than two portions in a batch won't cook very well. The calamari will release their juices before they're able to get any colour or roasted goodness.

TARTARE SAUCE

180ml mayonnaise (see page 274)

1 tsp Dijon mustard

Juice and zest of 1 lemon

¼ tsp Tabasco or hot sauce

2 tbsp finely chopped dill pickles

1 tbsp capers

½ red onion, finely chopped

1 tbsp flat-leaf parsley, chopped

1 tbsp fresh tarragon, chopped

1 tbsp fresh dill, chopped

Salt and black pepper

CALAMARI

400g calamari tubes and tentacles,
   cleaned and scored

1 egg white, lightly whisked

40g white sesame seeds

40g black sesame seeds

500ml avocado oil

Sea salt flakes and black pepper

1 lemon, cut into wedges

1 small handful fresh mint, chopped

1 small handful flat-leaf parsley,
   roughly chopped

1 First, make the tartare sauce by combining the mayonnaise, Dijon mustard, lemon juice and zest, Tabasco sauce, pickles, capers, onion, parsley, tarragon, dill and seasoning. Leave the mix in the fridge for an hour or so to infuse.

2 Drain any excess liquid from the calamari, pat them dry and place in a mixing bowl.

3 Season the calamari liberally with salt and pepper.

4 Add the egg white to the tubes and mix them vigorously for 3 or 4 minutes. The egg white and the calamari juices should create a paste coating the squid.

5 Now dip each piece of calamari covered in egg white into the white and black sesame seeds to cover.

6 Heat the oil in a large pan and shallow fry for 4 minutes, flipping with a slotted spoon. Be careful, the oil will spit. When ready, drain the calamari on paper towel.

7 Place the calamari in a clean mixing bowl while they're still hot, give them a final sprinkle of salt flakes, a big squeeze of lemon juice and cover them with the herbs.

8 Give them a quick toss to spread the herbs and serve immediately with the tartare sauce, or just as is.

GOES WELL WITH: Edamame Bean and Radish Salad, Stir-fried Spring Onions and Pak Choi.

GARLIC SQUID WITH SHRIMP PASTE AND OYSTER SAUCE

See page 213

Serves 2

Embrace the shrimp paste. When you read the ingredients on this list, they might scare you. I assure you, you have never tasted calamari with this much depth. It's next level.

4 tbsp avocado oil

1 head garlic, broken apart, cloves peeled and loosely chopped

1½ tbsp whole black peppercorns, pounded in a pestle and mortar until cracked

1 tsp shrimp paste

500g or 4 whole squid, cleaned, and cut into rings and tentacles

6 large spring onions, cut into 5cm pieces

3 tbsp oyster sauce

1 tsp Thai chilli paste

1 lime, cut into wedges

1 Get the avocado oil scorching-hot in a large pan. Add the garlic and peppercorns to fry for a minute or so.

2 Add the shrimp paste and use a wooden spoon to break it up and stir it around for 30 seconds.

3 Tip the squid into the pan and stir-fry it until it begins to caramelise. The garlic and the peppercorns will be dark and bittersweet by this stage.

4 Add the spring onions, oyster sauce and chilli paste and stir-fry until the spring onions are wilted. Serve immediately with wedges of lime.

GREAT ON ITS OWN AS A STARTER.

THAI PRAWN CAKES WITH THAI MAYO

Serves 4

This Thai sauce doesn't actually exist in Thailand; it's my take on mayonnaise we used to make at Ginja restaurant in Cape Town in my linecook days. It uses all the ingredients the Thai use to season their food, but in a mayonnaise, which is not Thai at all.

600g raw prawn tails, cleaned,
  half whole, half chopped

2 large handfuls fresh coriander,
  roughly chopped

1 red chilli, deseeded and
  finely chopped

Juice and zest of 2 limes

1 tsp minced garlic

1 thumb ginger, finely grated

125ml mayonnaise

1 small handful basil, picked and
  stems discarded

1 spring onion, finely chopped

1 tbsp fish sauce

2 tbsp coconut oil

1 Place the whole prawns, one handful of coriander, chilli, lime zest, garlic and ginger in a food processor and whizz until the mixture is fine.

2 Tip the mix out into a bowl. Mix through the chopped prawns and season with a big pinch of salt.

3 Place a bowl of water next to your work area and dip your hands in to wet them before forming 12 little prawn cakes. Leave them in the fridge to firm up for half an hour.

4 Now make the Un-Thai'd sauce by blitzing the remaining coriander, mayonnaise, basil, spring onion, lime juice and fish sauce with a stick blender in a small jug. If you're fancy, you could strain this through a sieve, otherwise just pop it in the fridge to infuse while you cook the prawn cakes.

5 Heat a couple of tablespoons of coconut oil in a large frying pan and add the prawn cakes. Make sure there is enough space between them for you to turn them easily.

6 Let them cook for about 4 minutes on each side, then transfer them to serving plates, or a platter.

7 Serve them with a twist of lime and the Un-Thai'd Sauce in a dipping bowl.

GOES WELL WITH: Edamame Bean and Radish Salad, Stir-fried Spring Onions and Pak Choi.

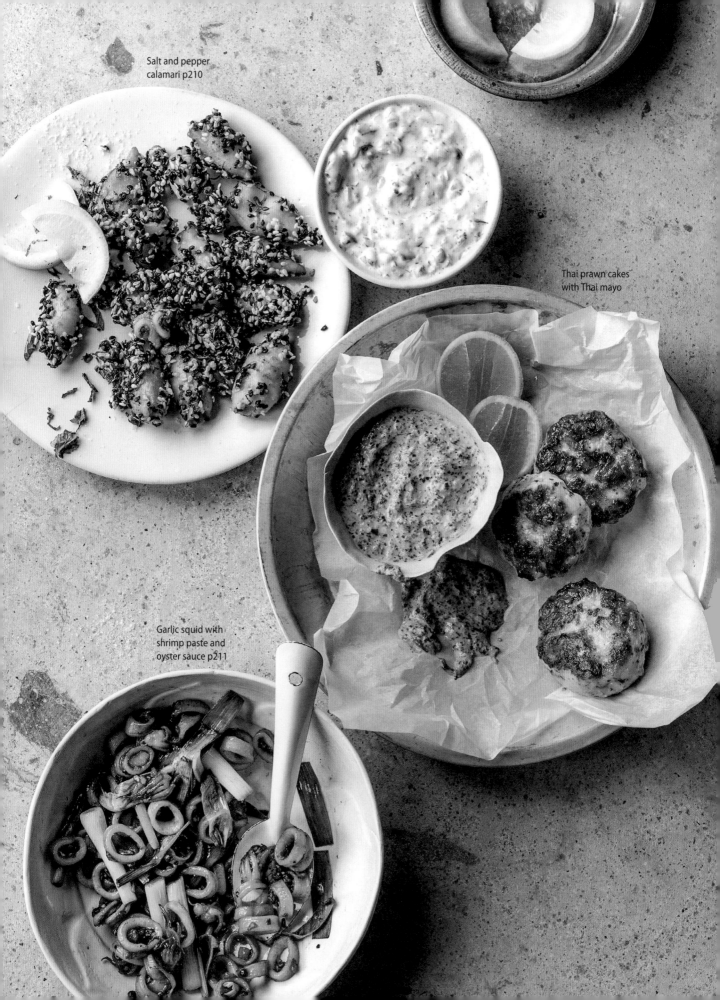

Salt and pepper
calamari p210

Thai prawn cakes
with Thai mayo

Garlic squid with
shrimp paste and
oyster sauce p211

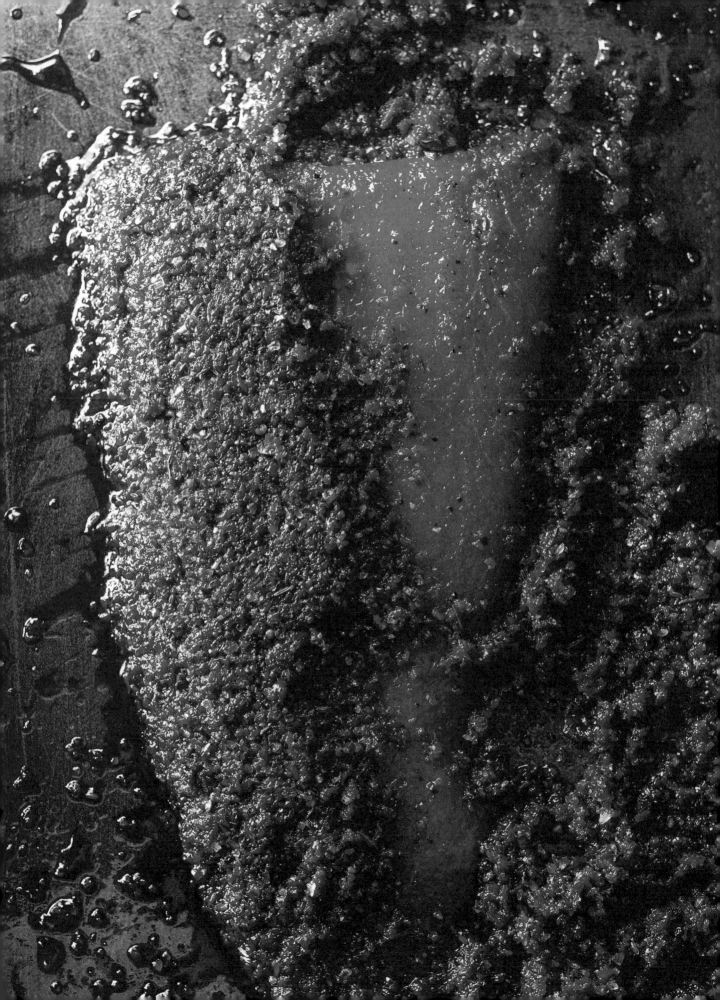

HOT-SMOKED FISH PLANK

See page 217

Makes 1.2kg, serves 10 as a starter

Plank-smoking is big in North America, but I've recently found plank sets at a number of online stores in the UK, South Africa and Australia. It is a much easier way to smoke fish, and it seems suppliers are upping their game in terms of the type of planks you can get. Over and above the traditional cherry and cedar woods, you can now find alder, maple, hickory and white oak, all in the same set.

1.2kg side of salmon, yellowtail or
  barramundi, scaled, pin-boned
1 plank of cherry, cedar, alder,
  maple, hickory or white oak
  (130mm x 280mm x 14mm)
Zest and juice of 1 big waxy lemon
1 large handful fresh dill, finely chopped
½ tsp salt
½ tsp black pepper
3 tbsp olive oil
Mayonnaise, to serve
Lemon, to serve
2 large handfuls watercress, to serve

1   Preheat a BBQ to medium heat (for this one you can also use a Weber or a gas grill).
2   Place the fish, skin-side down, on the plank.
3   Mix the lemon zest, juice, dill, salt, pepper and olive oil together, and spread the mix evenly over the top of the fish. Use your hands if you have to.
4   Place the plank (fish-side up!) directly on the grill and close the BBQ, leaving it to cook for 15 minutes.
5   After 15 minutes, move the plank directly onto a trivet and serve the fish with a dollop of mayonnaise, a twist of lemon and watercress.

'BEETEN' SALMON

See page 217

Makes 1.2kg, serves 10 as a starter

250g coarse salt
1 tbsp whole black peppercorns, cracked
1 tbsp dill seeds
1 tbsp caraway seeds
2 bay leaves, crushed
Zest of 1 lemon
250g raw beetroot, peeled
  and quartered
1.2kg salmon fillet, pin-boned
250ml mayonnaise (see page 274)
100g rocket
3 limes, cut into wedges

1   Put all the ingredients, except the salmon, mayonnaise, rocket and lime wedges, in a food processor and whizz it until the beets have broken down and you have chunky red paste.
2   Place the salmon in a slightly oiled dish big enough to fit the whole side in, pat dry, then cover it with the marinade.
3   Place a tray on top of the fish to weigh it down, and fill the top tray with anything heavy (wine bottles, bricks, bags of salt, sugar, whatever) and leave it in the fridge for 24 hours.
4   After 24 hours, gently scrape the marinade off the fish, wiping it clean with a wet cloth, and patting it dry with a dry one.
5   The next step requires the sharpest knife you have in the house. Place the fish skin-side down on a cutting board and slice it from side to side down to the skin, then use the blade to cut the slices from the skin and place them neatly on a serving platter. The end result will give you many slices, and one huge piece of skin left on the board.
6   Serve the salmon with mayonnaise, rocket and lime wedges.

SARDINES WITH WARM CHORIZO AND TOMATO DRESSING

Serves 4

8 fresh whole sardines, cleaned

1 tsp smoked paprika

4 tbsp olive oil

80g chorizo, casing removed and finely chopped

2 garlic cloves, finely chopped

Juice and zest of 2 lemons

100g cherry tomatoes, quartered

1 large handful flat-leaf parsley, roughly chopped

Lemon wedges, to serve

Salt and pepper

1 Season the sardines with salt, pepper and smoked paprika.

2 Heat a large pan up to a medium heat and add 2 tablespoons of olive oil.

3 Add the sardines and fry them for 4 minutes on each side to crisp the skin.

4 Once they are cooked, remove them from the pan and add the remaining olive oil to the pan.

5 Add the chorizo and sauté it until it has rendered most of its fat and is beginning to crisp up.

6 Now add the garlic, lemon juice and zest, and let them sizzle for a minute.

7 Finally, add the cherry tomatoes and fire up the pan as hot as possible while the tomatoes cook.

8 Arrange the fish on a platter with some lemon wedges and spoon the dressing over before serving.

GOES WELL WITH: Gomen Wat.

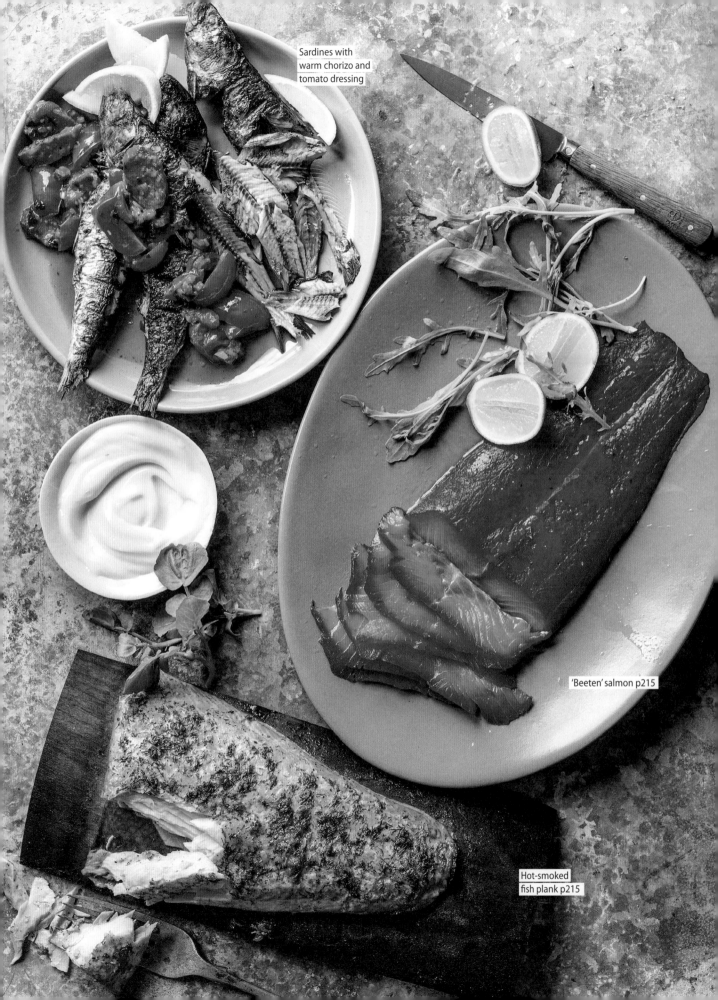

Sardines with warm chorizo and tomato dressing

'Beeten' salmon p215

Hot-smoked fish plank p215

PERSIAN-STYLE STUFFED FISH BAKE

Serves 6

5 tbsp olive oil

1 onion, thinly sliced

3 tbsp tamarind paste

4 garlic cloves, minced

1 big handful coriander,
   roughly chopped

1 big handful flat-leaf parsley,
   roughly chopped

1 big handful tarragon, very
   roughly chopped

1 whole fish (salmon, trout, Cape
   salmon, yellowtail, etc), about 1kg
   when filleted, scaled and boned

2 limes, quartered

Salt and black pepper

Extra olive oil for cooking

1 Heat your oven up to 180°C and grease a baking sheet with a little olive oil.
2 Combine the oil, onion, tamarind, garlic and herbs in a mixing bowl.
3 Place five 25cm pieces of string on the baking sheet and lay one fillet of fish, skin-side down, across the strings.
4 Use your hands to pack the herb mixture onto the fillet, then place the other fillet on top, skin-side up.
5 Now wrap the strings around the two fillets and tie them tightly together.
6 Heat 3 more tablespoons of olive oil to a very high heat in a large frying pan, then carefully lift the fish into the pan to fry on each side for five minutes to crisp up the skin.
7 Use a spatula or two, or just tip the pan to slide the fish back onto the baking tray, then pop it in the oven for 10 minutes.
8 When it has finished cooking, slice it into portions with a sharp knife and serve.

BAKED FISH WITH ALMOND AND PEPPERS

Serves 4

4 small trout fillets, boned

4 tbsp butter

40g sliced almonds

2 garlic cloves, chopped

1 tbsp chopped thyme leaves

1 red pepper, finely chopped

4 leathery sundried tomatoes,
   finely diced

Zest and juice of 1 lemon

Salt and pepper

1 Preheat your oven to 180°C.
2 Place the fillets skin-side down on a baking tray and season them with salt and pepper.
3 Heat the butter to a medium heat, add the almonds and sauté them until you can smell the nuttiness coming from the pan.
4 Now add the garlic, thyme and red pepper and sauté until they soften.
5 Add the sundried tomatoes and the lemon zest and juice. Stir for a minute until well mixed, then remove from the heat and pack the mix as a 'crust' over the four fillets of trout.
6 Bake them in the oven for 10 to 15 minutes and serve immediately.

GOES WELL WITH: Cauliflower Colcannon, Salsa Verde, Mayonnaise.

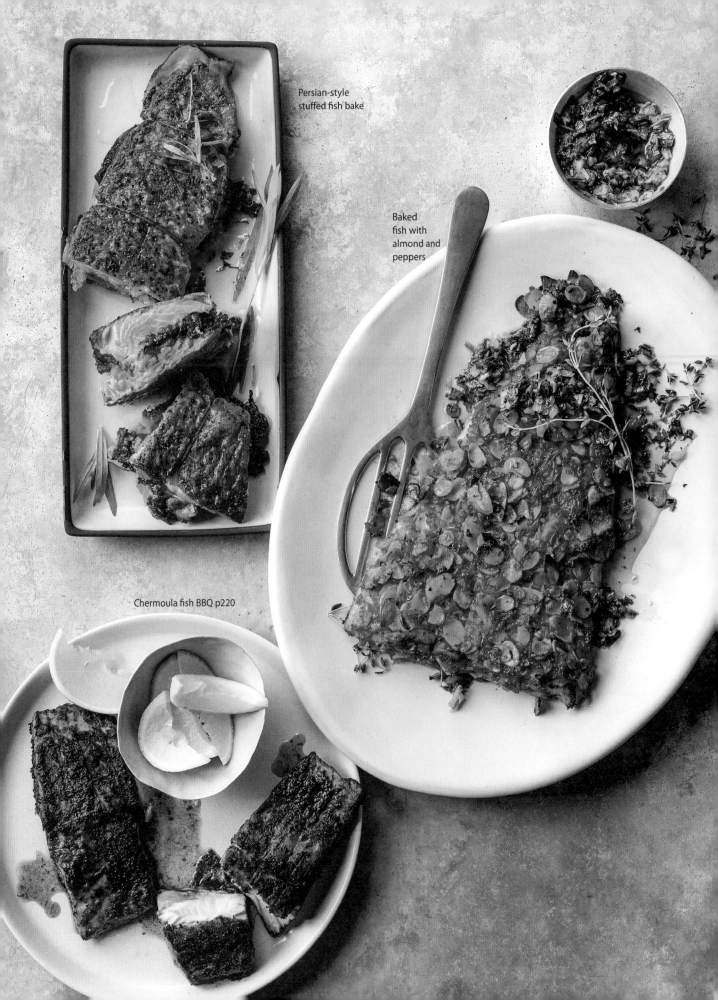

Persian-style
stuffed fish bake

Baked
fish with
almond and
peppers

Chermoula fish BBQ p220

CHERMOULA FISH BBQ

See page 219

Serves 4

Juice of 2 fat lemons
1 garlic clove, peeled
1 tbsp tomato paste
250ml olive oil
½ tsp coarse salt
½ tsp dried red chilli
1 handful fresh coriander
1 handful flat-leaf parsley
2 tbsp ground coriander
2 tbsp ground cumin
1 tbsp paprika
1½ tbsp turmeric
4 x 180g fillets or steaks of oily fish

1   Whizz everything except for the fish in a food processor, then tip the paste into a frying pan and fry it on a medium heat until it is nicely caramelised and oil has split from the mixture.

2   Light up a barbecue and get it to a high heat.

3   Divide the marinade between the fish pieces and baste them all over, before laying them out on an oiled sandwich grid and fastening it closed.

4   Place the grid over the hottest part of the fire and cook the fish for 5 minutes before turning it. Leave it for another 5 minutes, then keep turning it until you see the little white bits of protein coming out between the flecks of the fish – that means it is done.

5   Now remove the fish from the grid, carefully using any sharp tool that will help you do so without breaking the meat apart, and serve.

GOES WELL WITH: Berbere Cauliflower with Tarator.
For the full recipe for Chermoula, see page 288.

'BARBECUE MAY NOT BE
THE ROAD TO
WORLD PEACE,
BUT IT'S A START.'
– ANTHONY BOURDAIN

EGGS

Eggs are wonderful: versatile, delicious and nature's perfect multivitamin. For so long the falsely convicted felon of the food world, the wholesome egg has been welcomed back onto the recommended eating lists like a returning hero. I could write a whole book on eggs. For now this section will do.

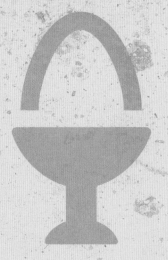

BRIE AND MUSHROOM FRITTATA

A frittata or crustless quiche is a great way to include egg and vegetables in your breakfast or lunch. We make ours in an oven-proof pan. This way you can fry the ingredients that you want in your frittata, pour in the eggs and pop it straight into the oven to cook. Only one dirty pan.

See page 225

Serves 1

3 extra-large eggs
4 tbsp cream
1 tbsp butter
100g sliced mushrooms of any kind
5 thick slices Brie (or Camembert)
Salt and pepper

1 Preheat your oven to 180°C.
2 In a bowl, whisk together the eggs and cream with some salt and pepper.
3 In a frying pan that can go in the oven, melt the butter over a medium heat.
4 Add the mushrooms and sauté them until golden-brown.
5 Now pour the egg mixture over the mushrooms, top with the sliced Brie and pop the pan into the oven for about 5 minutes or until the eggs are cooked through.
6 Serve immediately.

AVOCADO, MARINATED PEPPER AND CREAM CHEESE EGG ROLL

See page 225

Serves 1

This is one of my favourite egg roll toppings. To be honest, this combo was one of my go-tos for pizza toppings… sigh.

1 basic egg roll (see page 228)
3 or 4 pieces marinated red peppers
½ avocado, thickly sliced
1 dollop cream cheese (optional)
1 slice lemon
Salt and pepper

1 Make the egg roll and wait for it to cool.
2 Layer the toppings down the middle.
3 Finish it off with a twist of lemon, a crack of black pepper and a sprinkling of salt before rolling it up and tucking in.

TOMATO, SALAMI, PECORINO AND BASIL OMELETTE

Serves 1

You could totally use Cheddar instead of pecorino for this one. If you do use Cheddar, I would triple the quantity to make sure that what you miss in salty flavour you make up in gooey goodness.

2 large eggs

1 finger of butter

4 slow-roasted or pan-fried cherry tomatoes

4 slices salami

Small handful grated pecorino

5 leaves fresh basil

Salt and pepper

1 Turn the grill in your oven on to high (so it has time to warm up while you get your other bits together) and place one rack as close to the heating element as possible.

2 Put a small omelette-sized pan on a fairly high heat

3 In a small bowl, mix the eggs with some salt and pepper.

4 Add a knob of butter to the pan and the moment it has melted, add the eggs.

5 Using a wooden spoon or spatula, move the mixture around, exposing as much of the mix as possible to the base of the pan, but without leaving any gaps.

6 Once the egg has formed a reasonably solid base, but is still very runny on top, remove it from the heat.

7 Add the cherry tomatoes and salami and cover with the grated cheese, then place the whole pan under the grill.

8 Watch and wait as the eggs puff up and the cheese starts to bubble and melt. The moment your cheese starts going brown and bubbly, remove it from the oven.

9 Scatter with basil leaves and extra cheese, if you have any, and devour it.

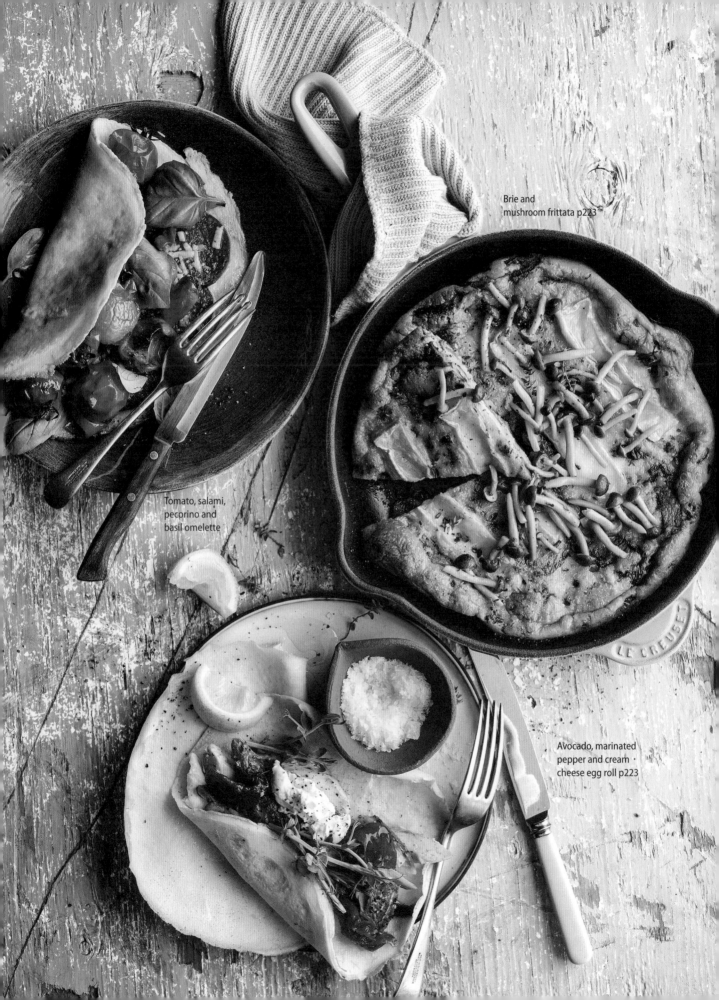

Brie and
mushroom frittata p223

Tomato, salami,
pecorino and
basil omelette

Avocado, marinated
pepper and cream
cheese egg roll p223

BOILED EGGS

Eggs!

1 Heat a saucepan of water to a gentle simmer. If the heat is too high, the eggs will crack, but if it's too low, you won't be able to time the cooking properly.
2 Once the water is at a gentle simmer, carefully lower the eggs into the pot.
3 Leave them to cook as long as needed (see opposite), then remove them from the water and put them straight into iced water to stop the cooking process.
4 Peel hard-boiled eggs underwater to avoid them breaking apart.

POACHED EGGS

Makes 1 perfect poached egg

2 tbsp apple cider vinegar
1 large egg

The quest for the perfect poached egg starts in the store or at the market. The freshest eggs poach the best because they hold their shape in the poaching liquid. Older eggs, while still fine to eat, tend to fill the pot with a web of egg white that would make a baboon spider blush.

1 Fill a small saucepan with water, add a splash of apple cider vinegar, and bring to a very light simmer (slightly fewer bubbles than lightly sparkling water).
2 Break the egg into a ramekin or small bowl. Now swirl the water to create a gentle whirlpool in the saucepan, lower the ramekin into the middle of the whirlpool and gently tip out the egg.
3 As the egg poaches, use a slotted spoon to flip it every minute or so.
4 Cook your egg as long as needed (see opposite).
5 If you intend on serving a number of eggs at the same time, remove them 1 minute before the allotted time. Use a slotted spoon to move each egg to a bowl of iced water to make sure they stop cooking instantly. If you want to be fancy, you can pick all the bits of loose egg white off the eggs. Either way, before serving, drop them back into the water to warm through for a minute or so.
6 When the eggs are ready, use a slotted spoon to remove them from the water. Dab them dry by tipping them onto a clean towel then back into the spoon, before sliding them onto the plate.

EGG POACHER 'POACHED' EGGS

Serves 4

A dash of any oil
4 large eggs

If you're a big-time foodie, you might judge me for putting this in here. Truth is, I don't care. It might be vintage, but you just don't get better-shaped, more perfectly cooked eggs than eggs cooked in these things. Your eggs also don't need to be laid yesterday. And a five-year-old could make them.

1 Fill an egg-poaching pan with 2cm of water. Place the pan over a medium heat and bring to a simmer.
2 Lightly oil the poaching cups and warm the cups in the pan.
3 Crack an egg into each cup, cover the pan and cook. A medium egg will cook in 3 to 4 minutes.

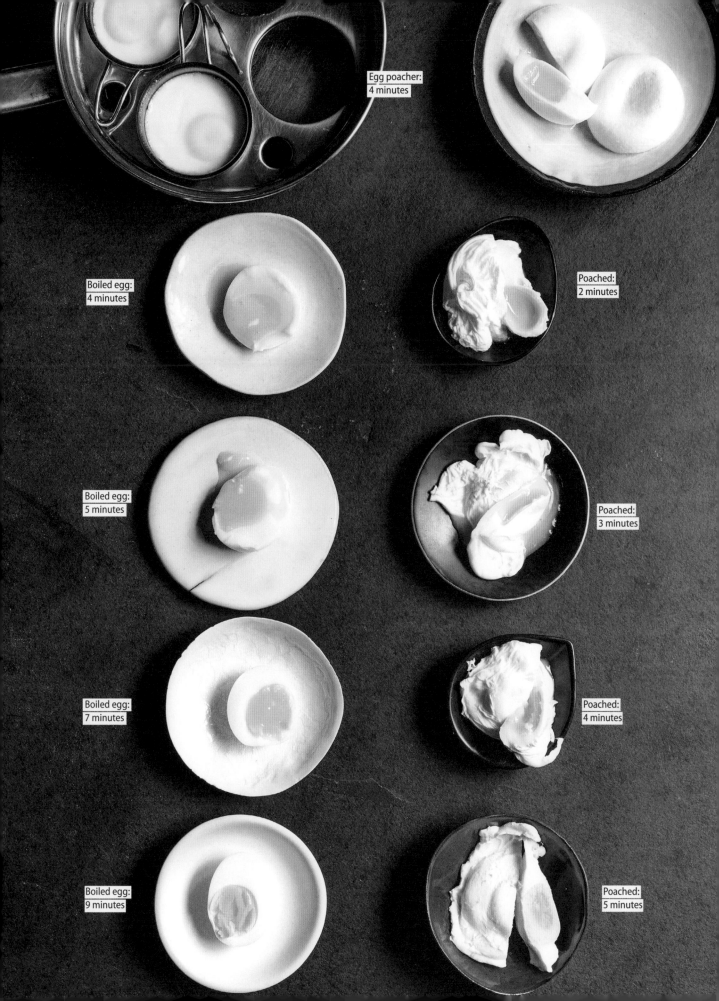

Egg poacher:
4 minutes

Boiled egg:
4 minutes

Poached:
2 minutes

Boiled egg:
5 minutes

Poached:
3 minutes

Boiled egg:
7 minutes

Poached:
4 minutes

Boiled egg:
9 minutes

Poached:
5 minutes

BASIC EGG ROLL

Serves 1

2 large eggs
1 finger of butter

An egg roll is a thin omelette that you can fill with almost anything for breakfast, food on the go or lunchtime wraps. The versatility of this recipe is endless. Egg rolls can also double up as a 'pancake' for hungry children (or adults).

1 Whisk the eggs very well together until they are light and foamy.
2 Heat a frying pan with some butter and allow to get up to a medium heat.
3 Pour the egg mixture into the pan and swish it around so that the mixture covers the bottom of the pan.
4 Cook the egg gently until it sets. Using a spatula, flip it over and let the egg cook gently on the other side.
5 Remove from the heat and fill with your choice of filling. Here are some ideas: smoked salmon, cream cheese and avocado with a squeeze of lemon and cracked black pepper; Black Forest ham, basil pesto, cream cheese and rocket; crispy bacon, Brie, sautéed cherry tomatoes and basil – try this with warm ingredients.

DANISH-STYLE CURRIED EGG MAYO

Serves 4

8 hard-boiled eggs, peeled and chopped
120ml mayonnaise
2 tsp curry powder
A small squeeze of lemon to taste
1 handful chopped chives
Salt and pepper

1 Mix all the ingredients together in a mixing bowl and pop it into the fridge for an hour to let the flavours infuse.
2 Serve on slices of cucumber or seed crackers (or whatever you're into).

SCRAMBLED EGGS

Serves 1

3 extra-large eggs
a big whack of salt
1 tbsp butter

Chopped spring onions or chives are best added into scrambled eggs while they are still raw. They release an amazing freshness and flavour during the cooking that is unbeatable. Another great flavour in scrambled eggs is a good sprinkling of smoked paprika.

1 Crack the eggs into a bowl and beat them along with the salt.
2 Now melt some butter in a pan on a medium heat and pour in the eggs.
3 Stir continuously with a spatula until the eggs are firm and steaming.
4 At this point, you could add any other ingredients that you like.
5 Mix your flavouring through and serve immediately.

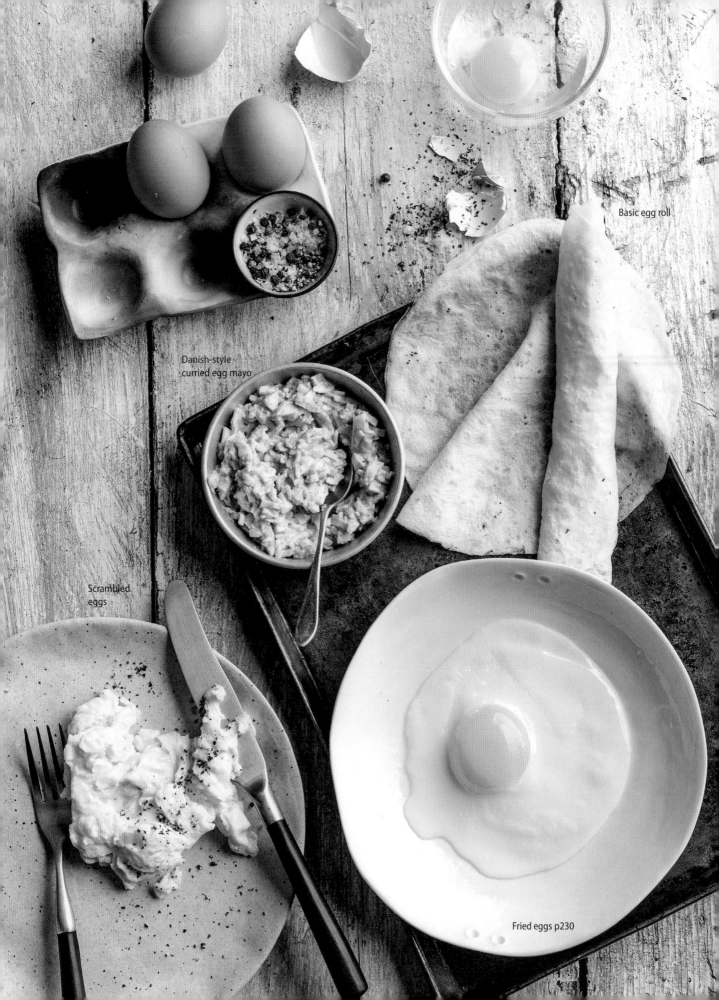

Basic egg roll

Danish-style
curried egg mayo

Scrambled
eggs

Fried eggs p230

THE BEST EGG MAYO

Serves 4

8 hard-boiled eggs, peeled and
  chopped
125ml mayonnaise (see page 274)
1 tsp Dijon mustard
2 spring onions, finely chopped
½ tsp salt
1 tsp black pepper
1 big pinch paprika

1 Mix all the ingredients together in a mixing bowl and pop it into the fridge for an hour
   to let the flavours infuse.
2 Enjoy it for breakfast, lunch or dinner as a topping on anything you like!

FRIED EGGS

See page 229

*When I fry eggs sunny-side up, I always find it hard to get the top of the egg cooked. To
counter this, I use a pan with a fitted lid, and when the base of the egg is cooked, I remove
the pan from the heat and pop the lid on to create a mini oven. This provides just enough
indirect heat to cook the top of the egg while keeping it, well, sunny.*

1 tbsp butter
2 extra-large eggs

1 Place a large pan onto a very low heat and melt the butter.
2 Once the butter begins to bubble, crack the eggs into the pan.
3 Let them tick away – perfect eggs take longer – until the white protein on top of the
   egg has cooked but before the yolk is completely done.
4 For sunny-side up, you can take them off the heat and put the lid on for a minute or
   two just to firm up the top of the eggs.
5 For over-easy, flip them gently and leave for about 30 seconds.

FERTILISERS

I call 'gut-healthy foods' fertilisers because, when you're looking after your gut lining and your gut biome, fertilising them is pretty much what you're doing. Given that your gut is about the size of a tennis court and it's where all the action happens, you may want to consider it Wimbledon Centre Court. Every day you're playing the game of your life, so best to keep it in shape. Water it, fertilise it, look after it daily.

There are two types of fertiliser:

Bone broth: rich with all the nutrients and minerals your body needs to build and protect your gut lining.

Word on the street has it that consuming bone broth is better for you than taking supplements, because the nutrients in bone broth are more bioavailable (which means you digest them properly). Personally, I think bone broths are better than supplements because they taste like food.

You can use your broth as the base for soup or gravy, or it can be drunk as is. If you're drinking it neat, try adding a little lemon juice, black pepper and chilli sauce to spice it up.

Fermented foods and drinks: rich with nutrients as a result of the fermentation process.

Foods like natural yoghurt, sauerkraut and kimchi, and drinks like kefir and kombucha, help repopulate or feed your gut bacteria.

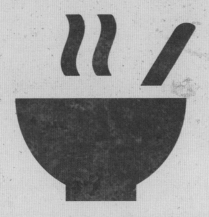

BASIC BROTH

See pages 237, 239, 241

Makes about 2 litres

1½kg beef, pork, chicken or fish bones
200g carrots, cut into chunks
2 stalks celery, cut into chunks
1 onion, cut into chunks
2 leeks, cut into chunks
3 litres water (or more)
4 sprigs parsley
2 sprigs thyme
1 bay leaf
5 peppercorns

1 Heat your oven to 220°C.
2 Place the bones in a roasting pan and roast for 30 minutes until well browned, turning occasionally (no need to oil or season).
3 When the bones are brown, add the carrots, celery, onion and leeks to the pan and roast for a further 5 minutes. Give everything a good stir before it goes into the oven.

Skip the first three steps for fish broth.

4 Transfer everything from the roasting pan into a large pot, ensuring you scrape out all the flavourful sticky bits.
5 Add the remaining ingredients to the pot and cover with water. You could fill the entire pot.
6 Bring to a boil, then drop the heat to a gentle simmer, and leave it to simmer uncovered for about 4 hours (30 minutes for fish broth), skimming off any scum that rises to the surface.
7 Once you hit 4 hours (30 minutes for fish), strain the stock through a fine sieve or muslin cloth and leave it to cool.
8 If the broth is still very bland, you can reduce it until the volume decreases and the flavour intensifies.
9 You can use it immediately or freeze for later use. It will keep in the freezer for months.

OXTAIL STEW

Serves 4

1.25kg oxtail, cut at each joint
4 tbsp olive oil
2 leeks, chopped
2 carrots, chopped
2 celery stalks, chopped
3 tbsp tomato paste
250ml red wine
1 handful thyme sprigs
1 large sprig rosemary
2 fresh bay leaves
2 cloves
1 x 400g can whole peeled tomatoes
500ml basic beef broth (see above)
Salt and pepper

1 Preheat your oven to 160°C.
2 Season the oxtail with salt and pepper, then seal them off in the oil in a medium oven-proof pot. Fry in batches that cover one layer of the pot only, until dark-brown all over.
3 Once all the oxtail pieces are done and removed, add the leeks, carrots and celery to the same fat, and sauté them until golden-brown.
4 Add the tomato paste and sauté until it begins to catch at the bottom of the pot.
5 Pour in the wine. As it boils, use a wooden spoon to scrape the sediment at the bottom of the pot into the sauce.
6 Add the thyme, rosemary, bay leaves and cloves, and simmer until the wine has reduced by half.
7 Now add the oxtail, tomatoes and broth or stock, and top up with water or stock to cover the meat.
8 Bring it all to the boil then put the lid on and pop it in the oven for 3 hours.
9 After 3 hours, the meat should be falling off the bone and the stew will be ready to serve.
10 If you'd like the sauce a bit thicker, you can strain it off into a smaller pot and reduce it down to a thick, intense gravy.

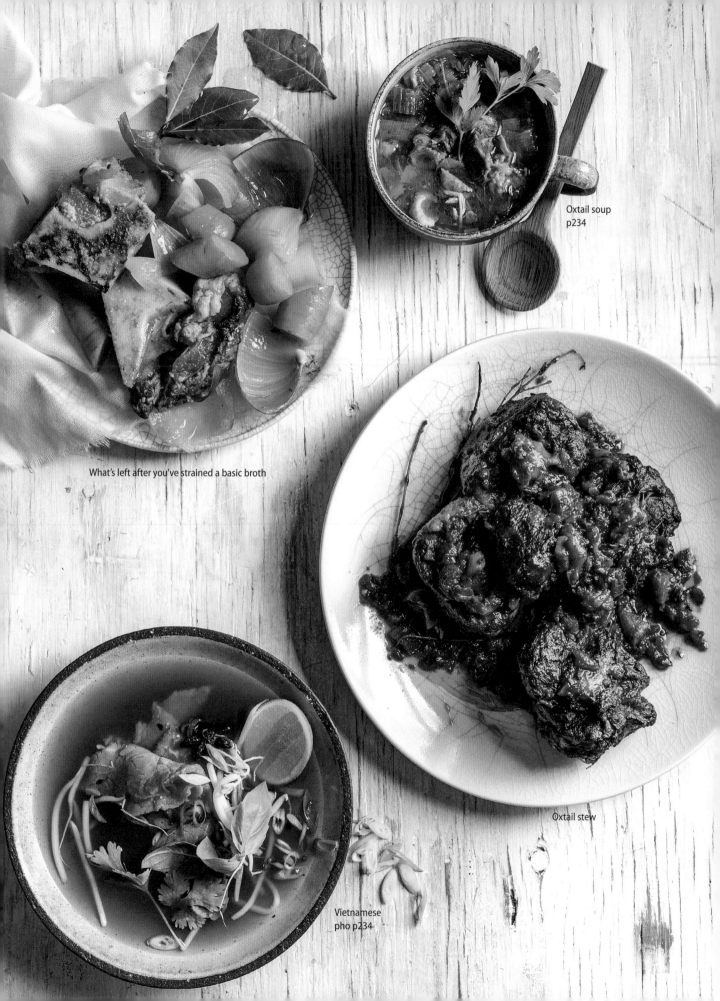

Oxtail soup
p234

What's left after you've strained a basic broth

Oxtail stew

Vietnamese
pho p234

VIETNAMESE PHO

Serves 4

Pho is the sneakiest way to get everyone eating broth without them even noticing. All your guests can make their own bowls of colourful garnish, then smother their creations in steaming hot broth. It's visually, gastronomically and nutritionally epic.

See page 233

PHO BROTH

1 large onion

1 thick thumb of ginger, whole

1½ litres basic beef broth (page 232) or beef stock

6 star anise

2 cinnamon sticks

4 cloves

1 tsp coriander seeds

1 tsp black peppercorns

2 tbsp fish sauce

2 tbsp lime juice

GARNISH

400g raw beef fillet, very thinly sliced

200g bean sprouts

3 spring onions, thinly sliced

1 small handful chopped fresh coriander

1 small handful roughly chopped basil leaves

1 fresh red chilli, thinly sliced

2 limes cut into quarters

Fish sauce, to serve

Hot chilli sauce, to serve

1 Start off by charring the onion and the ginger directly on the gas hob, like you would a pepper.
2 In the meantime, heat your broth up to a simmer in a medium-sized pot.
3 Then add all the spices, charred onion and ginger to the broth and leave to tick away for about 45 minutes. It should reduce, enhancing the flavours and infusing with the aromatics.
4 While the broth is simmering, get all of your garnishes ready and lay them out on the table in separate bowls. You can leave the chilli sauce and the fish sauce in the bottles.
5 When the garnishes and the broth are ready, get everyone seated around the table and tell them to fill their bowls with their favourite garnishes.
6 Now get them to fill their bowls to the brim with steaming broth, and enjoy.

OXTAIL SOUP

Serves 4

This is the most fantastic thing to do with leftover oxtail stew.

See page 233

2 fingers butter

2 large leeks, finely chopped

2 portions of oxtail stew; meat flaked, bones discarded (page 232)

1½ litres basic beef broth (page 232)

2 bay leaves

3 sprigs thyme

1 handful flat-leaf parsley, roughly chopped

40g watercress

1 Melt the butter in a large pot and gently fry the leeks in it until they soften.
2 Now add the oxtail, beef broth, bay leaves and thyme and bring to the boil.
3 As it begins to boil, reduce the heat and allow it to simmer for 20 minutes.
4 After 20 minutes, remove the soup from the heat and remove the bay and thyme.
5 Throw in the parsley and give it a quick stir before serving immediately with a handful of watercress in each portion.

CHICKEN SOUP FOR THE SOUL

See page 237

Serves 4

Chicken soup for the soul says it all. This is basically a repeat of the original broth-making process, but you are doubling up on the nutrients and flavour. You could add anything else you like to this. Chilli, bacon, cream or mushrooms will be great.

**400g boneless chicken thighs,
  thinly sliced**

1 stick celery, cut into bite-sized chunks

3 large leeks, sliced into thick discs

**1 massive carrot cut in half, lengthways
  and then into 1cm thick pieces**

**1½ litres basic chicken broth (page 232)
  or stock**

1 bay leaf

**1 small handful flat-leaf parsley,
  roughly chopped**

Juice of 1 lemon

Salt and black pepper

1   Place everything apart from the seasoning, parsley and lemon juice into a medium-sized pot.

2   Pump the heat up until it all hits a rolling boil, then drop it down to a gentle simmer.

3   Leave it like that for about an hour, topping up with water if it reduces too much (only top it up to the level at which you started, otherwise you'll dilute it).

4   By this point the chicken should be tender and the vegetables should be soft.

5   Add the parsley and lemon juice, season with salt and pepper to taste, and serve.

CHICKEN AND COCONUT SOUP

Serves 4

It might be the combo of old school and new school that makes this dish so good. After all, chicken has been the low-fat go-to for decades, and coconut is officially the hottest health food since wholewheat bread. But I reckon it's down to the combined sensations of silky coconut cream on the palate and Thai heat and aromatics whacking you in the mouth.

2 tsp coconut oil

150g any wild mushrooms, sliced

1½ thumbs fresh ginger, peeled and thinly sliced

2 garlic cloves, minced

2 stalks lemongrass, smashed

1 red pepper, sliced into strips

1 tsp Thai chilli paste (or more if you like it hotter)

750ml basic chicken broth (page 232)

375ml light coconut milk

2 tbsp fish sauce

Juice of ½ lime

4 small chicken breasts, finely sliced

1 handful fresh coriander, roughly chopped

3 spring onions, thinly sliced

1   Get the oil nice and hot in a medium-sized pot and fry the mushrooms until they're soft and beginning to caramelise.

2   Now add the ginger, garlic, lemongrass and red pepper and stir them for a couple of minutes until they become aromatic and the peppers are soft.

3   Then, add the chilli paste and give it a quick stir. No more than a minute.

4   Quickly add the chicken broth, coconut milk, fish sauce and lime juice and bring to a boil.

5   Reduce to a low heat and leave to simmer for about 10 minutes.

6   When you're almost ready to eat, add the chicken and leave it to cook for about 5 minutes.

7   Finally, throw in the fresh coriander and spring onions for a burst of freshness, and serve immediately.

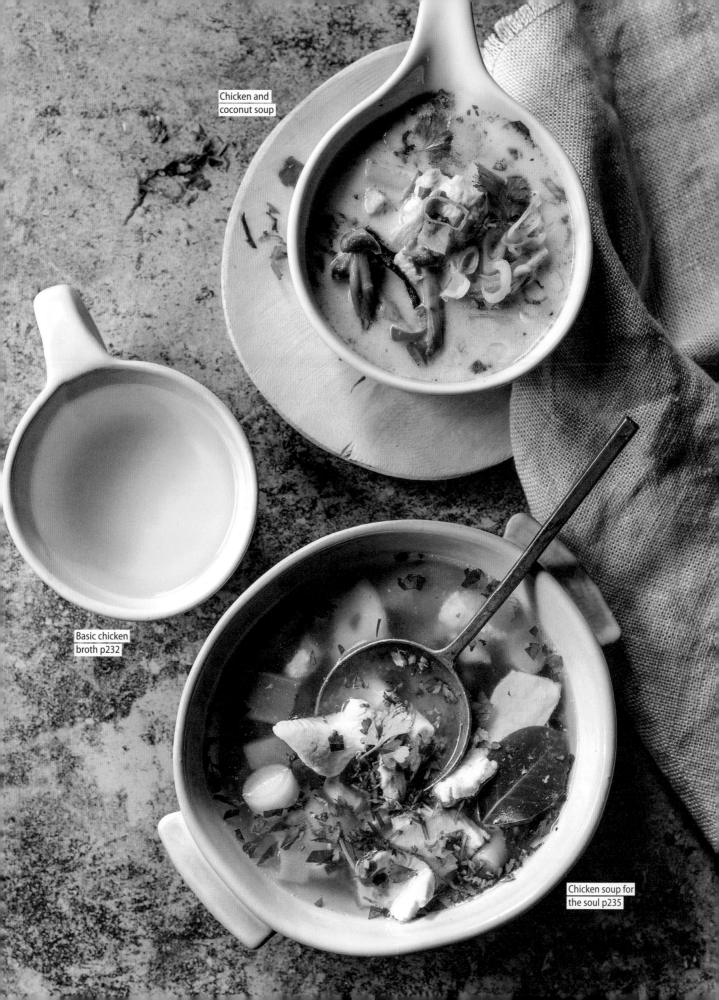

Chicken and coconut soup

Basic chicken broth p232

Chicken soup for the soul p235

PORK RAMENLESS

Serves 4

Ramen is a traditional Japanese dish that typically uses Chinese-style wheat noodles, but this recipe lacks the key ingredient, hence the name.

1 tsp sesame oil

80ml soy sauce

2 garlic cloves, thinly sliced

500g pork steaks

2 tsp coconut oil

2 tsp finely grated ginger

1 tsp Chinese five spice

1 red chilli, finely sliced

1½ litres basic pork broth (page 232)

250ml water

200g button mushrooms, quartered

150g mange tout, halved

2 medium-boiled eggs, cut lengthways

200g bean sprouts

50g toasted sesame seeds

1 For the pork marinade, combine the sesame oil, half of the soy sauce and half of the garlic in a mixing bowl.

2 Add the pork steaks, mix them together and leave them to marinate for 20 minutes.

3 Heat the coconut oil in a large saucepan over medium heat and add the ginger, five spice, chilli and remaining garlic, and cook for 2 minutes until they become aromatic.

4 Now add the pork broth, water and remaining soy sauce and bring it to the boil.

5 Once it begins to boil, reduce the heat and leave to simmer for 15 minutes.

6 Meanwhile, get a griddle pan very hot and grill the pork steaks for 3 minutes on each side. Leave them to rest before cutting them into strips.

7 Back to the broth, assuming 15 minutes have passed, add the mushrooms and mange tout and cook until tender.

8 To serve, divide the bean sprouts among serving bowls. Place the sliced pork and egg on top of the sprouts, fill each bowl with the broth. Finish it off with a sprinkling of sesame seeds.

KIMCHI JJIGAE

Serves 4

Kimchi Jjigae is a Korean soup that is usually made with water, not broth. The water is flavoured with strips of pork and shredded kimchi and then bulked up with tofu. In this case, we've swapped water for pork broth and skipped the tofu, leaving you with more nourishment and a punchier flavour.

2 tbsp sesame oil

350g pork belly, cut into bite-sized pieces

320g kimchi

1 brown onion, thinly sliced

1 tsp salt

1 garlic clove, minced

1 tbsp gochugaru (Korean hot
   pepper flakes)

1 tbsp gochujang (Korean pepper paste)

1 tsp black pepper

1 tbsp soy sauce

1 litre basic pork broth (page 232)

2 spring onions, chopped

1 Add the sesame oil to a medium-sized pot. Bring to a medium heat and throw in the pork, stirring every now and then until it is nice and caramelised.

2 Now add the kimchi to the pork and cook for 5 minutes, stirring constantly.

3 Then add the onion, salt, garlic, gochugaru, gochujang, black pepper and soy sauce to the pot and stir.

4 Add the broth, bring it to the boil, then leave it to simmer for 15 minutes.

5 Check the flavour. If it could be more intense, reduce the broth as you like.

6 When you're ready to serve, pump up the heat and drop the spring onions in as you take the broth off the heat. Serve immediately.

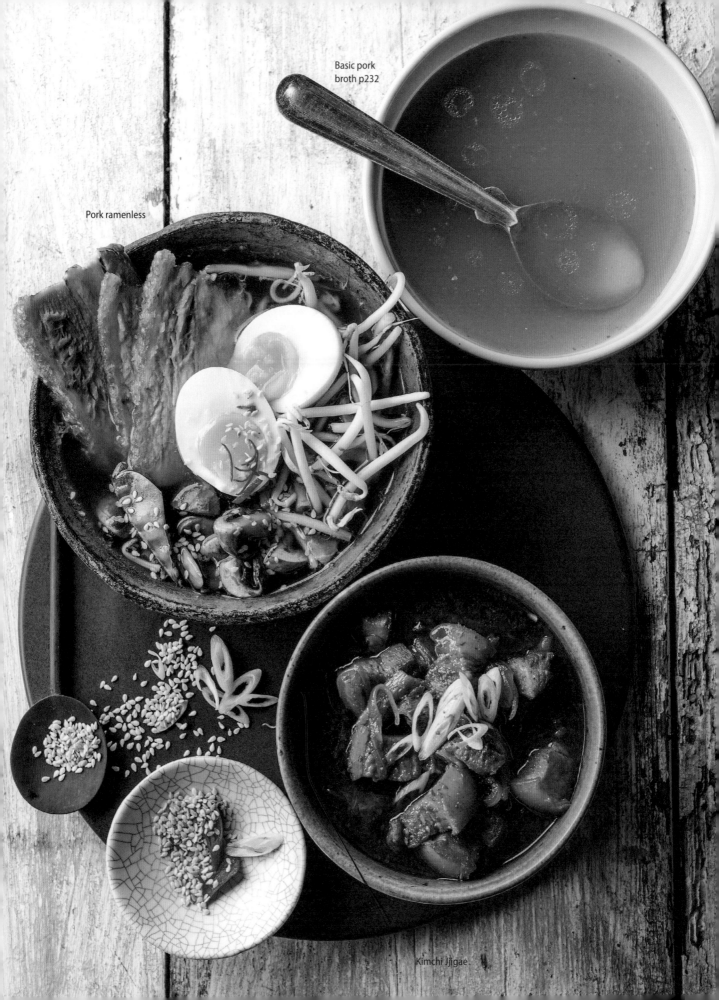

Pork ramenless

Basic pork
broth p232

Kimchi Jjigae

MALAYSIAN LAKSA

Serves 4

Laksa is a hot and spicy coconut curry usually soured with either fresh limes or tamarind, depending on where it comes from. The key to a good laksa is in the paste you use. There's a recipe in the condiment section of this book, but you could speed things up by buying one, if you have a brand you trust.

3 tbsp coconut oil

160ml laksa paste (see page 308)

1 litre basic chicken broth (page 232)

4 kafir lime leaves

4 small chicken breasts, thinly sliced

400g raw large shrimps, peeled and deveined

270ml light coconut milk

1 handful fresh mint, roughly chopped

1 handful fresh coriander, roughly chopped

2 spring onions, thinly sliced

Lime juice, to taste

Fish sauce, to taste

200g bean sprouts

1 lime, cut into wedges

Sliced fresh chilli, to serve

1 Heat the coconut oil in a large saucepan over high heat and fry the laksa paste until it begins to caramelise.

2 Add the chicken broth and kafir lime leaves and bring it up to the boil.

3 Lower the heat. Add the chicken and the shrimps and leave them to cook for 5 minutes.

4 Now add the coconut milk and simmer gently until it is heated through.

5 Throw in the herbs and the spring onions and immediately remove from the heat.

6 Season with fresh lime juice and fish sauce to get a balance of sour and salty.

7 Divide the soup among serving bowls and top with bean sprouts.

8 Serve as soon as possible with lime wedges and fresh chilli.

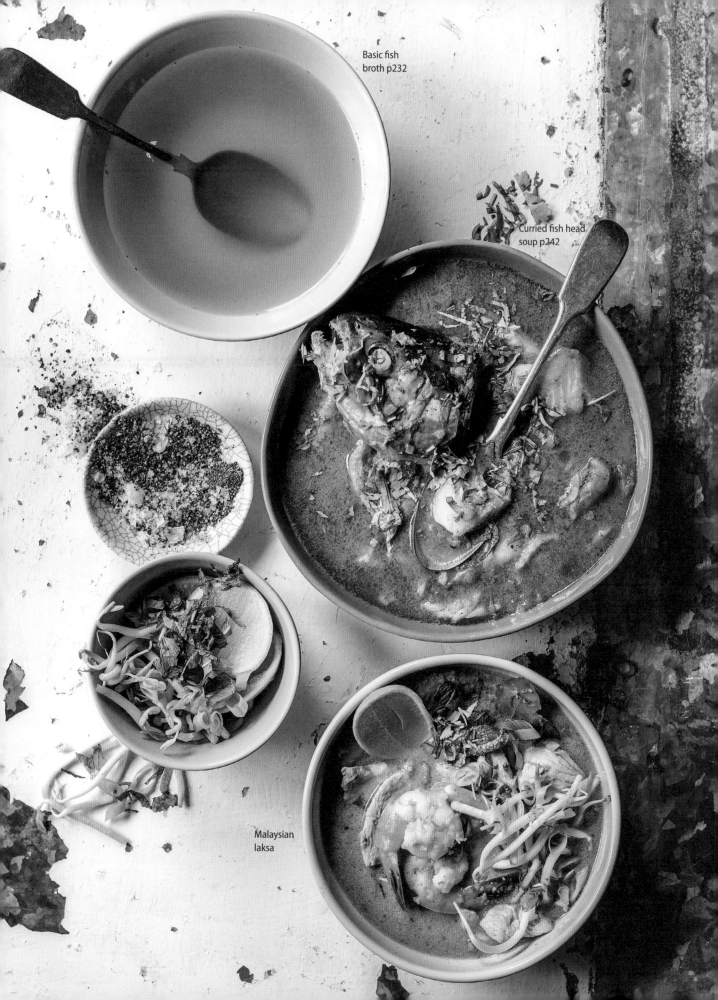

Basic fish
broth p232

Curried fish head
soup p242

Malaysian
laksa

CURRIED FISH HEAD SOUP

See page 241

Serves 4

Fish head curry ticks a lot of boxes for me. It's cheap as chips, has heaps of flavour and it turns heads… When you're ordering your fish, make sure you get the bones and the head in a separate pack, and for free of course. Use the bones for the broth, the fillets for grilling, and the head and whatever is left for this lip-smacker.

4 tbsp coconut oil

1 onion, finely chopped

1 tbsp cumin seeds

1 tsp mustard seeds

1 tsp fenugreek seeds

½ tsp ground cinnamon

3 tsp ground coriander

½ tsp ground turmeric

2 thumbs ginger, peeled and sliced

4 cloves garlic, finely chopped

1 tsp chilli powder

1 red chilli, finely chopped

200ml passata

250ml coconut milk

1 litre basic fish broth (page 232)

250g fish head, scaled and washed

400g white fish meat, scaled, boned, cut into 2cm cubes

1 handful fresh coriander, roughly chopped

Fish sauce, to taste

Lime juice, to taste

1 Heat the coconut oil in a large saucepan over a medium heat and fry the onion until golden-brown.

2 Add the cumin, mustard seeds, fenugreek, cinnamon, ground coriander, turmeric, ginger, garlic, chilli powder and fresh chilli, and stir to release the aromas.

3 Now add the passata, coconut milk and broth, and bring it all to the boil. Simmer the sauce until it has reduced by a third and thickened slightly.

4 Add the fish head and cubes and reduce the heat to a gentle simmer for 10 minutes to cook the meat through.

5 Simmer for the last 5 minutes then add the fresh coriander and season to taste with fish sauce and lime juice before serving.

KEYS TO KRAUT-ING (AND FERMENTING IN GENERAL)

Clean your hands

Always wash your hands before getting stuck in, but make sure you wash the soap off your hands too, otherwise your antibacterial soap will kill whatever you are trying bring to life.

Get your hands dirty

'Massaging' means squeezing the food between your hands, using the salt (and spices) as a grinding aid to help break down the cell walls and release the juices. The vegetables will generally hold their shape, but release enough juices to fill the gaps in a jar or crock.

Salt is science, not seasoning

The salt quantity is not for flavour, it is for controlling the fermentation. If you have a vegetable you want to ferment in a 'kraut' style, aim for a salt ratio of 2% of the weight of the stuff you're fermenting. In colder climates (not South Africa and Australia), 1.5% will work.

For a brine, if you're not going to salt the vegetable, but would rather just submerge it in salty liquid and hope for the same result, use a 5–7% salt-to-water ratio. Less for colder climates, more for hotter climates. Brining is often easier on the brain because you can make 1 litre of brine with 1 litre of water and 70g of salt, then just pour it over whatever you're fermenting as you go without weighing your veggies at every step.

Use the right vessel

Always decant your kraut into a ceramic sauerkraut crock or 'fermenting container' (or just a glass jar) and push the goods beneath the surface of the liquid, whether you are brining or krauting. The glass or masonry dish will keep the mix at a consistent temperature. They are also easier to clean and they don't hold on to the smells of your previous batches. There's nothing like the legacy stench of a failed sauerkraut batch to make you lose your appetite.

Air is the enemy

When you pack the kraut into a jar, crock or any vessel, it needs to be packed so tightly that no air bubbles (or as few as possible) exist. The top needs to be pushed down with a weighted lid that forces the juices to come up the sides of whatever you're fermenting. This creates a barrier of water between the kraut and the outside environment. Not doing this often results in mouldy kraut, which is not good. If it isn't wet enough, you can top it up with a little bit of 7% brine.

Temperature is your throttle

You can slow down the fermentation by keeping it cool, and you can speed it up by leaving it somewhere warmer. The risk of fast fermentation is that things could go a little too crazy, spoiling your batch.

Krauts live forever

I have eaten four-year-old kraut and it was nice. But if you go longer than four years, don't stress. According to the Encyclopedia of Microbiology, scientists recently uncovered a 300-year-old fermentation pit in Fiji; it had fermented breadfruit in it that was 'quite palatable'.

Don't cook kraut – unless you really want to

Cooking kraut kills the microbes, leaving it as mere mortal cabbage. It is still tasty to eat cooked, so if you're not eating it for its nutritive qualities (and you have a lot in supply), go for it.

Trust no-one

Don't let it freak you out that rotting food is actually the greatest preservation method. To think of all the science it took to develop preservatives, when all we needed to do was add salt and let the food rot. Not a whole lot of profit in that.

Get creative

There is a misconception that we need to be brave, take a deep breath, close our eyes and force down a regular dose of fermented foods for our sins. These foods are pungent, often overpowering in flavour and quite tough to eat on their own. Added to salads, sliced into salsas and other relishes, they have the potential to add an acidic kick and remarkable depth to a variety of different meals. Don't be brave, be creative. Pickles are your new secret weapon.

SAUERKRAUT

See page 247

Makes 500g

500g cabbage, finely shredded
10g salt (2% weight of the vegetable)

1 Massage the ingredients together and pack them into a fermentation dish or crock.
2 Leave in a cool dark place for 4 weeks. It is now ready to decant into a fridge container or to be eaten directly from the crock.

TURMERIC KRAUT

See page 247

Makes 500g

500g cabbage, finely shredded
10g salt (2% weight of the vegetable)
1 tbsp grated fresh turmeric (or 1 tbsp ground turmeric)
1 tsp freshly ground black pepper

1 Massage all the ingredients together and pack them into a fermentation dish or crock.
2 Leave in a cool dark place for 4 weeks. It is now ready to decant into a fridge container or to be eaten directly from the crock.

CUMIN CARROT KRAUT

See page 246

Makes 500g

300g cabbage, finely shredded
200g carrots, finely grated
2 tbsp cumin seeds
1 tbsp grated ginger
1 tbsp minced garlic
1 tsp ground turmeric
10g salt (2% weight of the vegetable)

1 Massage all the ingredients together and pack them into a fermentation dish or crock.
2 Leave in a cool dark place for 4 weeks. It is now ready to decant into a fridge container or to be eaten directly from the crock.

FENNEL KRAUT

See page 246

Makes 500g

200g fennel bulb, finely sliced
300g cabbage, finely shredded and outer leaves reserved
10g salt (2% weight of the vegetable)
½ tsp black pepper

1 Massage all the ingredients together and pack them into a fermentation dish or crock.
2 Leave in a cool dark place for 4 weeks. It is now ready to decant into a fridge container or to be eaten directly from the crock.

KIMCHI

See page 247

Makes 1kg

All of the keys to kraut apply to kimchi too. Make sure you refresh your memory on page 243.

1 head Chinese cabbage, halved
   lengthways
60g fine salt
1 clove garlic, minced
2 thumbs ginger, grated
3 tbsp fish sauce
2 tbsp rice vinegar
3 tbsp gochugaru (Korean chilli flakes)
1 tsp sugar (it ferments, don't worry)
10 radishes, shaved (1 daikon shaved)
 4 spring onions, finely sliced

1. Pack the cabbage into a baking dish or roasting pan and cover it with salt, ensuring all the pieces are evenly coated.
2. Add just enough water to cover the cabbage, and weigh it down with a plate or smaller bowl to ensure all the cabbage is immersed in the water.
3. Leave it to soak for 2 hours.
4. Rinse the cabbage under clean running cold water until all the salt is washed away and squeeze any excess water out before cutting into 3cm chunks.
5. Mix all the ingredients (except the radishes and spring onions) and rub into the cabbage, trying to ensure even distribution.
6. Now add the radishes and spring onions and mix well.
7. Pack the cabbage as tightly as possible into a jar with a tight-fitting lid to compress the ingredients. The tighter the better, as you want as little air in the jar as possible.
8. Open every few hours and press down further – the liquid will increase as the cabbage weeps – this is the good stuff, so don't throw it away.
9. Leave at room temperature for at least 7 days, after which you can refrigerate it.

PICKLED GARLIC

See page 247

Makes 100g

14g fine salt (7% of water volume,
  in weight)
200ml water
100g peeled garlic cloves

1. To make the brine, dissolve the salt in the water, bring it to the boil, then remove from the heat and let it cool down to room temperature.
2. Evenly divide the ingredients between the jars and top with the brine.
3. Seal the jars with lids and leave them in a cool dark place for 2 weeks or longer.
4. Once you've cracked one open, store it in the fridge for up to 300 years…

FERMENTED BEETROOT AND TURNIP

See page 246

Makes 500g

35g salt (7% of water volume,
  in weight)
500ml water
250g turnip, cut into chunks
250g beetroot, cut into chunks

1. To make the brine, dissolve the salt in the water, bring it to the boil, then remove from the heat and let it cool down to room temperature.
2. Pack the veg as tightly as possible into as few jars as possible and top with the brine.
3. Seal the jars with lids and leave them in a cool dark place for 2 weeks or longer.
4. Once you've cracked one open, store it in the fridge as long as you feel comfortable.

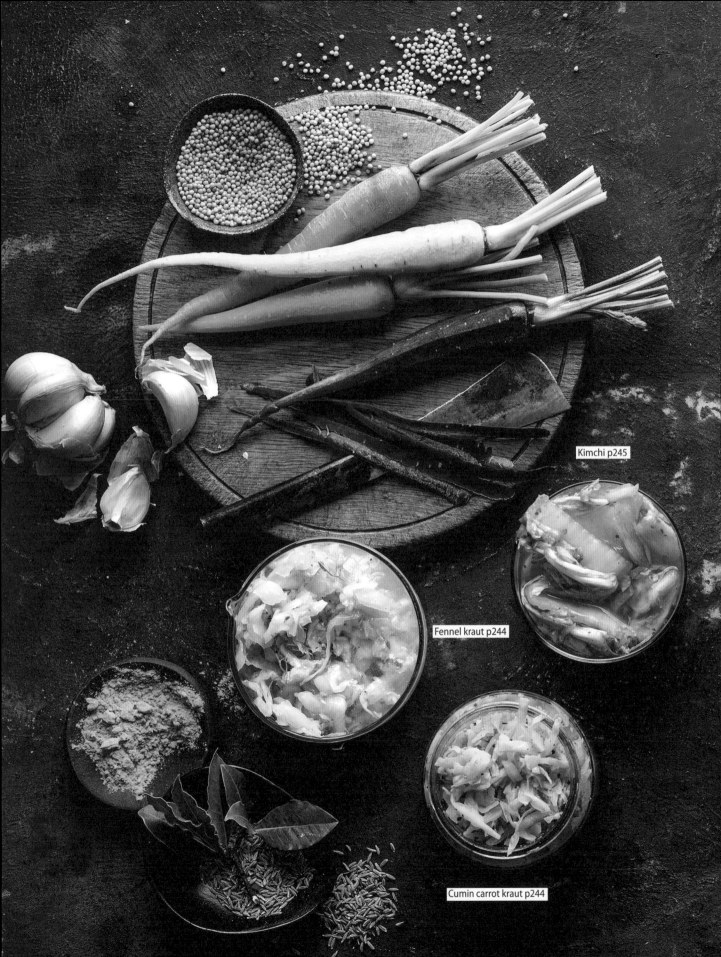

Kimchi p245

Fennel kraut p244

Cumin carrot kraut p244

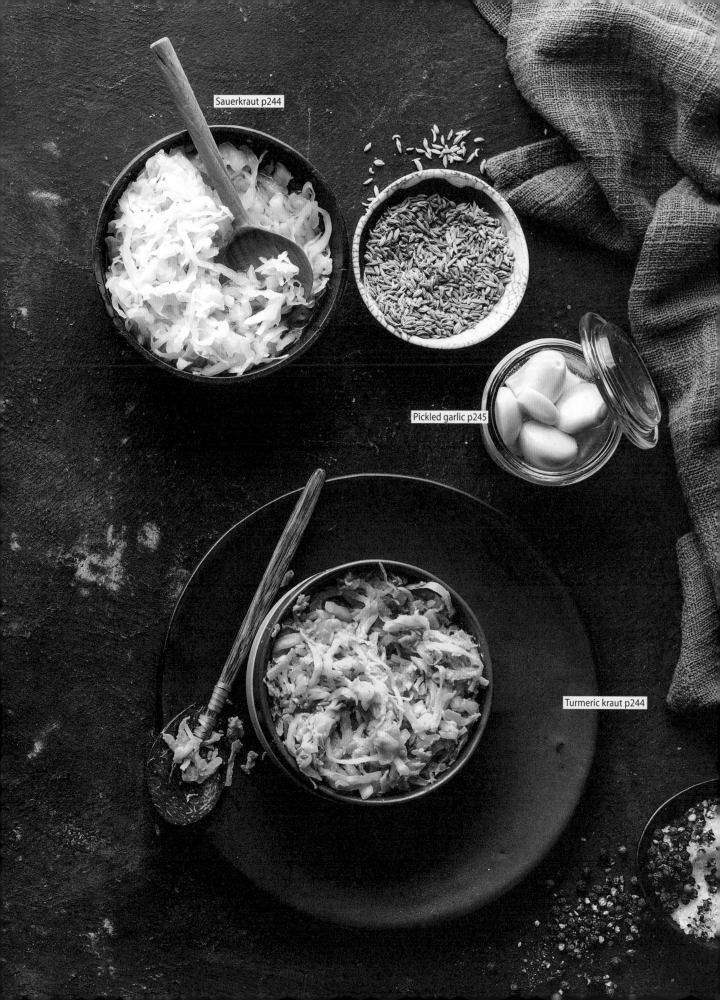

Sauerkraut p244

Pickled garlic p245

Turmeric kraut p244

CAULIFLOWER PICKLE

Makes 400g

500ml apple cider vinegar
180ml water
6 bay leaves
2 garlic cloves
1 tarragon sprig
1 tsp dill
1 tsp mustard seeds
1 tsp sea salt
1 tsp black peppercorns
400g cauliflower florets

1 Place the vinegar, water, bay leaves, garlic, tarragon, dill, mustard seeds, salt and peppercorns in a large pot and boil for 10 minutes.
2 Add the cauliflower and boil for another 4 minutes.
3 Fill the jars with the pickle and ensure that the vegetables and spices have been divided equally.
4 Store them in a dark place for 3 days before opening. Then store them in the fridge as long as you feel comfortable.

CELERY PICKLE

Makes about 500g

35g salt (7% of water volume,
 in weight)
500ml water
10 celery stalks, about 500g,
 cut crosswise in 5cm pieces
1 tbsp whole black peppercorns

1 To make the brine, dissolve the salt in the water, bring it to the boil, then remove from the heat and let it cool down to room temperature.
2 Evenly divide the ingredients between the jars and top with the brine.
3 Seal the jars with lids and leave them in a cool dark place for 2 weeks or longer.
4 Once you've cracked one open, store it in the fridge as long as you feel comfortable.

DILL PICKLE

Makes about 2 x 750ml jars

105g salt (7% of water volume, in weight)
1½ litres water
12 small cucumbers, about 9cm long
 and 3cm thick
2 heads fresh-blooming dill, stems
 trimmed (or 4 tbsp dill seed)
1 handful fresh dill
4 fresh vine leaves
4 dried red chillies

1 To make the brine, dissolve the salt in the water, bring it to the boil, then remove from the heat and let it cool down to room temperature.
2 Evenly divide the ingredients between the jars and top with the brine.
3 Seal the jars with lids and leave them in a cool dark place for 2 weeks or longer.
4 Once you've cracked one open, store it in the fridge as long as you feel comfortable.

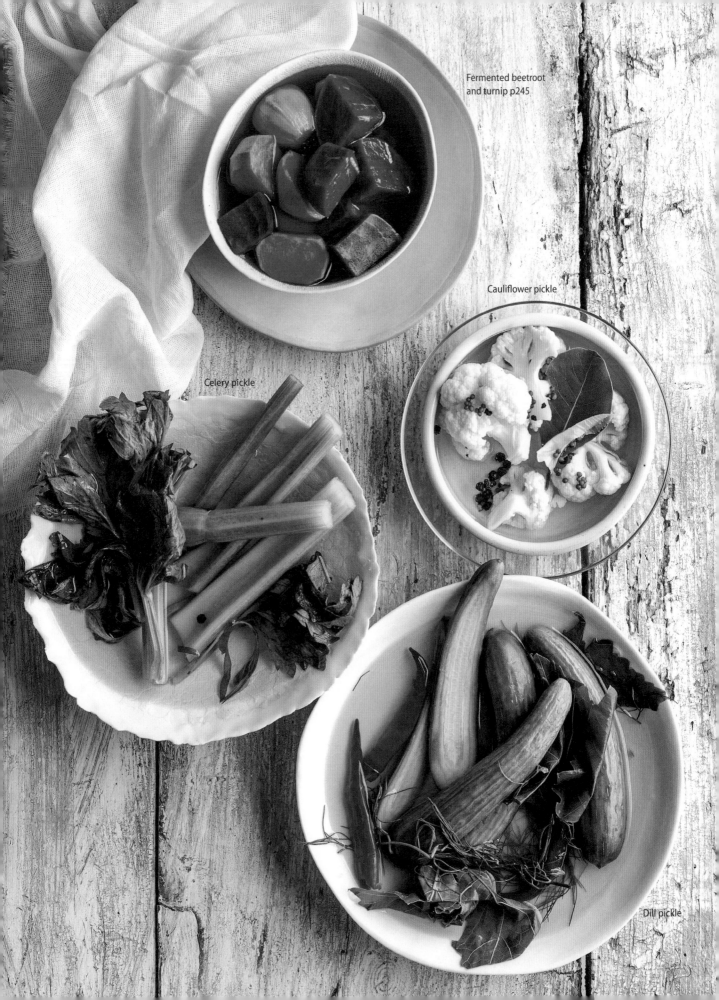

Fermented beetroot
and turnip p245

Cauliflower pickle

Celery pickle

Dill pickle

INDIAN LEMON AND LIME PICKLE

Makes 2kg

1kg lemons, quartered
1kg limes, quartered
60g sea salt
5 tbsp avocado oil
2 tsp mustard seeds
½ tsp fenugreek seeds
20 fresh curry leaves
2 tsp cayenne pepper
1 tsp ground turmeric
125ml fresh lime juice
125ml fresh lemon juice

1 Place the lemons, limes and salt in a large mixing bowl. Rub the fruit with salt inside and out.
2 Transfer to a jar and pack them tightly to fit. Cover with a lid and place the jar in a warm place that gets sunlight often, for 1 week. Shake the jar daily.
3 After a week, heat the avocado oil in a pan over a medium heat. Add the mustard seeds, fenugreek seeds and curry leaves. Cook for 2 minutes.
4 Transfer to a food processor and blend into a paste. Add the cayenne pepper, turmeric, lime juice and lemon juice. Mix well and pour the mixture into the jar with the fermented lemons and limes.
5 Seal the jar with a lid and refrigerate for a week before using. It can be enjoyed for up to a year.

SALTED LEMONS

Makes 2kg

125g sea salt
2kg lemons, quartered and 4 juiced
4 bay leaves
1 tbsp black peppercorns
2 tbsp olive oil

1 Line the bottom of the jar with 1 tablespoon of salt.
2 Mix the salt and lemons in a large mixing bowl, massaging the salt well into the lemon pieces.
3 Tightly pack the lemons into a jar, skin facing outwards, with bay leaves and peppercorns between each layer.
4 Pour in the juice and top with olive oil until everything is covered to protect it from air.
5 Seal the jar with a lid and leave in a cool, dark place for a minimum of 1 month before using.
6 Refrigerate once opened.

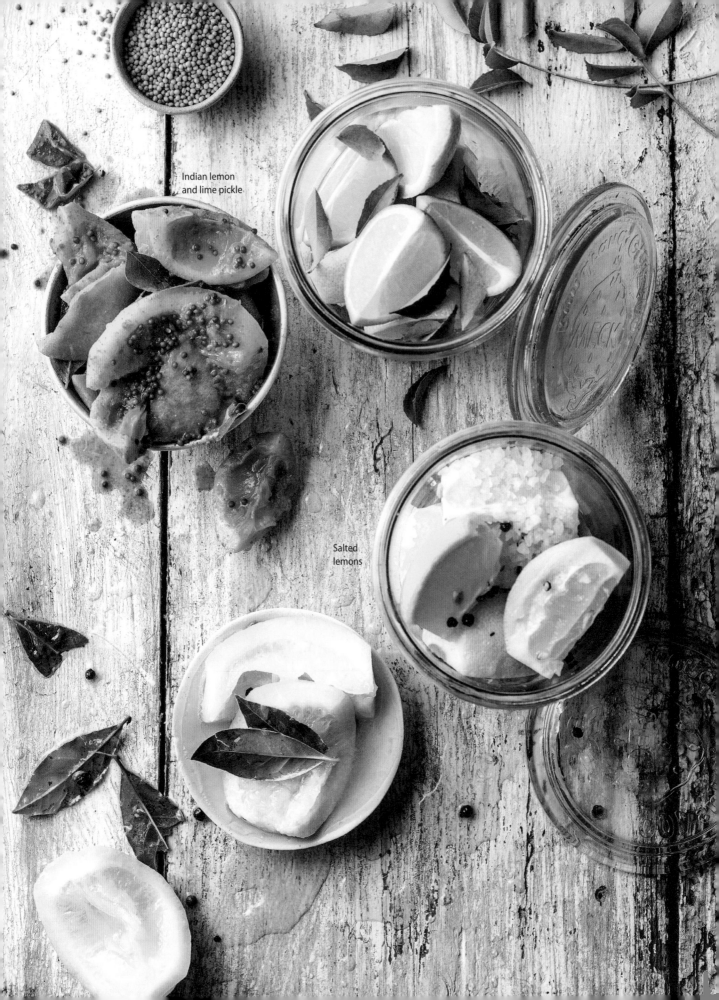

Indian lemon
and lime pickle

Salted
lemons

MILK KEFIR

Makes 1 litre

100g kefir grains

1 litre milk

1 You will need a glass jar (approximately 1 litre).
2 Put the kefir grains into the jar.
3 Slowly add the milk while stirring the mixture with a wooden spoon.
4 Cover lightly and allow 12 to 24 hours for culturing, depending on room temperature and the flavour you are after.

KEFIR CREAM CHEESE

500ml milk kefir

1 Put the milk kefir into a sieve lined with either cheesecloth, a paper coffee filter or a clean tea towel.
2 Allow to stand and drain over a bowl for 6 to 12 hours, or until it has the texture of cream cheese.

GOLDEN SHAKE

1 serving

250ml milk kefir

½ tsp maca powder

1 crack of black pepper

¼ tsp Ceylon cinnamon

1 pinch salt

½ tsp turmeric

1 tsp chia seeds

½ tsp honey

1 Combine all the ingredients in a blender and blitz until smooth.

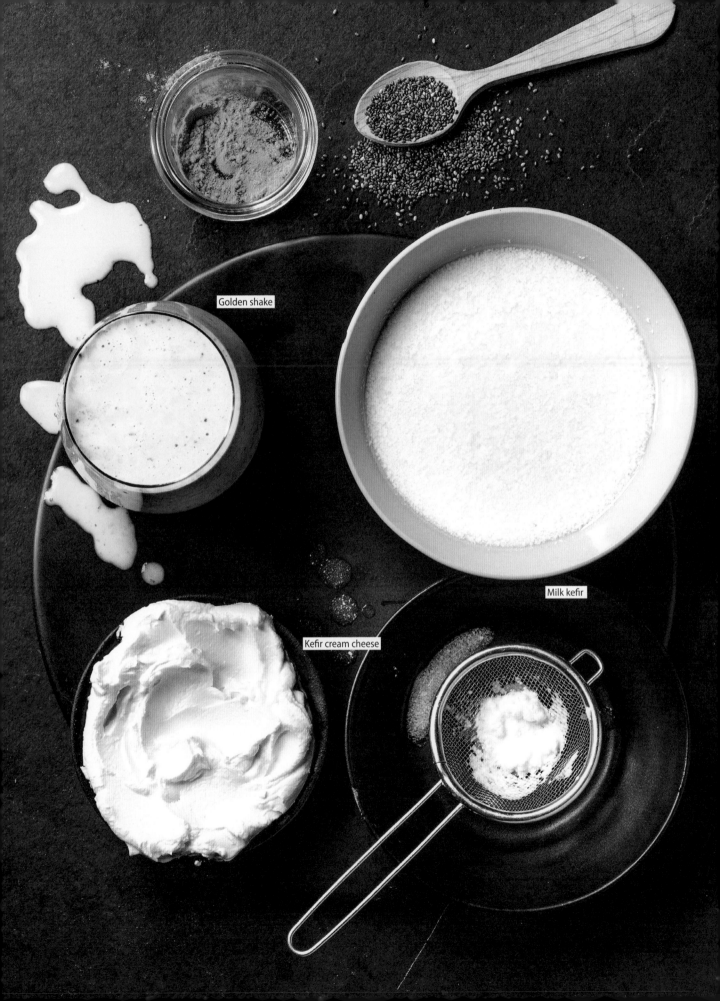

Golden shake

Kefir cream cheese

Milk kefir

UNDERSTANDING KOMBUCHA

Classic kombucha is a slightly fizzy fermented black tea with Eastern origins. As a result of fermentation, it is rich in nutrients, which for our purposes makes it fit for regular consumption (unless you are actively losing weight).

Unlike beer or wine, which makes use of yeast alone, the fermentation aid in kombucha is a jelly-like mushroom called a scoby, short for symbiotic colony of bacteria and yeast (see opposite page). If you buy kombucha from a health shop, you can make your own scoby, provided the stuff you're buying is high-enough quality. Or you could get one from a friend who brews it. Either way, making your own scoby and kombucha is preferable when following a low-carb diet, because it allows you more control over the sugar content – plus it's considerably less expensive.

The fermentation process is the key, converting sugar into nutrients and bacteria, but it isn't an exact science, with timings dependent on different climates, room temperatures and other factors. You can tell your kombucha isn't fermented enough if it's still sweet to the taste. Remember, without sufficient fermentation, you're simply drinking a sugary drink – not what we're looking for! You will know your kombucha is ready to drink when it tastes sour – almost free from any kind of sweetness. If you want to get technical, you could test it for sugar content, but that's unnecessary for even an enthusiastic kombucha fan.

For the above reasons, I always advise that people master the art of making their own kombucha rather than buying the stuff from a shop. Sweetness sells – a trick the kombucha dealers often use. For more on this interesting topic, see realmealrevolution.com.

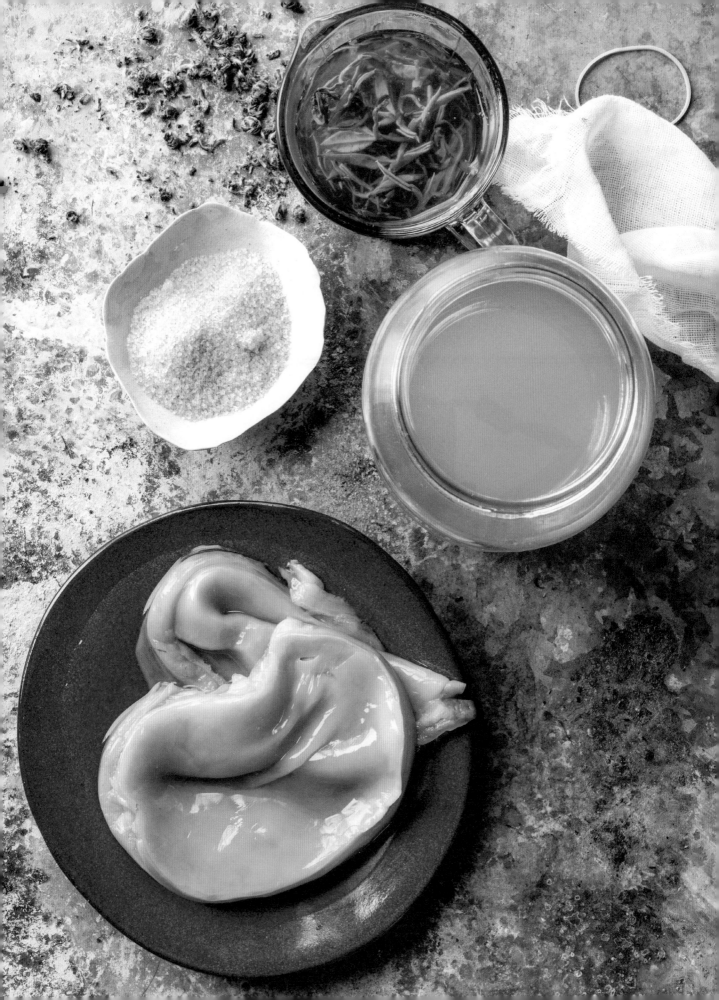

MAKING THE SCOBY

2.5 litres water

6 tea bags (Ceylon, Earl Grey or any Asian black tea)

190g white sugar

1 bottle (350-500ml) store-bought live kombucha

UTENSILS

1 x 3 litre jar

1 x 400ml jar (or any small jar)

Muslin cloth

1 Make sure the jars are clean and sterilised when you use them.

2 Boil the water (either in the kettle or in a pot).

3 Place the tea bags and sugar into the larger jar.

4 Pour the boiling water over the tea and the sugar, stir gently and leave to brew and cool (essentially making one huge cup of tea).

5 Once the tea is cool, remove the tea bags.

6 Pour in the bottle of kombucha. Remove some of the tea to make space if necessary.

7 Cover the opening of the jar with the muslin cloth and fasten it with an elastic band.

8 Leave the jar at room temperature for about two weeks.

9 A thick layer of jelly-like scoby will form either at the bottom or around the opening of the jar. It should be the same texture as thick, overcooked lasagne sheets.

10 To harvest the scoby, use a pair of tongs to lift it into the small (clean, sterile) jar and cover it with some leftover 'tea' from your main batch. You can leave it in the tea for up to two weeks before using it to make your next batch.

NOTE: The tea that is left in your big jar is your first batch of kombucha. You can bottle it, decant it into jugs or just leave it in the jar.

MAKING THE KOMBUCHA (USING YOUR OWN SCOBY)

3 litres water

6 tea bags (for more tannin and caffeine use Asian black tea, Earl Grey or Ceylon; for caffeine-free, use rooibos)

190g white sugar

1 scoby

250ml kombucha (from a bottle or previous batch)

1 x 3 litre jar

1 Make sure your jar is clean with no detergent residue.

2 Boil the water.

3 Place the tea bags, sugar and any flavour combinations (see below) into the jar.

4 Pour in the boiling water, stir gently to dissolve the sugar, and leave to brew and cool (making one huge cup of tea).

5 Wait until the mixture is cold.

6 Add the scoby and the reserved kombucha.

7 Cover it with a cloth and leave to ferment for a week in winter and three days in summer.

SOME FLAVOUR COMBINATIONS

Always add the flavours just before you add the hot water to brew the tea.

Apple Add a whole apple, cut into pieces. A week before you're going to drink it, pour 250ml of kombucha out and add 250ml of apple juice. Watch it fizz.

Pineapple Use the skins of the pineapple if you don't want to sacrifice the flesh. A week before drinking, tip out 250ml of kombucha and replace it with 250ml of pineapple juice.

Lemon and bay Add the zest of one big lemon and two fresh bay leaves.

Lavender and lemongrass 1 stick lemongrass cut in half lengthways and 6-8 lavender heads.

Cranberry 250ml dried cranberries. A week before drinking, tip out a cup of kombucha and replace it with a cup of cranberry juice.

Rosemary and lemon 20cm twig rosemary and the zest of 1 big lemon.

Chai 4 additional chai tea bags.

Pomegranate 250ml dried pomegranate rubies. A week before drinking, tip out a cup of kombucha and replace it with a cup of pomegranate juice.

Ginger 3 or 4 thumbs of fresh ginger sliced lengthways into matchsticks.

Cinnamon 2 sticks cinnamon, or more depending on your palate.

Hibiscus 1 handful dried hibiscus flowers.

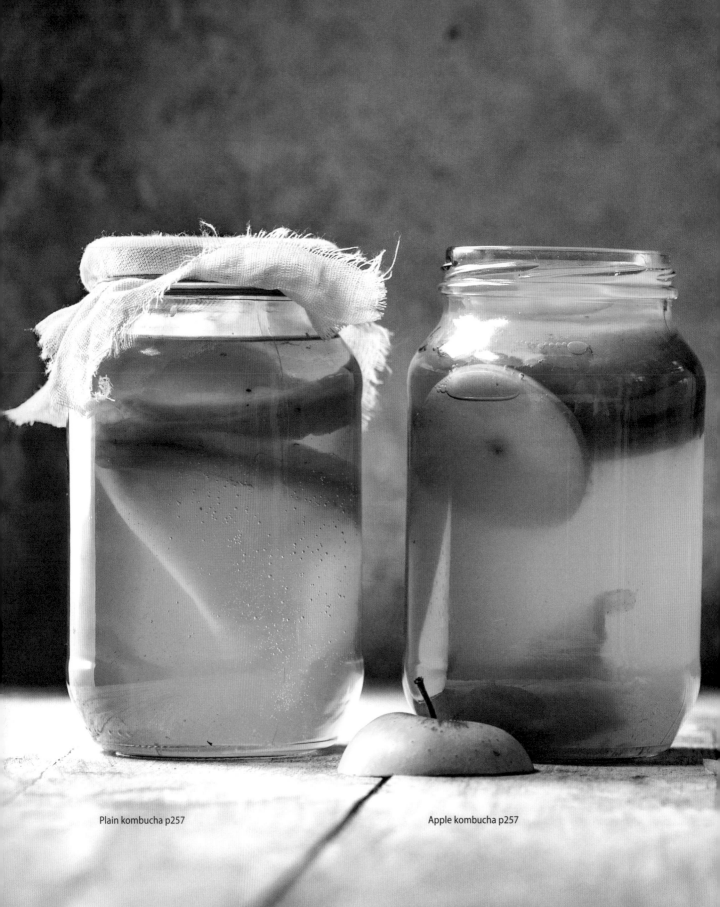

Plain kombucha p257

Apple kombucha p257

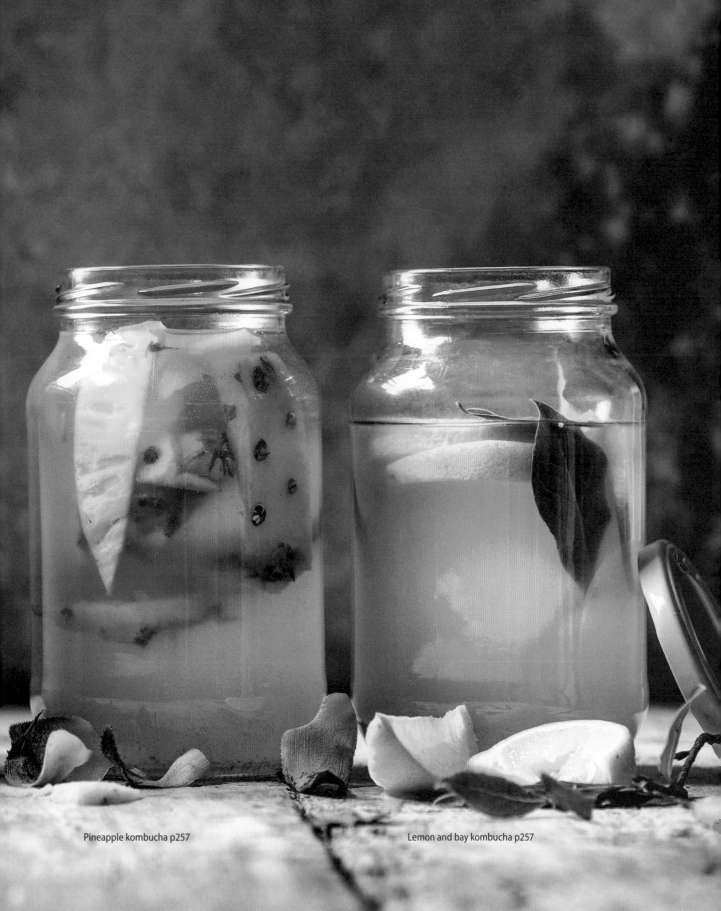

Pineapple kombucha p257

Lemon and bay kombucha p257

'AFTER A **GREAT DINNER** ONE CAN **FORGIVE ANYONE,** EVEN ONE'S RELATIVES.'

– OSCAR WILDE

STAPLES

Even if you have no idea what you are going to cook in the coming week, these should be on your list.

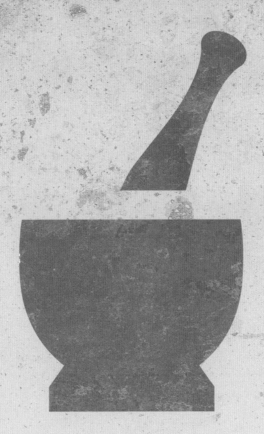

SEED CRACKERS ROUGH AND SMOOTH

The same ingredients can give totally different results if you just add in one step and a little extra water.

100g pumpkin seeds

100g sesame seeds

60g flaxseeds

100g sunflower seeds

1 tsp salt

3 tbsp psyllium husks

400ml (rough) or 600ml (smooth) water

1 Preheat your oven to 150°C. If you have a fan oven, make sure the fan is on.

2 For smooth crackers, grind the pumpkin, sesame, flax and sunflower seeds in a spice grinder before continuing to the next step.

3 Combine all the dry ingredients, then pour in the water and mix well before leaving it to stand until it is thick and pliable – about 10 minutes.

4 Spread the mixture out as thinly as possible on a baking tray lined with a silicone mat or baking parchment (silicone paper). You may need two trays. The mix should have no holes in it.

5 Bake the crackers for 1 hour, then, if they are not completely dry, check them every 5 minutes (from the 1-hour point). You may need to rotate them away from the hot spots in the oven.

6 They usually take about 1 hour 20 minutes to cook. Once they are lightly browned and crisp, take them out of the oven and leave them to cool.

7 Once cooled, break them into any size you like and store in an airtight container.

THE BEST SESAME AND ALMOND CRACKERS

300g almond flour (or ground almonds)

1½ tsp salt

160g sesame seeds

2 large eggs (whisked until frothy)

1 tbsp olive oil

1 Preheat your oven to 180°C.

2 Grease a baking tray well, or line a baking tray with baking paper.

3 In a large bowl, mix together the almond flour, salt, sesame seeds, eggs and oil. It will form a thick dough, so you may need your hands to give it a good mix.

4 Divide the dough in half and place one half of the dough on a sheet of baking paper, with another sheet over the top.

5 Using a rolling pin, roll the dough out until it is as thin as possible without breaking. The paper is not essential, but it makes it a lot easier to roll out.

6 Once it is as thin as you can get it, remove the top layer of the paper and slide the biscuit layer onto the baking tray.

7 Using a knife or a pizza slicer, slice the dough into 6cm squares, but don't try to separate the slices, just make grooves in the dough. They will break apart easily once they are baked.

8 Bake in the oven for 10 to 12 minutes until the biscuits are golden-brown.

9 Repeat with the other half of the dough.

10 Cool and serve immediately or store in an airtight container.

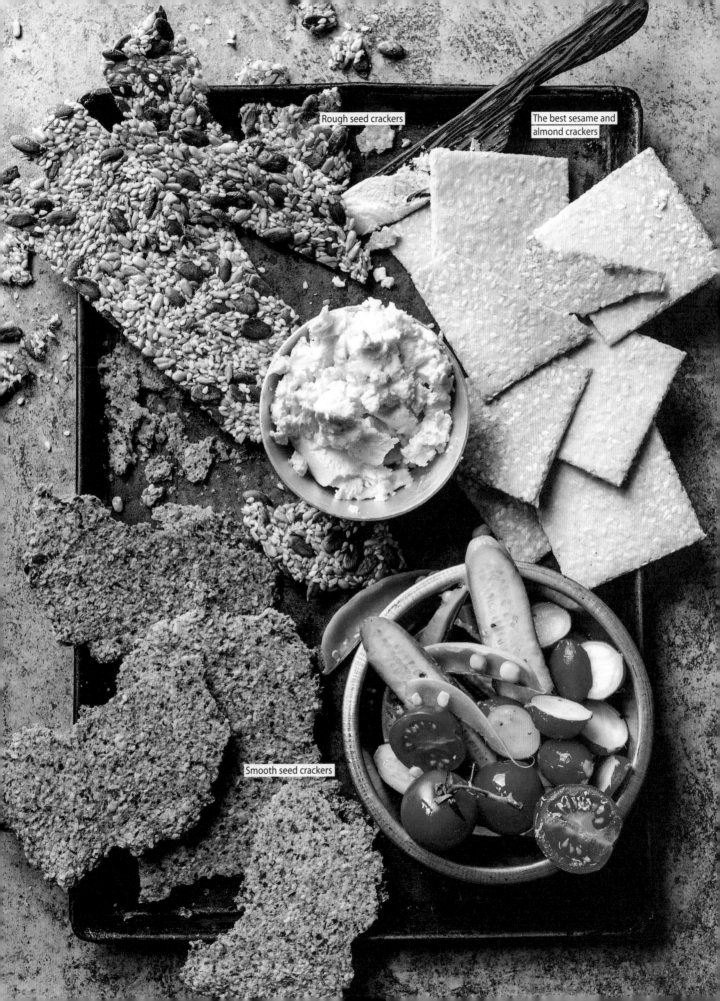

Rough seed crackers

The best sesame and almond crackers

Smooth seed crackers

BABA GANOUSH – AUBERGINE DIP

Makes 500ml

3 medium aubergines

3 cloves garlic, minced

2 tbsp lemon juice (you can add more if you like)

3 tbsp tahini

80ml olive oil, plus more for serving

1 large handful flat-leaf parsley

Coarse salt and black pepper

1 Preheat your oven to 200°C and pop the aubergines in. No oil. No seasoning.
2 After 1 hour and 30 minutes, they should be black or at least charred and soft (you could do this in a barbecue if you want an extra smoky flavour).
3 Gently pop them in a bowl and cover them to sweat in their own heat for 20 minutes.
4 Once they are cool, gently slit them open and use a spoon to scoop out the meat. Transfer the meat to another clean bowl. If a few black bits get in, that's cool; it will add to the charred flavour.
5 Add the garlic, lemon juice, tahini, olive oil and salt and blitz with a stick blender.
6 Finally, stir through the parsley and season to taste with salt and pepper.
7 Balance the flavours by adding more lemon juice if it's too bland, or more oil if it's too acidic.

GOES WELL WITH: Berbere Cauliflower with Tarator, Greek Kale Salad with Tahini Dressing, Persian-style Stuffed Fish Bake.

OLIVE TAPENADE

The key to this recipe is the quality of the olives, not the skill of the chef. If the olives you buy are the kind you could eat for days, the tapenade you make will be the same.

200g good-quality pitted black olives

2 medium anchovy fillets

2 tbsp capers

1 clove garlic, peeled

Juice of 1 lemon

½ tsp finely chopped fresh thyme

80ml olive oil

1 Pulse everything in a food processor until the mix is chunky, then store in a jar in the fridge until you need it for up to two weeks.

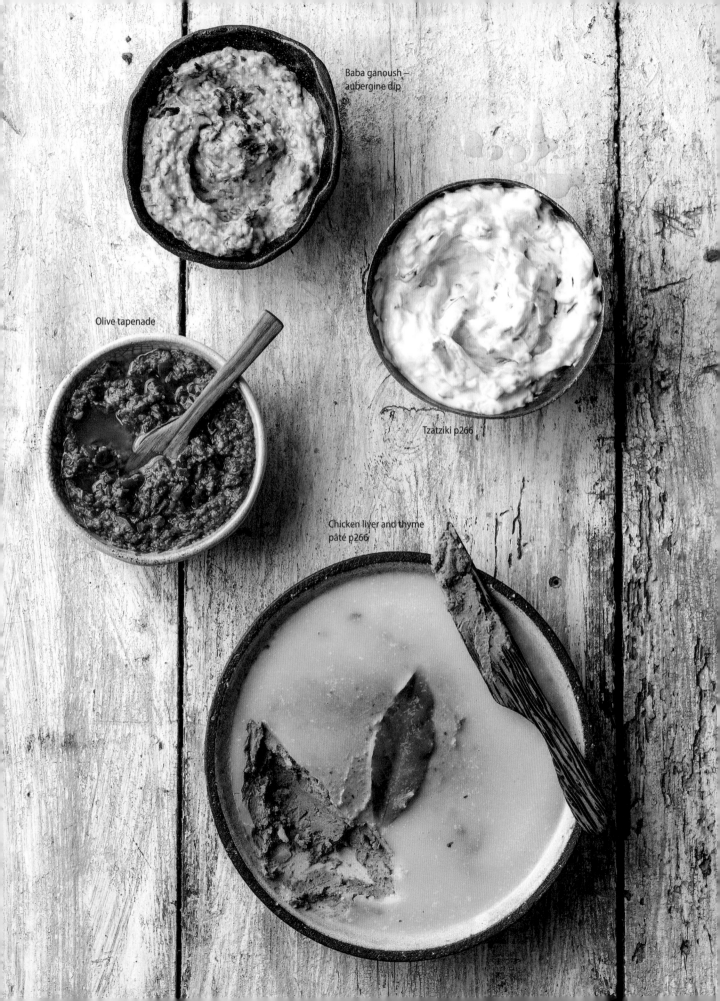

Baba ganoush – aubergine dip

Tzatziki p266

Olive tapenade

Chicken liver and thyme pâté p266

CHICKEN LIVER AND THYME PÂTÉ

See page 265

Makes 700g

120g butter
2 medium onions, thinly sliced
150g streaky bacon, thinly sliced
1 bay leaf
2 cloves garlic, minced
1 small handful thyme sprigs
500g chicken livers (rinsed and
    patted dry)
80ml dry sherry
80ml cream
75g softened butter
1 small handful parsley, chopped
Salt and pepper
Bay leaves, to garnish (optional)
Butter or duck fat, melted, to cover

1 Melt the butter in a deep frying pan and add the onions, bacon and bay leaf. Fry gently on a medium heat until the onions are golden and very soft.
2 Add the garlic and thyme and continue to cook for another 3 minutes.
3 Turn up the heat, then add the chicken livers. Fry them until they are soft but still a little pink.
4 Add the dry sherry and cook for a minute until the alcohol has burned off.
5 Then add the cream and cook for another minute.
6 Pour the contents of the pan into a food processor and blitz until the mixture is smooth. Add the softened butter and the parsley, season generously with salt and pepper and blitz until it is all combined.
7 If you want to go the extra mile, you could now push this mixture through a sieve for that extra smooth pâté. I only do that every now and then.
8 Now pour the mixture into pâté dishes.
9 For that classic finish, place bay leaves on the top of each pâté and pour a thin layer of melted butter or duck fat over it. This layer stops the pâté from oxidising and helps to preserve the lovely blush-pink colour.
10 Refrigerate until the pâté is cold all the way through.

TZATZIKI

See page 265

Makes 2 cups

1 medium English cucumber
400ml Greek yoghurt
2 tbsp lemon juice
2 cloves garlic, minced
1 glug of olive oil
Salt and pepper

1 Cut the cucumber in half lengthways and use a spoon to scrape the seeds out.
2 Grate the cucumber on either the fine or thick grain, whichever blows your hair back.
3 Now roll the cucumber up in a clean dishcloth or some muslin cloth and use all your might to wring every last drop of moisture out of it.
4 Mix the cucumber along with everything else into the yoghurt, and season to taste.
5 Leave it in the fridge for at least 1 hour to infuse properly, then splash over extra olive oil before serving.

SAUCES, SEASONINGS & CONDIMENTS

This section contains an arsenal of sauces, seasonings and condiments that you can add to just about anything. Most of these are classics, and learning to make them will dramatically enhance your portfolio of impressive cooking skills. These recipes are also dotted throughout the book, included in the methods of the dishes they are cooked with – consider this your easy reference resource.

Note: there's no gimmick or cheat to these sauces; they're just awesome recipes to complement low-carb cooking.

WHIPPED FETA DIP

Makes 250ml

150g cream cheese
100g feta cheese
Juice and zest of 1 lemon
1 medium spring onion, chopped
1 bunch chives, finely chopped
Salt and pepper

1 Whizz the cream cheese, feta and lemon zest in a food processor until they are smooth.
2 Now fold in the spring onion and chives and season with salt and pepper.
3 Serve immediately or leave it for 1 to 2 hours to let the flavours of the chives and spring onion develop.

SALSA VERDE

Makes 300ml

½ red onion, finely chopped
2 tbsp red wine vinegar
4 anchovies, minced
40g flat-leaf parsley, finely chopped
40g basil, finely chopped
2 tbsp capers, minced
150ml olive oil

1 Mix everything in a bowl and leave it to infuse for a few hours in the fridge.

HARISSA

Makes 250ml

250ml olive oil
3 garlic cloves, roughly chopped
1 tbsp red chilli, deseeded
  and chopped
5ml ground caraway seeds
2 tsp ground cumin
1 tsp ground coriander
1 pinch salt
3 tbsp tomato paste
180ml olive oil
1 tbsp sweet paprika
1 handful fresh coriander

1 Warm a quarter of the oil, though not too hot, then add the garlic, chilli, caraway, cumin, coriander and salt.
2 Gently fry the ingredients in the oil until they become fragrant, probably about 3 or 4 minutes.
3 Add the tomato paste and sauté gently for a few more minutes.
4 Add the remaining olive oil and stir it through, then remove them from the heat and scrape the contents of the pan into a narrow container (the jug that comes standard with a stick blender is a great option).
5 Now add the sweet paprika and fresh coriander to the mixture and blend well with a stick blender.
6 This should keep for a month in the fridge.

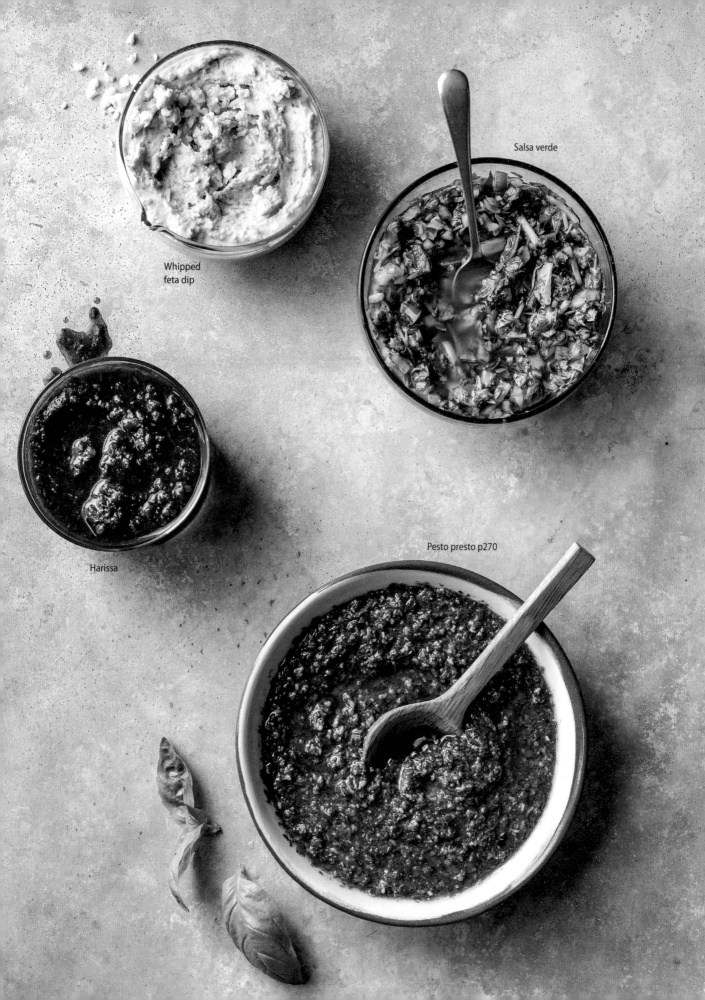

Whipped
feta dip

Salsa verde

Harissa

Pesto presto p270

PESTO PRESTO

Makes 250ml

We learned to make pesto on my second day of college. My lecturer, Chef G, gave us the secret ratio. It's literally as easy as one-two-three: one part pine nuts, two parts Parmigiana Reggiano, three parts basil (in weight, not volume). Olive oil to loosen it, lemon juice to add a sour tang, and garlic to give you a nice punch. In other words, the ratio is the base; the other three you need to add as you feel. If you don't have feelings, do this:

1 garlic clove
25g pine nuts, lightly toasted
75g fresh basil leaves
Juice of 1 large lemon
125ml olive oil
50g Parmigiana Reggiano, finely grated
Salt and pepper

1   Whizz the garlic, pine nuts, basil and lemon juice in a food processor until they are chopped to your desired consistency.
2   Now add the olive oil and grated Parmigiano Reggiano and pulse it 3 or 4 times.
3   Check the acidity and the seasoning. If it's a little bland, you probably need to add more lemon juice; if it's too acidic, more olive oil.
4   Pour into a jar, cover with a layer of olive oil, and store in the fridge for up to 2 weeks

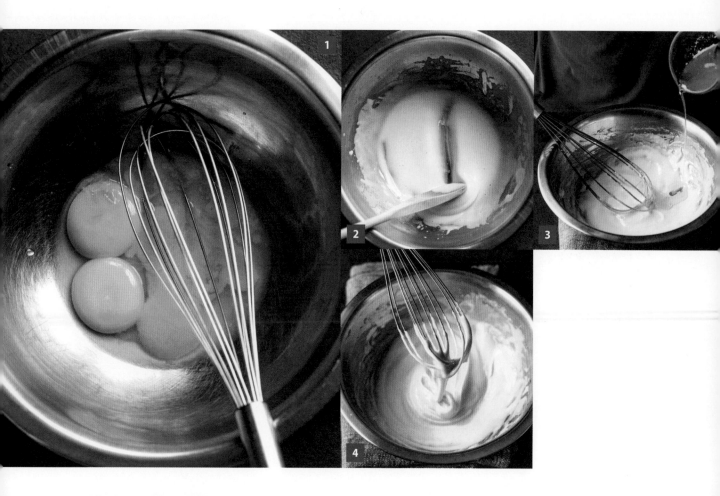

HOLLANDAISE

Makes 375ml

250ml clarified butter
1 tbsp water
3 egg yolks
Juice of 1 fat, juicy lemon
1 pinch cayenne pepper
Salt and white pepper

Theses rules apply to hollandaise and béarnaise:
★ *Never refrigerate.*
★ *Never reheat.*
★ *Make as much as you need right now – it's hard to reuse.*

To make the clarified butter, melt 350g butter in a small saucepan and bring it to a simmer. Use a spoon or ladle to skim the froth and milk solids from the surface until you are left with a clear 'clarified' butter. This should take about 10 minutes.

1   To make the hollandaise, place the water, egg yolks and lemon juice in a mixing bowl on top of a small saucepan of boiling water.
2   Whisk the mixture until it is light and fluffy, then remove from the heat.
3   While whisking continuously, pour in the clarified butter, 2 tablespoons at a time. Be sure to fully incorporate each new addition of butter before adding the next.
4   Once all of the butter is in, add the cayenne pepper and season with salt and white pepper to taste. You should be left with the consistency of… hollandaise. If it's too thick, whisk in drops of lemon juice or hot water to thin; if it's too thin, whisk in more clarified butter.

VINAIGRETTE

See page 275

Makes 250ml

I've used the classic vinaigrette ratio of 1 part vinegar to 3 parts oil. But all vinegars and oils have different strengths and they must be mixed accordingly – so make sure you taste and adjust. If it's too acidic, whisk in some more oil; if it's too flat, whisk in some more vinegar.

4 tbsp red wine vinegar
1½ tbsp Dijon mustard
180ml olive oil
Salt and pepper

1 Start with the 1:3 vinegar: oil ratio – plus mustard.
2 In a medium mixing bowl, whisk together the vinegar and the mustard.
3 While continuing to whisk, slowly pour in the oil until it's all incorporated and emulsified.
4 Use as is or season with salt and pepper.

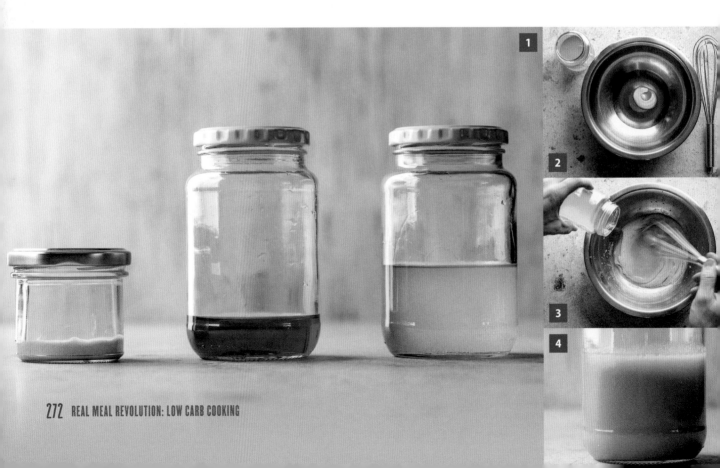

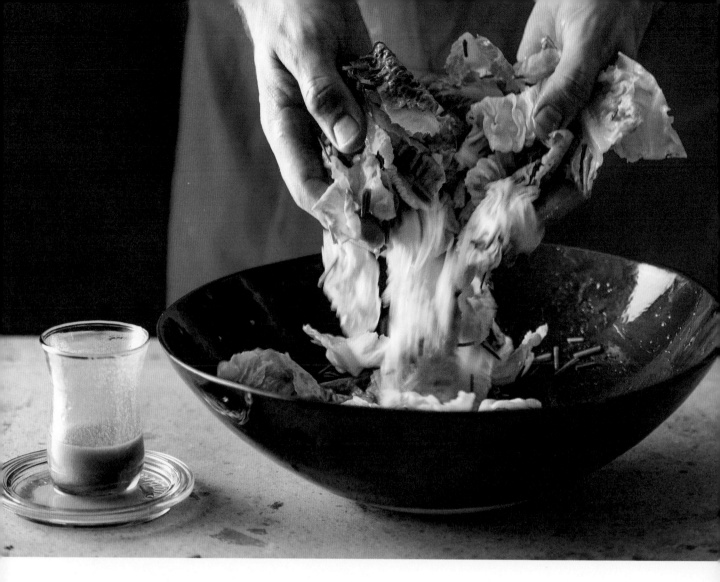

THE IMPORTANCE OF TOSSING

This might seem like an unnecessary lesson to add in here, but I've seen many people fail at the easiest of salad recipes by missing this step.

While it looks very nice in photos to drizzle a salad with some exciting dressing, it actually tastes better if the whole salad is tossed in its dressing.

When I lived in France, we didn't even make salads. We just took butter lettuce, snipped in chives and tossed it all in vinaigrette – that was the salad. With good olive oil, strong mustard and vinegar, that's all a salad needs to be amazing.

A dressing can often separate before it gets to the salad, which, in the absence of a tossed salad, means the first people to pour the dressing over theirs will get straight oil with no kick, while the last to arrive will only get the harsh vinegar with no oil to soften it.

Remember: toss the salad. That way, everyone gets to taste everything.

MAYONNAISE

Makes 500ml

3 extra large egg yolks
1 tbsp Dijon mustard
Juice of 1 lemon
300ml avocado oil or
   melted coconut oil
150ml olive oil
Salt and pepper

1   Whizz the eggs, mustard and lemon juice in a food processor until smooth.
2   Mix the avocado/coconut oil with the olive oil. The blend should be room temperature or just warmer.
3   While the food processor is whizzing away, slowly pour in the oil, glug by glug, making sure the sauce is fully emulsified and the oil is fully incorporated before adding the next glug.
4   Season to taste with salt and pepper and add more lemon juice if it needs some acidity.
5   Store in the fridge for up to two weeks.

EPIC BLUE CHEESE DIP

Makes 250ml

70g blue cheese like Stilton,
   Gorgonzola, Roquefort, etc
100ml buttermilk
80g cream cheese
1 handful parsley, chopped
1 handful chives, finely chopped

1   Blitz everything with a stick blender in a small jug and chill before serving.

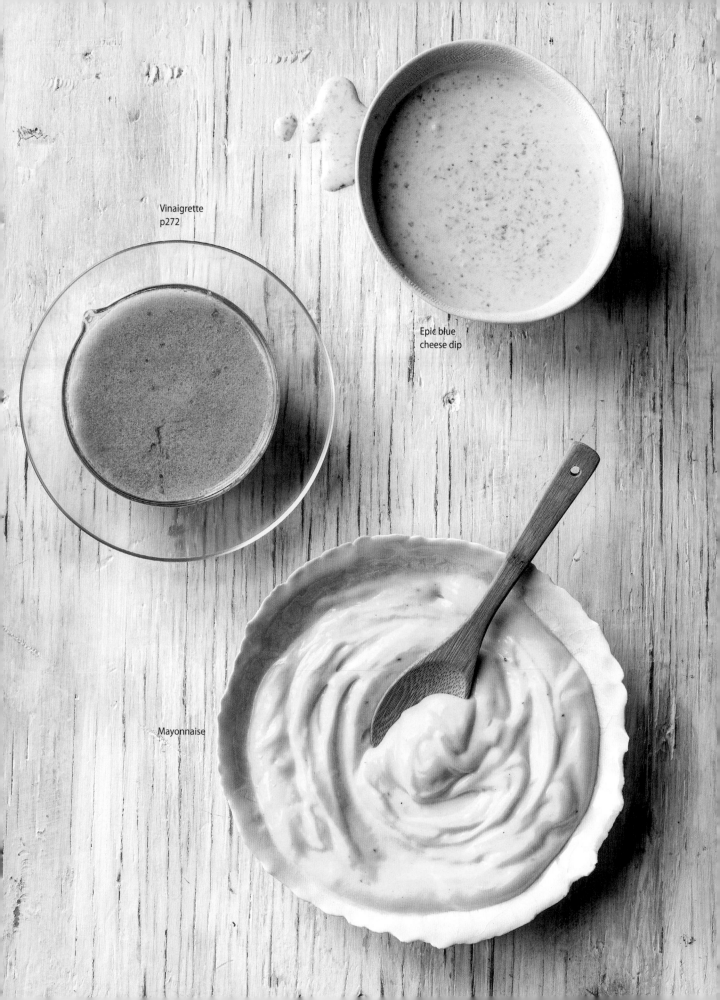

Vinaigrette
p272

Epic blue
cheese dip

Mayonnaise

SUNDRIED TOMATO AND HERB BUTTER

300g butter, cubed and softened

1 tbsp orange zest

1 garlic clove, crushed

100g sundried tomatoes, chopped

1 handful basil, roughly chopped

1 pinch salt and pepper

1 In a food processor, whizz all the ingredients together until a soft, smooth butter is formed.

2 Using foil, roll the butter into a thick log/cigar and pop it in the freezer to set.

3 Next time you need to add some love to your favourite sauce or a grilled steak, simply slice off a disk of butter and place it on top, or stir it into whatever sauce you're making.

ANCHOVY BUTTER

2 tbsp capers, roughly chopped

4 medium anchovy fillets, roughly chopped

300g butter, cubed and softened

1 tbsp lemon zest

1 handful parsley, roughly chopped

1 pinch salt and pepper

1 In a food processor, whizz all the ingredients together until a soft, smooth butter is formed.

2 Using foil, roll the butter into a thick log/cigar and pop it in the freezer to set.

3 Next time you need to add some love to your favourite sauce or a grilled steak, simply slice off a disk of butter and place it on top, or stir it into whatever sauce you're making.

GARLIC AND HERB BUTTER

300g butter, cubed and softened

1 handful parsley, chopped

1 handful chives, chopped

2 garlic cloves, crushed

1 pinch salt and pepper

1 In a food processor, whizz all the ingredients together until a soft, smooth butter is formed.

2 Using foil, roll the butter into a thick log/cigar and pop it in the freezer to set.

3 Next time you need to add some love to your favourite sauce or a grilled steak, simply slice off a disk of butter and place it on top, or stir it into whatever sauce you're making.

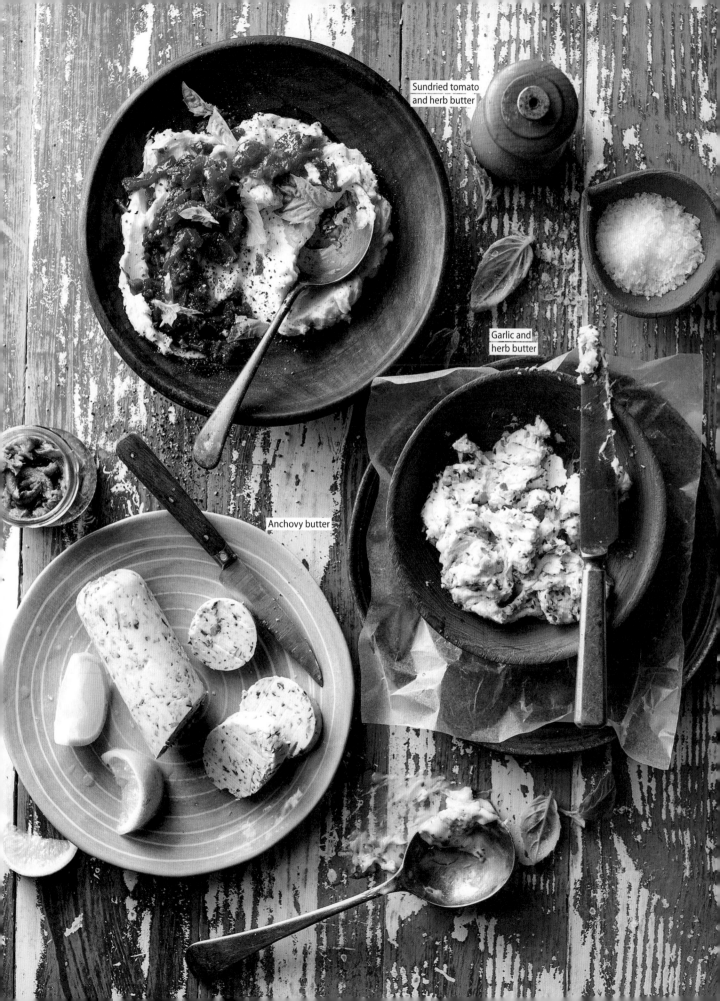

Sundried tomato
and herb butter

Garlic and
herb butter

Anchovy butter

GUACAMOLE

Makes 500g

2 avocados, peeled and pips removed

Juice of 1 lime

½ tsp salt

½ tsp ground cumin

½ red onion, finely chopped

1 jalapeño chilli, finely chopped (seeds removed for a mild version)

1 garlic clove, minced

2 tomatoes, deseeded and diced

½ a handful fresh coriander, roughly chopped

1 Place the avocados in a bowl and mash them roughly with a fork or potato masher.

2 Mix in the remaining ingredients and leave, covered, in the fridge for about 2 hours before serving.

KOREAN SALAD DRESSING

Makes 125ml

2 garlic cloves, minced

1 spring onion, chopped

¼ red onion, thinly sliced

4 tbsp soy sauce

2 tsp fish sauce

1 tbsp sesame oil

1 tbsp apple cider vinegar

2 tbsp gochugaru (Korean hot pepper flakes)

1 Mix everything together in a mixing bowl, then add whatever you're dressing to the bowl and mix together before serving.

CHARRED JALAPEÑO SAUCE

Makes 375ml

6 fresh ripe jalapeño peppers (red preferable, but not essential)

4 tbsp apple cider vinegar

250ml avocado oil

1 garlic clove

½ tsp fresh oregano, chopped

Salt and pepper

1 Hold the peppers directly in the flame of a gas hob and burn the skin, turning them until they are black all over.

2 While they are still hot, seal them in a sandwich bag or container and let them sweat until cool.

3 Once they are cool, use your fingers to pull off the stem, scrape out the seeds and scratch off the big pieces of skin. You want a little bit of char left behind, so don't get too serious here.

4 Drop them into a small jug with the remaining ingredients and blitz together with a stick blender.

5 You can serve this immediately, or leave overnight to reach the next level.

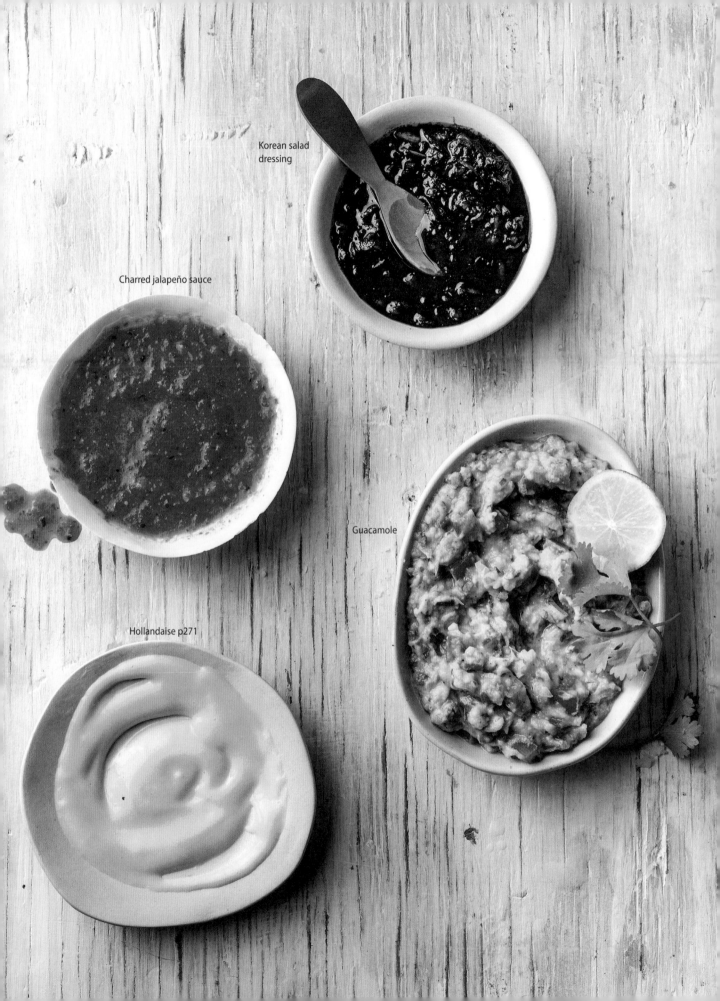

Korean salad dressing

Charred jalapeño sauce

Guacamole

Hollandaise p271

'WOE TO THE COOK
WHOSE SAUCE HAS
NO STING.'
— CHAUCER

CHOCOLATE MOLE

See page 283

Makes 500ml

This mole is perfect for a beef or chicken casserole.

4 tbsp avocado oil
½ tsp black peppercorns
½ tsp aniseed
½ tsp cumin seeds
3 cloves
1 cinnamon stick
2 onions, thinly sliced
5 garlic cloves, roughly chopped
2 tbsp almonds
2 tbsp pecans
2 tbsp hazelnuts
1 tbsp sesame seeds
1 litre chicken stock or broth
  (page 232)
½ tsp cayenne pepper
1 tsp sweet paprika
2 tbsp cocoa powder
Salt and black pepper

1 Heat the oil in a large pan over a medium heat and add the pepper, aniseed, cumin, clove and cinnamon stick to the pan. Cook for a minute until fragrant.
2 Add the onion and garlic to the pan and sauté until golden-brown.
3 Now add the almonds, pecans, hazelnuts and sesame seeds and toast until the sesame seeds are toasted.
4 Add the chicken stock, cayenne pepper, paprika and cocoa powder, and let it simmer until the liquid has reduced by half.
5 Tip the whole thing in a blender and whizz it until it forms a smooth paste, then pop it back onto the heat and let it simmer on a very low heat until you get a thick ketchup consistency.
6 Pour it over pretty much anything.

TIRADITO MARINADE

See page 283

Makes 125ml or enough for 500g fish

5 limes, juiced
1 red chilli, finely chopped
1 tsp amarillo paste (or any
  medium-strength chilli paste)
1 garlic clove, diced
4 tbsp olive oil
½ handful fresh coriander, roughly
  chopped
Salt and pepper to taste

1 Blitz everything except the coriander in a small jug with a stick blender.
2 Mix through the coriander and season to taste with salt and pepper.

CHEESE SAUCE

Makes 500ml

2 tbsp butter
1 onion, finely chopped
2 garlic cloves, minced
250ml dry white wine
500ml cream
200g grated Parmigiano Reggiano
  (or other strong cheese like any blue,
  Gruyère, Cheddar, raclette, etc)
1 big pinch ground nutmeg
Salt and black pepper

1 Melt the butter in a saucepan over a medium heat and add the onions to sauté until they are golden-brown.
2 Add the garlic and stir it around until it becomes fragrant, then add the wine.
3 While the wine is boiling away, use a wooden spoon to scrape any sediment off the bottom of the pan and into the sauce. That's your flavour right there.
4 Once the wine has almost evaporated, pour in the cream and let it reduce by a third, stirring occasionally.
5 Now throw in the cheese and stir well (you could even whisk it), until the cheese has melted and is well incorporated.
6 Add the nutmeg and season with salt and pepper.

MAGICAL MUSHROOM SAUCE

Makes 500ml or serves 4

350g mixed mushrooms – the wilder,
  the better
3 tbsp butter
3 garlic cloves, roughly chopped
1 tbsp thyme leaves
1 shot brandy
250ml white wine
250ml chicken stock (or veg if
  you're veg)
250ml cream
1 handful flat-leaf parsley, roughly
  chopped
Salt and black pepper

1 Cut the mushrooms into small chunks the size of halved button mushrooms.
2 Melt the butter in a large pan over a medium heat and wait for it to turn nutty and golden.
3 Immediately add the mushrooms, spreading them out evenly in the pan, but not stirring them.
4 After five minutes, turn the mushrooms to brown the other sides, and continue this until they are caramelised all over. If you stir them too early, they will release the juices and you will lose caramelisation.
5 Once they are all golden, add the garlic and thyme and stir well until fragrant.
6 Throw in the brandy and flambé it if you know how. Otherwise just wait for it to cook off.
7 Then add the wine and cook it down until the mixture is dry.
8 Next add the chicken stock and let it reduce by half.
9 Add the cream, reduce the heat to low and allow it to thicken, stirring occasionally.
10 Once thickened, season with salt and pepper and finish it off with the freshly chopped parsley.

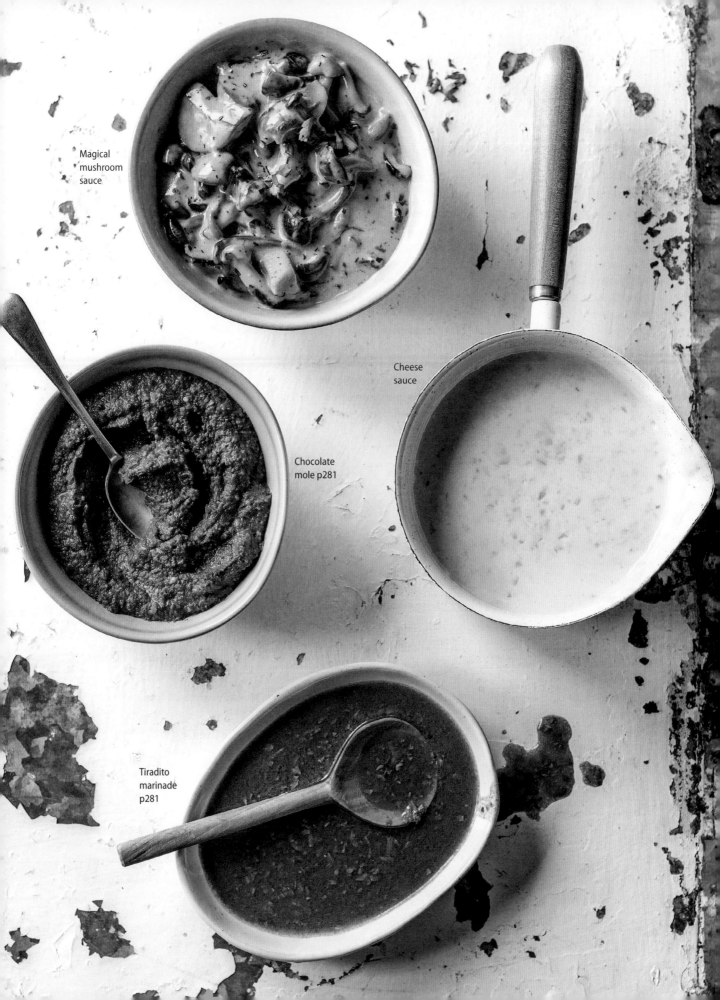

Magical
mushroom
sauce

Cheese
sauce

Chocolate
mole p281

Tiradito
marinade
p281

BRANDY AND PEPPERCORN SAUCE

Makes 250ml or serves 4

This recipe is best when it's made in the same pan you grilled a steak in. The brandy picks up all the burnt bits of meat and seasoning, which adds awesome depth. If you back yourself to do it, use the same pan while your meat rests.

4 tbsp Madagascan green peppercorns

2 tbsp butter

½ red onion, super-finely chopped

1½ tsp Dijon mustard

80ml brandy

250ml cream

1 bunch chives, finely chopped
   (optional)

Salt and pepper

1 First, crush half the peppercorns in a pestle and mortar, or chop them finely with a knife.

2 Melt the butter in a medium-sized pan over a medium heat and add the peppercorns (whole and chopped) and the red onion, and sauté them gently until the onions begin to caramelise.

3 Add the mustard and stir it around until it begins to stick to the bottom of the pan.

4 Now throw in the brandy and light it with a lighter to burn off the alcohol. If that scares you, just boil it until it has reduced by two-thirds. It'll give you the same end result – but, of course, flambéing looks cooler.

5 Add the cream, reduce the heat and simmer until the sauce has thickened.

6 As your last move before serving, season it with salt and pepper and stir through the fresh chives.

TRIPLE GARLIC SAUCE

Makes 250ml or serves 4

This sauce marries all three of garlic's flavour profiles: the bitter flavour of burnt bits of chopped garlic from being sautéed, the sweet pungency from being roasted and the burny freshness from minced raw garlic. It makes everything taste so much more, well, tasty.

2½ big heads of garlic (bigger cloves
   will make your life easier with this one)

2 tbsp butter

250ml dry white wine

1 tbsp lemon juice

5ml lemon zest

375ml cream

Salt and black pepper

1 Take the half head and mince half of it (quarter head), and roughly chop the other half (quarter head).

2 Then take the two whole heads and roast them following the steps for Roasted Garlic on page 286.

3 Melt the butter in a saucepan over a medium heat and add the chopped garlic to sauté for a few minutes.

4 As the garlic begins to caramelise, add the wine, lemon juice and zest, and let it reduce to a third of its volume.

5 Now add the cream and the roasted garlic flesh, and simmer until it has reduced and thickened nicely, maybe five minutes.

6 Remove it from the heat and blitz it with a stick blender.

7 Just before serving, put it back on the heat and stir in the minced garlic with some salt and pepper for seasoning, then serve immediately.

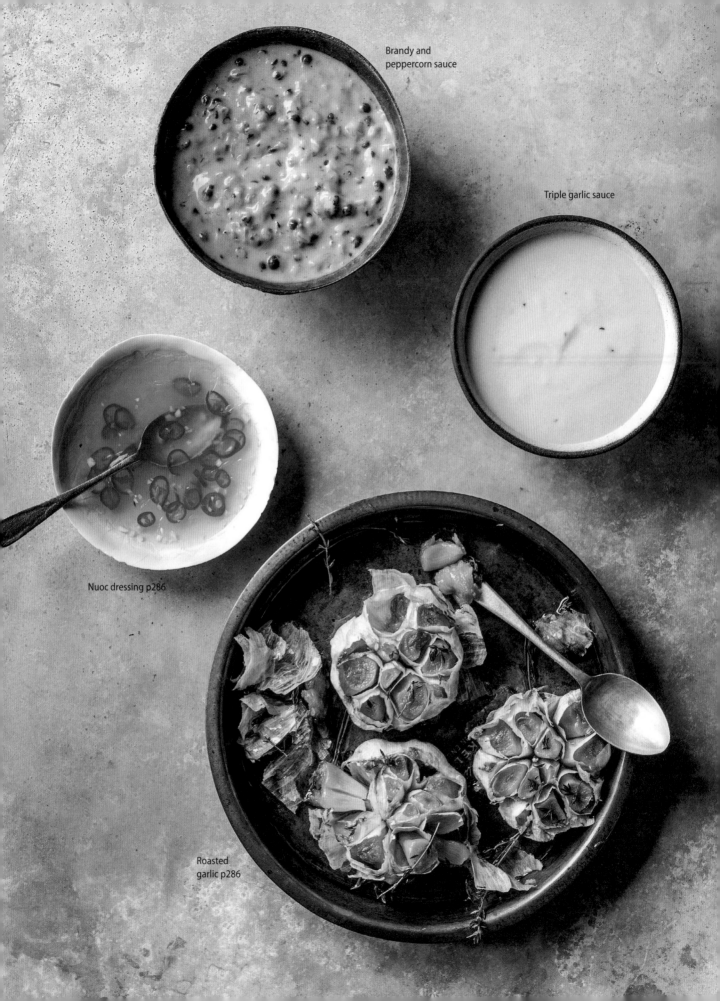

Brandy and peppercorn sauce

Triple garlic sauce

Nuoc dressing p286

Roasted garlic p286

NUOC DRESSING

See page 285

Makes 250ml or serves 4

Nuoc (pronounced 'nok', kind of) is the most important dressing and dipping sauce in Vietnamese cuisine – a general seasoning for everything.

1 tbsp lime juice
1 garlic clove, chopped
1 whole red chilli, deseeded and thinly sliced
1 tbsp rice vinegar
4 tbsp fish sauce
1 tbsp water

1　Mix everything together in a small bowl and serve.

ROASTED GARLIC

See page 285

3 heads of garlic, whole
3 sprigs thyme
Olive oil

1　Preheat your oven to 180°C.
2　Cut the top off the heads of garlic to expose the flesh.
3　Pour olive oil into the heads until they are 'full' of oil, and top each with a sprig of thyme.
4　Cover the heads in foil (individually or over the dish) and roast them for 1 hour. The cloves should be soft, brown and sweet.
5　When the heads have cooled down, unwrap and use a knife to break off the cloves, and then use your fingers to squeeze the flesh out of each clove into a jar or bowl.
6　Cover with olive oil and store in the fridge until needed.

COLOMBIAN HOT SAUCE

See page 289

Makes 375ml

This is the perfect sauce to pair with heavier dishes. It's super-refreshing and it packs a punch that will stand up to the highest level of richness.

1 habanero chilli (if you're soft like me, use a less aggressive chilli)
1 big handful fresh coriander, chopped
8 spring onions, chopped
2 big, ripe and juicy tomatoes
Juice of 2 big limes
2 tbsp apple cider vinegar
Salt and pepper

1   Blitz everything in a food processor then store in a jar. I'd avoid the stick blender for this one, because you're aiming for a slightly chunkier end result.

GREMOLATA

See page 289

Makes 2 tbsp (serves 4)

This is one of my favourite finishers for rich stews. Gremolata is traditionally used to freshen up osso buco (Italian braised veal shin) but you can use this for anything – sharpening a dish of calamari, spicing up an aioli, or dressing anything by just adding lemon juice and olive oil – remember the 1:3 ratio.

2 tbsp lemon zest, preferably microplaned
1 garlic clove, finely chopped
1 large handful flat-leaf parsley, roughly chopped

1   Mix all the ingredients together in a bowl.

SAUCES, SEASONINGS AND CONDIMENTS **287**

CHERMOULA

Makes 375ml

Juice of 2 fat lemons
1 garlic clove, peeled
1 tbsp tomato paste
250ml olive oil
½ tsp coarse salt
½ tsp dried red chilli
1 handful fresh coriander
1 handful fresh parsley
2 tbsp ground coriander
2 tbsp ground cumin
3 tsp paprika
1½ tbsp turmeric

1 Purée all the ingredients into a fine paste in a food processor or using a stick blender.
2 Put the mixture into a pan and cook for about 15 minutes until the oil begins to split from the mixture.
3 Store in a sterilised jar for up to a month in the fridge.

CHIMICHURRI

Makes 300ml

2 handfuls fresh parsley
1 small handful fresh oregano
1 small handful mint
1 small handful basil
1 garlic clove, minced
½ red onion, very finely chopped
2 tbsp red wine vinegar
180ml olive oil

1 There are two ways to do this. Either whizz everything except the olive oil in a food processor, then add the oil and pulse 3 or 4 times. Or chop everything very finely and mix together in a bowl.
2 Whichever road you go down, make sure you leave the mix in the fridge for 1 or 2 hours before serving.

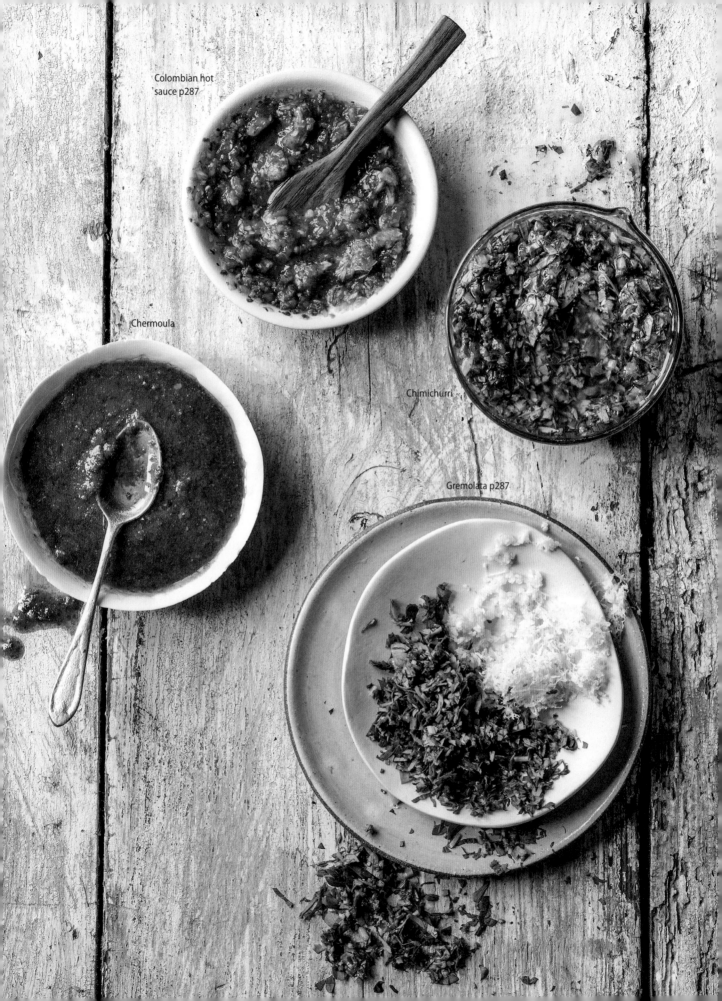

Colombian hot
sauce p287

Chermoula

Chimichurri

Gremolata p287

MONTER AU BEURRE

The only way I thicken sauce.

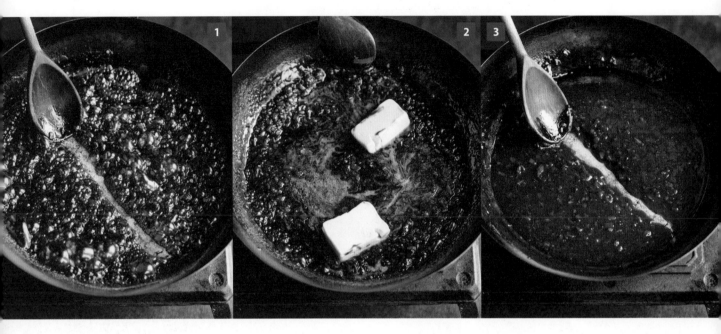

Thickening sauces without wheat or corn flour can be a challenge for the home cook, but I take a fairly dim view of using flour to thicken and advise against it wherever possible. Apart from using a roux at the beginning of a white sauce, or velouté, it really isn't necessary.

Naturally thickened sauces generally have a more intense flavour and are higher in nutrients. By naturally thickened, I mean sauces that are either reduced or are thickened with butter at the end.

This last method, the one I prefer, is called *monter au beurre*. The direct translation from French is to 'stir in butter', and that's exactly what you do. A lot of butter. By stirring cold butter into a highly reduced gravy, you give it a glassy shine, rich flavour and silky texture. It will split eventually, but for about 15 minutes it will be the most delicious thing you have ever tasted.

★ Reduce whatever sauce you have down to the point that it looks like it's bubbling like caramel (shot **1**).
★ Add a few knobs of hard cold butter (shot **2**).
★ Shake the pan around, or stir it, while moving it on and off the heat, until the butter has emulsified (shot **3**).
★ Serve immediately.

REDUCING

A sort of thickening…

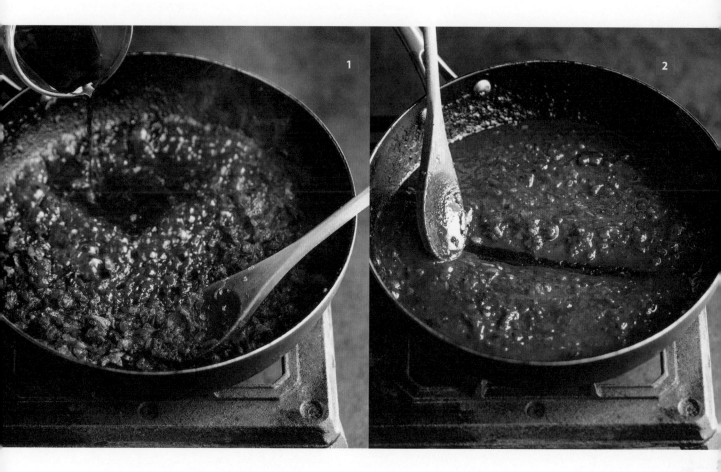

This is not really a method of thickening, but rather a method that guarantees you end up with a thick sauce. The secret is to use tomato paste at the beginning of the cooking process.

★ Sauté whatever vegetables you want in your sauce – onions, carrots, leeks, celery or peppers.
★ Stir in a spoonful of tomato paste and let it catch on the base of the pan, forming a sediment.
★ Add stock or red wine and let it boil. Use a wooden spoon to scrape the sediment off the bottom of the pan and mix it into the sauce (shot **1**).
★ If the sauce recipe calls for cream, stock, broth or any other liquid, add it in now, stirring.
★ When you are finished adding what needs to be added, you can just reduce the sauce by boiling away the liquid. Because of the tomato paste, it will thicken naturally as it reduces (shot **2**).

RED AND WHITE GRAVY

Makes 300ml

RED GRAVY

1 roasting tray with fat and seasoning
   leftover from a roast
1 onion, finely chopped
1 garlic clove
1 sprig rosemary or thyme
250ml red wine
400ml beef broth or stock (page 232)
4 knobs cold, hard butter

WHITE GRAVY

Use white wine instead of red wine
Use chicken broth instead of beef broth
Use 250ml cream instead of butter

1 Roast your meat in a roasting pan or dish that can be placed directly on the stove or gas hob.

2 Once your roast is done, remove the meat from the pan or dish and place the pan on a gas hob or stove on a medium heat. Get the fat and pan juices hot and sizzling.

3 Add the onion and sauté it, using the juices it releases to loosen the burnt bits from the bottom of the pan.

4 Once the onion is caramelised, add the garlic and rosemary or thyme, and stir about until it all becomes fragrant.

5 Now add the wine and reduce by half, continuing to scrape the bottom of the pan clean.

6 Once it has reduced by half, add the stock and reduce the entire contents of the pan down to a thick, sticky sauce.

7 For red gravy, keep it on a medium heat and drop in the butter, stirring constantly until fully emulsified. For white gravy, add the cream, bring it to the boil, and simmer until thick and buttery.

8 Season to taste and serve immediately.

JONNO'S BBQ MARINADE

Makes 125ml or enough for 500g meat

2 tbsp cumin seeds
2 tbsp fennel seeds
2 tbsp smoked paprika
2 garlic cloves, peeled
1 big handful fresh oregano, picked and
   roughly chopped
4 tbsp lemon juice
180ml olive oil

1 Pound the cumin and fennel seeds in a pestle and mortar to break them up. They don't need to be a fine powder, but there should be no whole seeds left.

2 Pop them, along with the remaining ingredients, into a small jug and blitz together with a stick blender.

3 Store in the fridge or use immediately to baste anything you like.

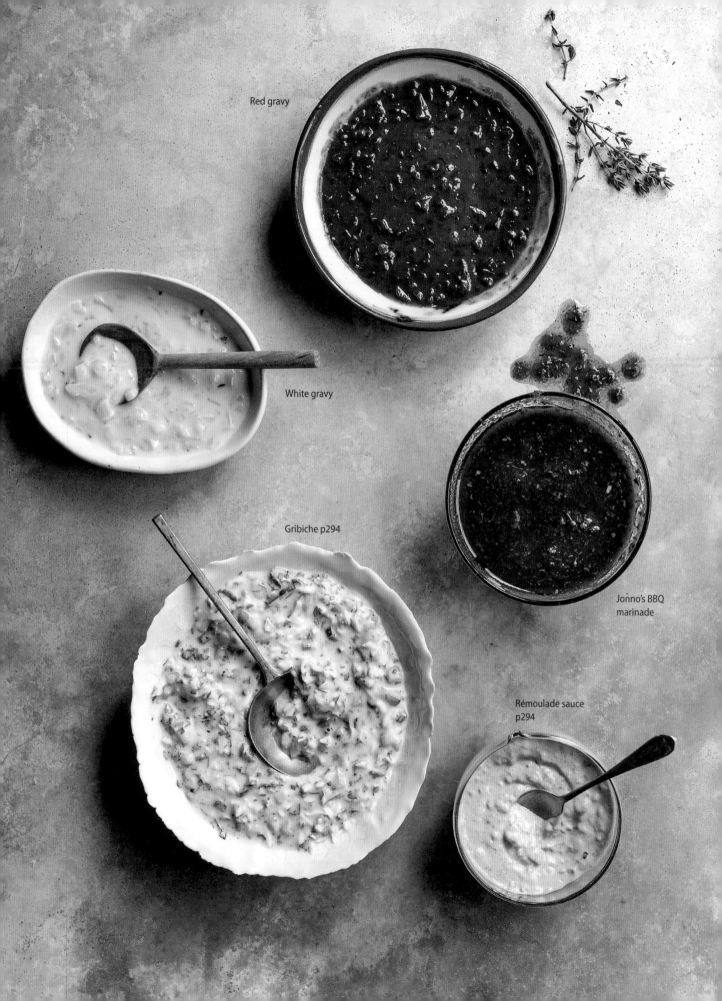

Red gravy

White gravy

Gribiche p294

Jonno's BBQ
marinade

Rémoulade sauce
p294

GRIBICHE

See page 293

Makes 600ml

4 hard-boiled eggs, yolks removed and
   whites finely grated
1½ tbsp Dijon mustard
2 tbsp white wine vinegar
4 tbsp olive oil
250ml avocado oil
8 cornichons (baby gherkins),
   finely chopped
1½ tbsp capers, finely chopped
2 tbsp fresh tarragon, chopped
2 tbsp chervil, chopped
2 tbsp flat-leaf parsley, chopped
Salt and black pepper

1 Add the boiled egg yolks, mustard and vinegar to a food processor and whizz until they are smooth.
2 With the blender running, slowly pour in the oils, a few tablespoons at a time. Wait for the oil to be completely incorporated (emulsified) before adding the next round.
3 Once you have added all the oil, you should have a creamy-looking mayo.
4 Now fold in the remaining ingredients and the grated egg whites, season and leave it to infuse for a couple of hours before serving with literally any savoury dish.

RÉMOULADE SAUCE

See page 293

Makes 250ml

180ml mayonnaise
5ml sherry vinegar (or tarragon
   vinegar)
½ celery stalk, finely chopped
1 tbsp Dijon mustard
1 tbsp wholegrain mustard
1 tbsp grated horseradish (creamed
   if you can't get fresh)
2 tsp capers, minced
1½ tsp sweet paprika
1 tsp Tabasco
Salt and pepper to taste

1 Mix all the ingredients together in a bowl and leave it to stand in the fridge for a couple of hours to infuse before serving.

REAL MEAL REVOLUTION: LOW CARB COOKING

TARTARE SAUCE

See page 297

Makes 250ml

180ml mayonnaise (see page 274)
5ml Dijon mustard
Juice and zest of 1 lemon
1 generous drop of Tabasco sauce
40g dill pickle, finely chopped
1 tbsp capers
½ red onion, finely chopped
1 tbsp flat-leaf parsley, chopped
1 tbsp fresh tarragon, chopped
1 tbsp fresh dill, chopped
Salt and black pepper

1   Mix all the ingredients together in a bowl, season to taste and leave it to stand in the fridge for a couple of hours to infuse before serving.

WET JERK

See page 297

Makes 250ml

8 spring onions, chopped
1 red chilli, stemmed and finely
   chopped
125ml avocado oil
Juice of 3 limes
3 garlic cloves, finely chopped
Small handful thyme leaves
Small handful basil leaves
Small handful coriander leaves
2 tbsp smoked paprika
2 tsp ground ginger
1 tsp cayenne pepper
½ tsp allspice
½ tsp ground cinnamon
½ tsp ground cloves
½ tsp ground nutmeg
½ tsp ground cumin
2 tsp black pepper
1 tsp salt

1   Whizz everything up in a blender and store in a jar in the fridge for up to two weeks.

CAESAR DRESSING

Makes 350ml

2 egg yolks

7 anchovies

Juice of 1 lemon

2 tsp Dijon mustard

1 garlic clove, peeled

2 tbsp mayonnaise

4 tbsp olive oil

125ml avocado oil

125ml finely grated Parmigiana
   Reggiano

Salt and black pepper

1   Whizz the yolks, anchovies, lemon juice, mustard, garlic and mayo in a food processor until super smooth.

2   With the blender running, slowly pour in the oils, a few tablespoons at a time. Wait for the oil to be completely incorporated (emulsified) before adding the next round.

3   When all of the oil is mixed in and you have a thick, creamy dressing, whisk in the cheese, season with salt and pepper, then leave in the fridge to infuse.

4   Be careful when you season this one, as the cheese and anchovies will provide plenty of salt already.

ROMESCO SAUCE

Makes 250ml

1 charred red pepper, thinly sliced
   (page 108)

1 garlic clove, finely chopped

40g flaked almonds, toasted

4 tbsp tomato paste

1 small handful flat-leaf parsley,
   leaves only

2 tbsp sherry vinegar

5ml smoked paprika

5ml cayenne pepper

125ml olive oil

Salt and black pepper

1   Place all the ingredients except the olive oil in a food processor and blend until fine.

2   With the blender running, slowly pour in the oil, a few tablespoons at a time. Wait for the oil to be completely incorporated (emulsified) before adding the next round.

3   Season with salt and pepper and keep it chilled until you're ready to serve.

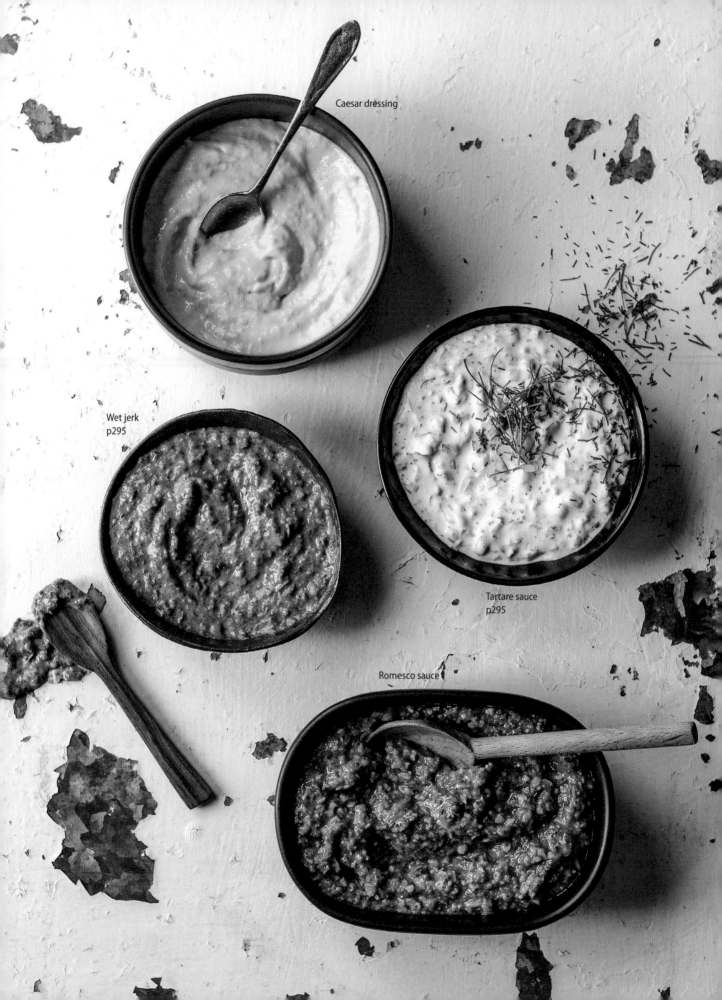

Caesar dressing

Wet jerk
p295

Tartare sauce
p295

Romesco sauce

TARATOR SAUCE

Makes 200ml

100g tahini
2 tbsp lemon juice
1 garlic clove, minced
1 pinch salt
water

My stepmum spent a few years in Lebanon as a child and this is her recipe. I love this sauce so much I asked her to make 5 litres of it to serve with the falafel at our wedding – there's nothing better. It goes well with anything from grilled fish to roast veg.

1 Whisk all the ingredients together in a small mixing bowl
2 While continuing to whisk, slowly add water, 2 tablespoons at a time, until your sauce has reach the desired consistency.
3 It should have the consistency of drinking yoghurt or thin cream.

BASIC CHINESE DRESSING

Makes 250ml

4 tbsp rice wine vinegar
4 tbsp soy sauce
1 tbsp ginger, grated
1 tsp garlic, minced
2½ tbsp sesame oil
125ml avocado oil
2 tbsp sesame seeds, toasted
1 spring onion, finely sliced

1 Place all the ingredients in a mixing bowl and whisk until well combined.

WAFU JAPANESE DRESSING

Makes 250ml

¼ onion, grated, with juice
80ml soy sauce
80ml rice vinegar
80ml avocado oil
1 tbsp white sesame seeds, toasted
1 tbsp black sesame seeds, toasted
½ tsp black pepper

1 Place all the ingredients in a mixing bowl and whisk until well combined.

GINGER AND MISO DRESSING

Makes 250ml

125ml rice wine vinegar
125ml white miso
4 tbsp fresh lime juice
4 tsp grated ginger

1 Place all the ingredients in a mixing bowl and whisk until well combined.

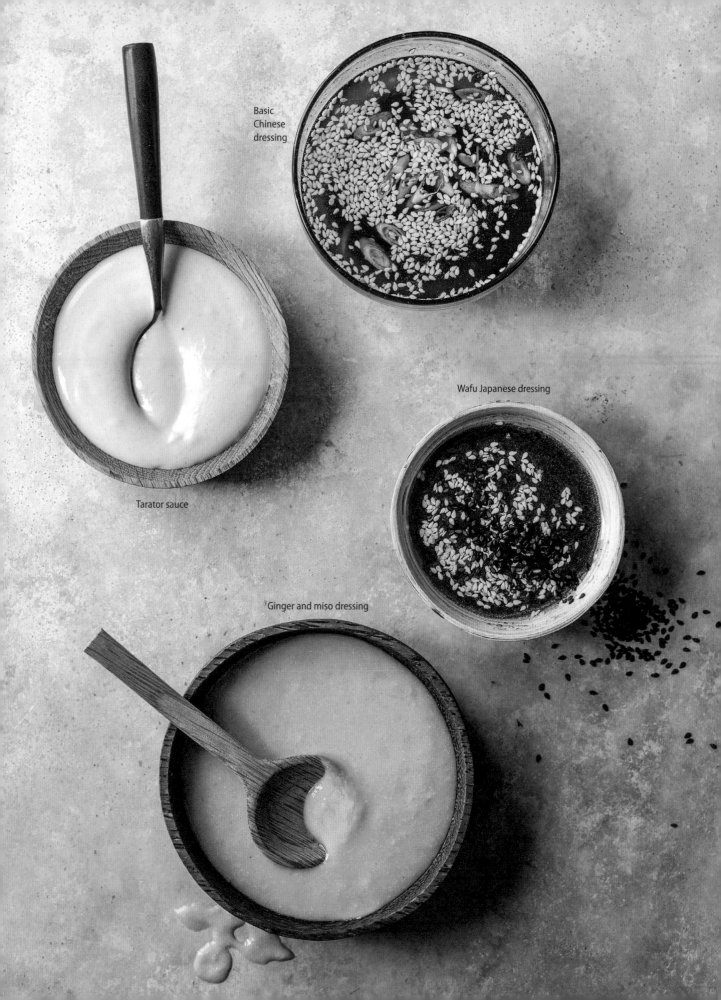

Basic
Chinese
dressing

Tarator sauce

Wafu Japanese dressing

Ginger and miso dressing

TATAKI MARINADE

Makes 125ml

6 tbsp soy sauce

4 tbsp mirin

2 spring onions, finely sliced

2 tbsp lime juice

2 tbsp grated ginger

2 cloves garlic, minced

1   Place all the ingredients in a mixing bowl and whisk until well combined.

NUTLESS SATAY MARINADE

Makes 125ml or enough for 500g meat

1 red onion, peeled and roughly
   chopped

5 garlic cloves, peeled

1 thumb ginger, peeled and roughly
   chopped

½ tsp ground white pepper

1 tsp ground coriander seeds

3 tsp ground fennel seeds

3 tsp ground cumin seeds

1 tsp dried shrimp paste

½ tsp ground turmeric

1   Place everything in a small jug and blitz with a stick blender, before adding it to
    your meat.

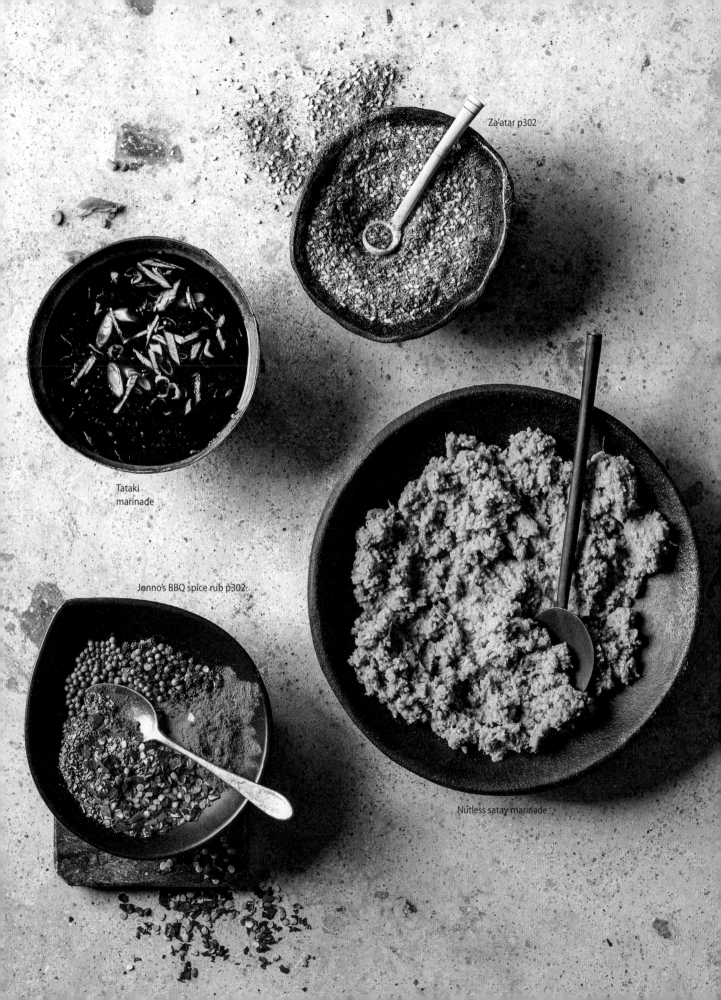

Za'atar p302

Tataki
marinade

Jonno's BBQ spice rub p302

Nutless satay marinade

JONNO'S BBQ SPICE RUB

See page 301

Makes 4 tbsp

5ml, whole black peppercorns
1 tbsp coriander seeds
1 tbsp dried chilli flakes
1 tbsp smoked paprika
1 tbsp mixed dried herbs
A huge pinch of salt

1 Add the ingredients into a pestle and mortar and give them a solid pounding. Or put them in a spice or coffee grinder.
2 To get the most even covering over your meat, sprinkle the rub onto a platter and dab the meat down on the rub on each side.

ZA'ATAR

See page 301

Makes 8 tbsp

2 tbsp dried marjoram
2 tbsp dried oregano
1 tbsp dried thyme
½ tsp coarse salt
1 tbsp ground sumac
2 tbsp white sesame seeds

1 Spoon the dried herbs, salt and sumac into spice grinder and pulse for a few seconds. Then stir through the sesame seeds and store in a jar until needed.

BERBERE SPICE PASTE

See page 305

Makes 180ml

100ml olive oil
Juice of 1 lemon
1 garlic clove, chopped
1½ tbsp ground coriander
1 tbsp ground cinnamon
1 tbsp sumac
1½ tsp ground cumin
½ tsp ground allspice
1 pinch ground nutmeg
1 pinch ground cardamom

1 Place all the ingredients in a small jug and blitz with a stick blender until smooth.

DRY JERK RUB

This is the perfect dry rub for any fish or chicken on the barbecue. It's also great for roasted vegetables. *See page 305*

Makes 80ml

2 tbsp salt
2 tsp onion powder
2 tsp ground allspice
2 tsp garlic powder
1 tsp dried red chillies
1 tsp black pepper
1 tsp ground nutmeg
1 tsp dried chives
1 tsp paprika
1 tsp ground ginger
½ tsp dried thyme
½ tsp ground cloves
½ tsp ground cinnamon

1 Place all the ingredients in a mixing bowl and stir until well combined.

THE EASIEST TOMATO SAUCE

See page 305

Makes 500ml

1 x 400g tin whole peeled or
  chopped tomatoes
125ml olive oil
1 onion, roughly chopped
2 celery stalks, roughly chopped
3 garlic cloves, peeled
1 bay leaf
1 handful fresh basil leaves
Salt and black pepper

1 Preheat your oven to 140°C.
2 Use your hands to squash and mix everything (except the basil, salt and pepper) together in a small baking dish. It should come halfway up the sides.
3 Cover it with foil and pop it in the oven for 90 minutes.
4 Remove the foil and pop it back in for 10 minutes under a hot grill to char a few bits.
5 Tip the contents into a jug or mixing bowl, add the basil and salt and pepper, and blitz with a stick blender until smooth.

PERSIAN TAMARIND SAUCE

Makes 250ml

3 tbsp olive oil

1 onion, thinly sliced

2 tbsp almonds, toasted and chopped

4 tbsp tamarind paste

3 garlic cloves, minced

½ handful finely chopped fresh coriander

½ handful tarragon, finely chopped

½ handful flat-leaf parsley, finely chopped

1 Heat the olive oil in a large pan over a medium-low heat and add the onions to caramelise for up to 30 minutes until they go dark and sticky.

2 Once they are dark, add the almonds, tamarind and garlic and cook gently for another 10 minutes.

3 Now remove from the heat and stir in the herbs.

4 Leave it to cool before using using it as a sauce, otherwise serve warm as a dip.

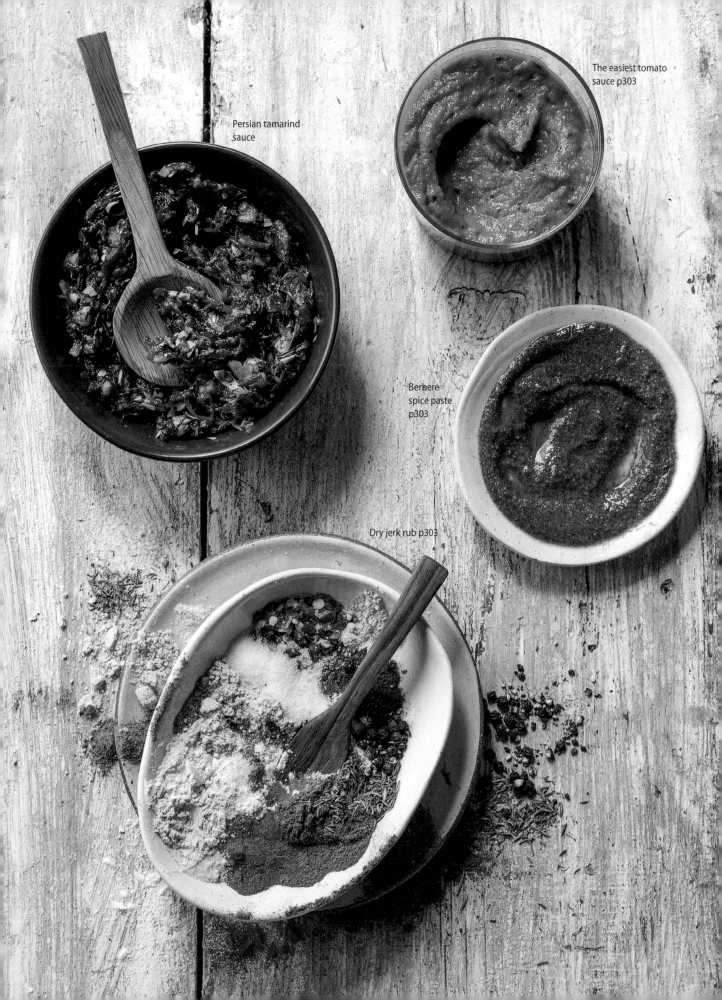

Persian tamarind
sauce

The easiest tomato
sauce p303

Berbere
spice paste
p303

Dry jerk rub p303

AVOCADO AND ZA'ATAR HUMMUS

Makes 250g

If you're using your own homemade za'atar, I recommend you go easy on the salt. That way you can get a lot more flavour into the hummus without letting it get too salty. Store-bought za'atar is always a little saltier for some reason.

1 large ripe avocado
2 big tbsp tahini
5ml za'atar
1 garlic clove, minced
Juice of 1 fat lemon
4 tbsp olive oil
salt

1 Whizz all the ingredients together in a food processor and leave for 1 to 2 hours in the fridge for the flavours to infuse.

BOURBON MISO MARINADE

Makes 250ml

100g miso
4 tbsp bourbon or
   Tennessee whiskey
1 tbsp chilli paste
2 tbsp apple cider vinegar
2 tbsp wholegrain mustard
1 tbsp minced ginger
1 small garlic clove, minced

1 Place all the ingredients in a mixing bowl and whisk until well combined. Store in the fridge until ready to use.

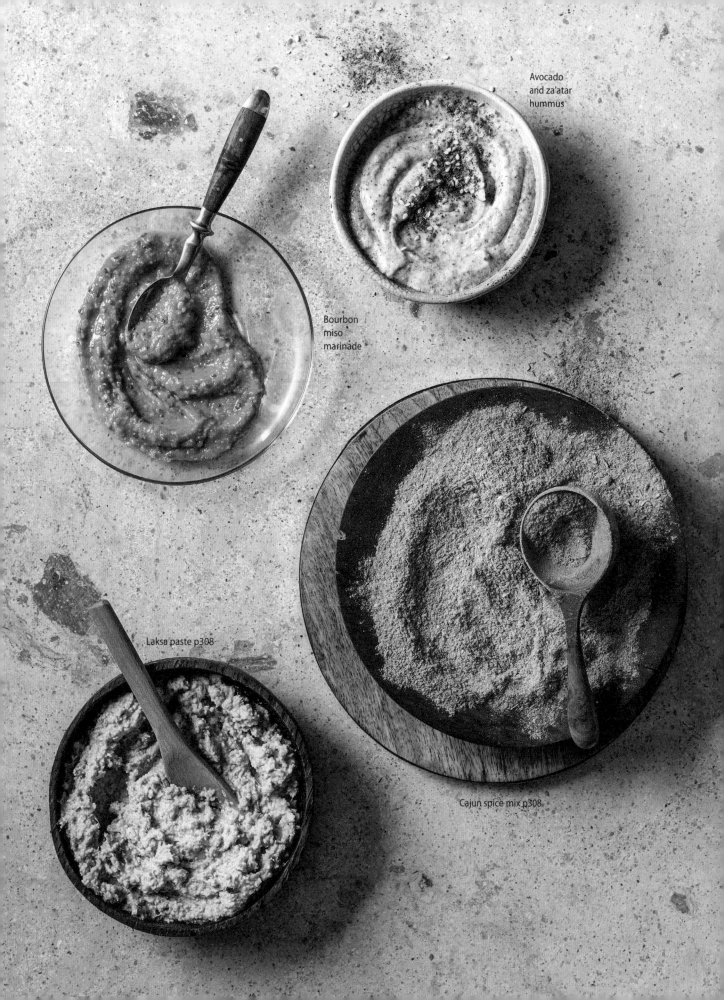

Avocado
and za'atar
hummus

Bourbon
miso
marinade

Laksa paste p308

Cajun spice mix p308

CAJUN SPICE MIX

See page 305

Makes 250ml

3 tbsp fine salt
3 tbsp cayenne pepper
3 tbsp black pepper
3 tbsp smoked paprika
3 tbsp garlic powder
2 tbsp onion powder
2 tbsp dried oregano
2 tbsp dried thyme

1 Mix all the ingredients in a bowl, then place in an airtight container and store in a cool dark place.

LAKSA PASTE

See page 305

Makes 250ml

1 tsp ground coriander
½ tsp ground turmeric
½ tsp sweet paprika
½ tsp ground cumin
6 dried red chillies, soaked in warm water till soft then drained
1 onion, chopped
2 lemongrass stalks, roughly chopped
3 thumbs ginger
60g cashew nuts
2 garlic cloves, finely chopped
1 tbsp shrimp paste
3 tbsp avocado oil

1 Toast the coriander, turmeric, paprika and cumin over medium heat in a large pan until they become aromatic, then let them cool completely.
2 Add the spices and the remaining ingredients to a food processor and blend them until you have a smooth paste.
3 Store in an airtight container and refrigerate for up to a week.

JOIN THE REVOLUTION
THE ONLINE PROGRAM THAT'S UNIQUE TO YOU

If you're reading this, you're probably interested in tasty, healthy eating. You also know that life often gets in the way of that ideal.

I'd like to invite you to take the next steps in discovering delicious low-carb meals with the help of my customised online program. The easiest route to a lifestyle of real food, it offers you more than 700 recipes and the following unique member benefits:

MEAL PLANS It all starts with a plan. We tailor-make these plans each week, making it as easy as possible for you.

MEAL TRACKER Analyse everything you eat, or choose not to. Everyone is unique, so we give you all the tools to become the best version of yourself.

COMMUNITY SUPPORT Meet a whole lot of like-minded people to share with and help, who will in turn help to take your life to the next level.

THE EASIEST WAY TO EAT DELICIOUS, REAL FOOD

Being a Real Meal member unlocks access to more than double the number of recipes, on-the-go lists, brand-new recipe videos and informative tutorials with me and my guests.

For buying the book, I'd like to offer you 50% off the joining fee. Please visit **www.realmealrevolution.com**, follow the prompts to sign up, and enter this code.

RMRLCCGIFT180716

Thank you so much for reading my book, and I hope to see you online.

Jonno

ACKNOWLEDGEMENTS

Thank you to my wife, Kate, and my kids, Imogen and Angus, for loving me and giving me a reason to write. Special thanks to Carmen, my research assistant, and to Rob, Penny, Morgan, Guss, Grant, Jason and my team at Real Meal Revolution for continuing to push the boundaries of what we're trying to achieve. More special thanks to Toby, our photographer, and Caro, our stylist, for knocking another shoot out the park. To Tim Richman and his team at Burnet Media for being such a pleasure to create books with, and to Duncan and the good people at Little, Brown for always having my back and investing in my work. Thank you. You're bloody legends.

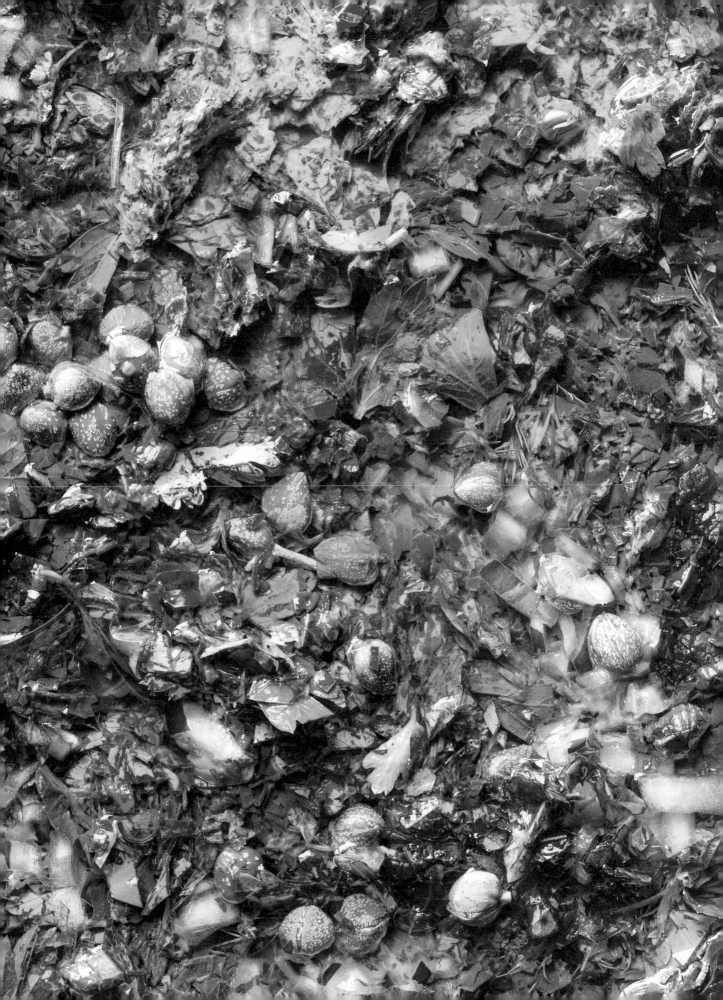

INDEX

First published in Great Britain in 2018 by Robinson

•

1 3 5 7 9 10 8 6 4 2

•

Copyright © Real Meal Revolution (Pty) Ltd, 2018

•

Photography Toby Murphy
Food styling Caro Gardner
Production Burnet Media

•

The moral rights of the author have been asserted.

•

All rights reserved.
No part of this publication may be reproduced, stored in a retrieval system,
or transmitted, in any form, or by any means, without the prior permission
in writing of the publisher, nor be otherwise circulated in any form of binding
or cover other than that in which it is published and without a similar condition
including this condition being imposed on the subsequent purchaser.

•

Important note
The recommendations in this book are solely intended as education
and information and should not be taken as medical advice.

•

A CIP catalogue record for this book
is available from the British Library.

•

ISBN: 978-1-47214-255-9

•

Typeset in Myriad Pro 8.5pt on 12.5pt
Printed and bound in China by C&C Offset Printing Co. Ltd

•

Papers used by Robinson are from well-managed forests and other responsible sources.

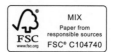

Robinson
An imprint of
Little, Brown Book Group
Carmelite House
50 Victoria Embankment
London EC4Y 0DZ

•

An Hachette UK Company
www.hachette.co.uk
www.littlebrown.co.uk

CONVERSION TABLE

Oven temperatures

°C	Fan °C	°F	Gas	Description
110	90	225	¼	Very cool
120	100	250	½	Very cool
140	120	275	1	Cool
150	130	300	2	Cool
160	140	325	3	Warm
180	160	350	4	Moderate
190	170	375	5	Moderately hot
200	180	400	6	Fairly hot
220	200	425	7	Hot
230	210	450	8	Very hot
240	220	475	8	Very hot

Weights for dry ingredients

Metric	Imperial	Metric	Imperial
7g	¼ oz	400g	14oz
15g	½ oz	425g	15oz
20g	¾ oz	450g	1lb
25g	1 oz	500g	1lb 2oz
40g	1½oz	550g	1¼lb
50g	2oz	600g	1lb 5oz
60g	2½oz	650g	1lb 7oz
75g	3oz	675g	1½lb
100g	3½oz	700g	1lb 9oz
125g	4oz	750g	1lb 11oz
140g	4½oz	800g	1¾lb
150g	5oz	900g	2lb
165g	5½oz	1kg	2¼lb
175g	6oz	1.1kg	2½lb
200g	7oz	1.25kg	2¾lb
225g	8oz	1.35kg	3lb
250g	9oz	1.5kg	3lb 6oz
275g	10oz	1.8kg	4lb
300g	11oz	2kg	4½lb
350g	12oz	2.25kg	5lb
375g	13oz	2.5kg	5½lb
		2.75kg	6lb

Liquid measures

Metric	Imperial	Aus	US
25ml	1fl oz		
50ml	2fl oz	¼ cup	¼ cup
75ml	3fl oz		
100ml	3½fl oz		
120ml	4fl oz	½ cup	½ cup
150ml	5fl oz		
175ml	6fl oz	¾ cup	¾ cup
200ml	7fl oz		
250ml	8fl oz	1 cup	1 cup
300ml	10fl oz/½ pint	½ pint	1¼ cups
360ml	12fl oz		
400ml	14fl oz		
450ml	15fl oz	2 cups	2 cups/1 pint
600ml	1 pint	1 pint	2½ cups
750ml	1¼ pints		
900ml	1½ pints		
1 litre	1¾ pints	1¾ pints	1 quart
1.2 litres	2 pints		
1.4 litres	2½ pints		
1.5 litres	2½ pints		
1.7 litres	3 pints		
2 litres	3½ pints		
3 litres	5¼ pints		

realmealrevolution.com

therealmealrevolution1

@realmealrevolution

therealmealrevolution